Colonoscopy and Polypectomy

Editor

CHARLES J. KAHI

GASTROENTEROLOGY
CLINICS OF NORTH AMERICA

www.gastro.theclinics.com

September 2013 • Volume 42 • Number 3

ELSEVIER

1600 John F. Kennedy Boulevard • Suite 1800 • Philadelphia, Pennsylvania, 19103-2899

http://www.theclinics.com

GASTROENTEROLOGY CLINICS OF NORTH AMERICA Volume 42, Number 3
September 2013 ISSN 0889-8553, ISBN-13: 978-0-323-18856-2

Editor: Kerry Holland
Developmental Editor: Donald Mumford

Gastroenterology Clinics of North America (ISSN 0889-8553) is published quarterly by Elsevier Inc., 360 Park Avenue South, New York, NY 10010-1710. Months of issue are March, June, September, and December. Business and Editorial Offices: 1600 John F. Kennedy Blvd., Suite 1800, Philadelphia, PA 19103-2899. Customer Service Office: 6277 Sea Harbor Drive, Orlando, FL 32887-4800. Periodicals postage paid at New York, NY and additional mailing offices. Subscription prices are $305.00 per year (US individuals), $153.00 per year (US students), $508.00 per year (US institutions), $335.00 per year (Canadian individuals), $617.00 per year (Canadian institutions), $423.00 per year (international individuals), $211.00 per year (international students), and $617.00 per year (international institutions). Foreign air speed delivery is included in all *Clinics* subscription prices. All prices are subject to change without notice. **POSTMASTER**: Send address changes to *Gastroenterology Clinics of North America*, Elsevier Health Sciences Division, Subscription Customer Service, 3251 Riverport Lane, Maryland Heights, MO 63043. Telephone: 1-800-654-2452 (U.S. and Canada); 314-447-8871 (outside U.S. and Canada). Fax: 314-447-8029. E-mail: journalscustomerservice-usa@elsevier.com (for print support); journalsonlinesupport-usa@elsevier.com (for online support).

Reprints. For copies of 100 or more, of articles in this publication, please contact the Commercial Reprints Department, Elsevier Inc., 360 Park Avenue South, New York, New York 10010-1710. Tel. (212) 633-3813, Fax: (212) 462-1935, E-mail: reprints@elsevier.com.

Gastroenterology Clinics of North America is also published in Italian by Il Pensiero Scientifico Editore, Rome, Italy; and in Portuguese by Interlivros Edicoes Ltda., Rua Commandante Coelho 1085, 21250 Cordovil, Rio de Janeiro, Brazil.

Gastroenterology Clinics of North America is covered in *MEDLINE/PubMed (Index Medicus)*, *Excerpta Medica*, *Current Contents/Clinical Medicine*, *Science Citation Index*, *ISI/BIOMED*, and *BIOSIS*.

Printed and bound by CPI Group (UK) Ltd, Croydon, CR0 4YY

Transferred to digital print 2013

Contributors

EDITOR

CHARLES J. KAHI, MD, MSCR, FACP, FACG, AGAF
Associate Professor of Clinical Medicine, Indiana University School of Medicine;
Gastroenterology Section Chief, Richard L. Roudebush VAMC, Indianapolis, Indiana

AUTHORS

RACHEL R. ABOU MRAD, MD
Division of Gastroenterology, Department of Internal Medicine, American University
of Beirut Medical Center, Beirut, Lebanon

JOSEPH C. ANDERSON, MD
Associate Professor of Medicine, University of Connecticut School of Medicine,
Farmington, Connecticut; White River Junction VAMC, White River Junction, Vermont; The
Geisel School of Medicine at Dartmouth Medical, Hanover, New Hampshire

AUDREY H. CALDERWOOD, MD
Assistant Professor of Medicine, Section of Gastroenterology, Boston University School
of Medicine, Boston, Massachusetts

JAMES CHURCH, MB, ChB, FRACS
Department of Colorectal Surgery, Digestive Diseases Institute, Cleveland Clinic,
Cleveland, Ohio

DEEPIKA DEVUNI, MBBS
Instructor, University of Connecticut School of Medicine, Farmington, Connecticut

MARTIN GOETZ, MD, PhD
Professor, Innere Medizin I, Universitätsklinikum Tübingen, Tübingen, Germany

VICTORIA GÓMEZ, MD
Department of Gastroenterology, Mayo Clinic, Jacksonville, Florida

SUSHOVAN GUHA, MD, PhD
Associate Professor and Director of Research, Department of Gastroenterology,
Hepatology and Nutrition, The University of Texas Medical School at Houston, Houston,
Texas

DAVID G. HEWETT, MBBS, MSc, PhD, FRACP
Associate Professor, School of Medicine, The University of Queensland, Brisbane,
Queensland, Australia

ZILLA H. HUSSAIN, MD
Dartmouth-Hitchcock Medical Center, Lebanon, New Hampshire

BRIAN C. JACOBSON, MD, MPH
Associate Professor of Medicine, Section of Gastroenterology, Boston University School of Medicine, Boston, Massachusetts

TONYA KALTENBACH, MD, MS
Attending Physician, Endoscopy Unit, Veterans Affairs Palo Alto and Stanford University, Palo Alto, California

MOUEN A. KHASHAB, MD
Assistant Professor of Medicine, Director of Therapeutic Endoscopy, Division of Gastroenterology and Hepatology, Department of Medicine, The Johns Hopkins Medical Institutions, Baltimore, Maryland

FELIX W. LEUNG, MD, FACG
Division of Gastroenterology, Department of Medicine, Sepulveda Ambulatory Care Center, Veterans Affairs Greater Los Angeles Healthcare System, North Hill, California; David Geffen School of Medicine at UCLA, Los Angeles, California

HEIKO POHL, MD
Dartmouth-Hitchcock Medical Center, Lebanon, New Hampshire; VA Medical Center, White River Junction, Vermont

GOTTUMUKKALA RAJU, MD
Professor of Medicine, Department of Gastroenterology, Hepatology and Nutrition, The University of Texas MD Anderson Cancer Center, Houston, Texas

AMIT RASTOGI, MD, FASGE
Director of Endoscopy, Kansas City VA Medical Center, Associate Professor of Medicine, University of Kansas, Kansas City, Missouri

DOUGLAS K. REX, MD
Division of Gastroenterology, Department of Medicine, Indiana University Health, Indiana University Hospital, Indianapolis, Indiana

ANDRES SANCHEZ-YAGUE, MD
Attending Physician, Endoscopy Unit, Veterans Affairs Palo Alto and Stanford University, Palo Alto, California; Attending Physician, Endoscopy Unit, Hospital Costa del Sol, Marbella, Spain

PAYAL SAXENA, BMBS(Hons), FRACP
Division of Gastroenterology and Hepatology, Department of Medicine, The Johns Hopkins Hospital Institutions, Baltimore, Maryland

ALA I. SHARARA, MD, FACG, AGAF
Professor and Head, Division of Gastroenterology, Department of Internal Medicine, American University of Beirut Medical Center, Beirut, Lebanon

HARMINDER SINGH, MD, MPH, FACG
Assistant Professor of Medicine and Director, GI Cancer Prevention and Research, Departments of Internal Medicine and Community Health Sciences, IBD Clinical and Research Centre, University of Manitoba, Winnipeg, Manitoba, Canada

ROY SOETIKNO, MD
Chief of Endoscopy, Endoscopy Unit, Veterans Affairs Palo Alto and Stanford University, Palo Alto, California

NIRAV THOSANI, MD, MHA
Chief Clinical Fellow, Department of Gastroenterology, Hepatology and Nutrition, The University of Texas Medical School at Houston, Houston, Texas

HALEH VAZIRI, MD
Assistant Professor of Medicine, University of Connecticut School of Medicine, Farmington, Connecticut

MICHAEL B. WALLACE, MD, MPH
Department of Gastroenterology, Mayo Clinic, Jacksonville, Florida

JEROME D. WAYE, MD
Clinical Professor of Medicine, Icahn School of Medicine at Mount Sinai, Director of Endoscopic Education, Mount Sinai Hospital, New York, New York

Contents

Technique Fundamentals

Douglas K. Rex

The primary goal of most colonoscopies, whether performed for screening, surveillance, or diagnostic examinations (those performed for symptoms or positive screening tests other than colonoscopy) is the detection of neoplasia and its subsequent removal by either endoscopic polypectomy or referral for surgical resection. Unfortunately, colonoscopy has proved to be a highly operator-dependent procedure with regard to detection. Variable detection results in some of the cancers that occur in the interval before the next colonoscopy.

David G. Hewett

 Video demonstrating cold snare polypectomy technique in small and diminutive polyps accompanies this article

Colonoscopic polypectomy is fundamental to effective colonoscopy. Through its impact on the polyp-cancer sequence, colonoscopic polypectomy reduces colorectal cancer incidence and mortality. Because it eliminates electrosurgical risk, cold snaring has emerged as the preferred technique for most small and all diminutive polyps. Few clinical trial data are available on the effectiveness and safety of specific techniques. Polypectomy technique seems highly variable between endoscopists, with some techniques more effective than others are. Further research is needed to investigate operator variation in polypectomy outcomes and establish an evidence base for best practice.

Andres Sanchez-Yague, Tonya Kaltenbach, Gottumukkala Raju, and Roy Soetikno

Advanced endoscopic resection techniques allow curative treatment of difficult colonic lesions and avoid the need for surgery in certain cases. If endoscopic resection is indicated, the choice of the most appropriate resection technique depends on lesion characteristics and endoscopist expertise.

Advances in Technique, Technology, and Neoplasia Detection

Amit Rastogi

Cap-assisted colonoscopy is a simple, practical, and inexpensive technique that serves several useful purposes in enhancing the performance of colonoscopy. It helps improve polyp detection by its ability to visualize otherwise blind mucosal areas on the proximal aspects of folds and flexures, although its effect on adenoma detection is inconsistent. By helping navigate the colon more efficiently, it facilitates intubation of the cecum faster, with lesser patient discomfort. Cap-assisted colonoscopy can be tried as a salvage procedure in cases of failed cecal intubation with regular colonoscopy and can be of assistance during polypectomy, especially for polyps located on the proximal aspects of folds.

 Videos of removal of a colon polyp during retroflexion in the right colon and retroview of a polyp accompany this article

A retroview in the colon permits an 11–25% increase in the adenoma detection rate when compared with a standard straight forward view during colonoscopy. This can often be accomplished in the rectum or the proximal colon by using dial controls and shaft manipulation to turn the tip of a standard colonoscope 180°. A special slim caliber instrument, the "Third Eye Retroscope" (a backward viewing device) has been developed which is inserted through the working channel of a colonoscope. New colonoscopes are being developed that have the capability of side vision with accompanying light illumination which, with wide angle lenses, provide an almost complete retroview of the colon.

Water-aided methods for colonoscopy include the established water immersion and the recent novel modification of water exchange. Water immersion entails the use of water as an adjunct to air insufflations to facilitate insertion. Water exchange evolved from water immersion to facilitate completion of colonoscopy without discomfort in unsedated patients. Infused water is removed predominantly during insertion rather than withdrawal. A higher adenoma detection rate has been reported with water exchange. Aggregate data of randomized controlled trials suggest that water exchange may be superior to water immersion in attenuating colonoscopy discomfort and optimizing adenoma detection, particularly in the proximal colon.

Chromocolonoscopy is the process of endoscopically examining the colon mucosa after it has been stained with dye. The goal is to allow the endoscopist to identify subtle features in the mucosa, such as morphologically flat polyps or crypt patterns. Studies examining the efficacy of chromocolonoscopy to identify adenomas missed by conventional colonoscopy have shown that although chromocolonoscopy increases polyp yield, most additional lesions are small in size. Staining can also help in differentiating neoplastic from non-neoplastic polyps. Perhaps the most useful aspect of chromocolonoscopy is increasing the yield for dysplasia in patients undergoing colonoscopy for inflammatory bowel disease surveillance.

Advancements in image technology have allowed recognition of mucosal architecture in more detail and may improve adenoma detection. This review provides a technical overview on individual imaging technologies and their effect on detection of adenomas. Only high-definition endoscopy has been shown to improve detection of small adenomas. None of the digital chromoendoscopy technologies improves adenoma detection. Limited studies on autoimmunfluorescence imaging in conjunction with high-definition endoscopy may improve detection of small adenomas.

Gastrointestinal endoscopy had major technological improvements and novel technologies in recent years. High-definition endoscopy has permitted an increasingly detailed view of the mucosa during colonoscopy. Filter techniques that enhance analysis of vessel and surface structures. Autofluorescence imaging relies on functional imaging of tissue alterations. Endocytoscopy is an ultrahigh-contact microscopy procedure for cellular analysis of the epithelium. Endomicroscopy is an adaption of laser scanning microscopy for real-time intravital surface and subsurface microscopy during endoscopy. With these technologies, endoscopy has moved from prediction of histology based on morphologic patterns toward visualization of cellular and subcellular details, providing real-time histology.

Quality and Outcomes

Adequate bowel preparation is essential for optimal colonoscopy. Suboptimal bowel preparation occurs in 25% to 40% of cases and is associated with canceled procedures, prolonged procedure time, incomplete examination, increased cost, and missed pathology. There are several effective formulations for colon cleansing with a good safety profile. Split dosing should be implemented whenever possible in an effort to enhance tolerance and adherence, and improve mucosal visibility and overall quality of the examination. In this review, modern bowel preparations are discussed including their mechanism of action, mode of use, safety, and how to optimize outcomes.

Colonoscopy is an excellent area for quality improvement because it is high volume, has significant associated risk and expense, and there is evidence that variability in its performance affects outcomes. The best end point for validation of quality metrics in colonoscopy is colorectal cancer incidence and mortality, but a more readily accessible metric is the adenoma detection rate. Fourteen quality metrics were proposed in 2006, and these are described in this article. Implementation of quality improvement initiatives involves rapid assessments and changes on an iterative basis, and can be done at the individual, group, or facility level.

There is substantial indirect evidence for the effectiveness of colonoscopy in reducing colorectal cancer incidence and mortality. However, several recent studies have raised questions on the magnitude of effect for right-sided colorectal cancers. Well-documented variation in outcomes when colonoscopy is performed by different groups of endoscopists suggests that the recent emphasis on the quality of the procedures should lead to improved outcomes after colonoscopy including reduction in incidence and mortality due to right-sided colorectal cancers.

Colonoscopy is a relatively invasive modality for the diagnosis and treatment of colorectal disease and for the prevention or early detection of colorectal neoplasia. Millions of colonoscopies are performed each year in the United States by endoscopists with varying levels of skill in colons that present varying levels of challenge. Although better scope technology has made colonoscopy gentler and more accurate, the sheer number of examinations performed means that complications inevitably occur. This article considers the most common complications of colonoscopy and advises how to minimize their incidence and how to treat them if they do occur.

The Future

Optimization of training and teaching methods in colonoscopy at all levels of experience is critical to ensure consistent high-quality procedures in practice. Competency in colonoscopy may not be achieved until more than 250 colonoscopies are performed by trainees. Such tools as computer-based endoscopic simulators can aid in accelerating the early phases of training in colonoscopy, and magnetic endoscopic imaging technology can guide the position of the colonoscope and aid with loop reduction. Periodic feedback and retraining experienced endoscopists can improve the detection of colonic lesions.

Gastrointestinal endoscopy is a rapidly evolving field. Techniques in endoscopy continue to become more sophisticated, as do the devices and platforms, particularly in colonoscopy and endoscopic resection. This article reviews new platforms for endoscopic imaging of the colon and discusses new endoscopic accessories and developments in endoscopic resection.

GASTROENTEROLOGY
CLINICS OF NORTH AMERICA

Preface

Colonoscopy and Polypectomy: Moving Forward in the Battle Against Colorectal Cancer

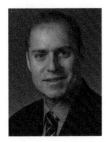

Charles J. Kahi, MD, MSCR
Editor

Why a new publication about colonoscopy and polypectomy?

A well-performed, high-quality colonoscopy prevents colorectal cancer and saves lives. Far from merely being a stagnant medical procedure, colonoscopy is an integrated scientific field in constant dynamic evolution. Recent progress has included advanced resection techniques, which have pushed the boundary of what can effectively and safely be accomplished during colonoscopy, new accessories and imaging technologies to allow better detection and characterization of colon neoplasms, improvements in bowel preparation to improve mucosal visibility and patient tolerability, more effective recognition and management of complications, new teaching and training approaches, and platform and device innovations. These positive developments have not been without accompanying controversy: recent evidence shows decreased colonoscopy protection against right-sided colorectal cancer, and increased recognition that this is largely due to operator-dependent factors, notably high variability in the detection and complete resection of precancerous polyps. Ongoing quality initiatives aim to identify and correct the causes of this variability and highlight the importance of fundamentals, such as optimal colonoscope withdrawal and mucosal inspection techniques, vigilance and recognition of non-polypoid and serrated neoplasia, and effective and complete polypectomy.

This volume aims to summarize these exciting developments in the field of colonoscopy, provide an overview of the current state of the art and current controversies and challenges, and hopefully inspire readers to share the passion, pick up the torch, and contribute to advancing the field.

It has been a personal pleasure and privilege for me to collaborate with some of the world's foremost experts in colonoscopy and polypectomy. I am indebted to them for their expertise, dedication, and inspiring teaching; this work would not have otherwise

Gastroenterol Clin N Am 42 (2013) xiii–xiv
http://dx.doi.org/10.1016/j.gtc.2013.05.016
0889-8553/13/$ – see front matter © 2013 Published by Elsevier Inc.

gastro.theclinics.com

been possible. Finally, I would like to thank Kerry Holland and the staff at Elsevier for their professional oversight of the publication process.

Charles J. Kahi, MD, MSCR
Indiana University School of Medicine
Indianapolis, IN, USA

Richard L. Roudebush VAMC
Gastroenterology Section
Indianapolis, IN, USA

E-mail address:
ckahi2@iu.edu

Dedication

This issue of *Gastroenterology Clinics of North America* is dedicated to the following people:

    Nadine, Joe, and Nicholas
    My parents
    My teachers and mentors

Optimal Withdrawal and Examination in Colonoscopy

Douglas K. Rex, MD

KEYWORDS

- Colonoscopy • Colorectal polyps • Adenoma detection rate • Withdrawal time

KEY POINTS

- Advanced colonoscopy skill must be demonstrated by measurement of quality indications, particularly the adenoma detection rate.
- High-level detection is associated with white-light examination technique that involves adequate time; meticulous probing of the proximal sides of folds, flexures, and valves; adequate colonic distention; and effort to clean up residual debris.
- Endoscopists should be able to recognize the full spectrum of pre-cancerous colorectal lesions, including subtle lesions such as flat and depressed conventional adenomas and serrated lesions.
- New approaches to reducing variable detection, including the use of systematic video recording of examinations, correction of visual gaze patterns, and development of insights into personality and behavioral factors that influence detection, warrant aggressive investigation.

INTRODUCTION

The primary goal of most colonoscopies, whether performed for screening, surveillance, or diagnostic examinations (those performed for symptoms or positive screening tests other than colonoscopy) is the detection of neoplasia and its subsequent removal by either endoscopic polypectomy or referral for surgical resection. Unfortunately, colonoscopy has proved to be a highly operator-dependent procedure with regard to detection,[1] and the consequences of this variation include occurrence of colorectal cancer in the interval before the next colonoscopy (so-called "interval cancers" or "post-colonoscopy cancers"). Many of the articles in this edition of Gastroenterology Clinics of North America are devoted to technical improvements in imaging that could potentially improve neoplasia detection or reduce the variation between examiners and detection. However, studies describing attempts to improve detection solely through technology improvements have generally shown lower detection gains,[2] than is achieved by taking the colonoscope out of the hands of a

Division of Gastroenterology, Department of Medicine, Indiana University Health, Indiana University Hospital, #4100, 550 North University Boulevard, Indianapolis, IN 46202, USA
E-mail address: drex@iupui.edu

Gastroenterol Clin N Am 42 (2013) 429–442
http://dx.doi.org/10.1016/j.gtc.2013.05.009
0889-8553/13/$ – see front matter © 2013 Elsevier Inc. All rights reserved.

low-level adenoma detector and giving it to a high-level detector. A high-level detector will commonly increase the percentage of patients with one or more adenomas detected by 3-fold to 6-fold[3–6] and the total number of adenomas detected by more than 10-fold.[3] The goal of this article is to help create colonoscopists who can achieve high-level detection of the full spectrum of cancerous and precancerous lesions in the colorectum.

PARIS CLASSIFICATION

Both malignant and precancerous lesions in the colon grow in a spectrum of shapes that range from overtly polypoid or fungating to lesions that have no elevated component and are entirely or mostly depressed below the level of normal mucosa. Without doubt, lesions that are flat or depressed are more difficult on average to detect and are more easily hidden from view behind folds and flexures, as well as overlooked even when brought into view, compared to the polypoid lesions. In order to study and communicate effectively regarding the spectrum of shapes of cancer and precancerous lesions, the Paris Classification was developed.[7]

In the Paris Classification (**Fig. 1**), lesions are divided into polyps (Type 1 lesions) and flat and depressed lesions (Type 2). Type 1 lesions may be pedunculated (1p) or sessile (1s) polyps. Among the polyps, the sessile polyps are substantially more common than pedunculated polyps.

Among the Type 2 lesions, the most common by far is the 2a lesion (**Fig. 2**), which is flat but elevated relative to the mucosal surface. The difference between a 1s lesion and a 2a lesion is that a 1s lesion projects into the lumen more than the diameter of a standard biopsy forceps of 2.5 mm and the flat 2a lesions project into the lumen less than 2.5 mm. 2b lesions are truly flat and are exceedingly rare. In my experience, most 2b lesions are serrated rather than conventional adenomas. Both the polypoid lesions (1p and 1s) and the flat lesions (2a and 2b) have a low prevalence of invasive cancer. Although there is a widely held impression that flat lesions are more likely to contain high-grade dysplasia and invasive cancer than polypoid lesions, literature on that issue is quite mixed, and some studies show that 2a lesions have the lowest prevalence of invasive cancer of all precancerous lesions.

Depressed lesions, designated as 2c and its variants in the Paris Classification (see **Fig. 1**) are some of the most dangerous lesions in the colorectum. These lesions are characterized by a depressed element that typically occupies most or a substantial part of the lesion surface and has a fairly sharp drop-off from the normal mucosa or elevated portion of the lesion to the depressed section. The shape of an individual lesion and its proper assignment in the Paris Classification can often be best achieved by surface dye spraying with dilute indigo carmine, which highlights lesion morphology. The prevalence of depressed lesions is quite low, approaching rarity, but the lesions are quite significant because in many series up to 50% contain high-grade dysplasia or invasive cancer. Correct recognition of depressed lesions is also important because if possible they should be resected en bloc and with inclusion of a rim of normal mucosa at the periphery.

The most common area of confusion is distinguishing a 2a plus 2c depressed lesion (**Fig. 3**) from a 2a lesion that has a slight valley on its surface (**Fig. 4**), commonly referred to as a "pseudodepression" or "2a dip." About 15% of 2a adenomas have such a dip and it does not predict an increased chance of advanced pathology.[8] The characteristic features are that the 2a dip occupies only a small portion of the surface area of the 2a adenoma, and the transition from the elevated portion into the valley is gradual in the 2a dip, as opposed to sharp in the 2a plus 2c depressed lesion.

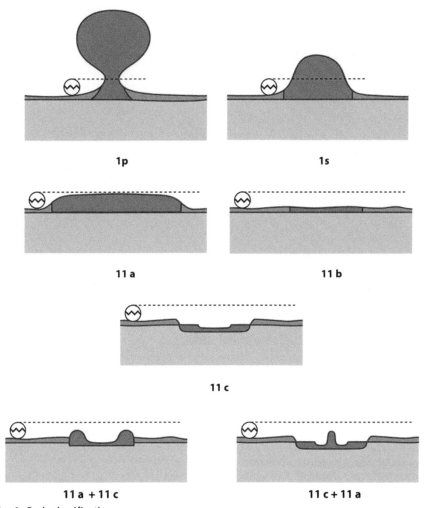

Fig. 1. Paris classification.

When 2a lesions extend over 1.0 cm in diameter, they are referred to as lateral-spreading tumors (LSTs). In the past, such lesions were often referred to as "carpet lesions" or just "sessile polyps." LSTs are further characterized as granular LST, meaning that the surface is bumpy, or nongranular LST, which has a smooth surface. Granular LSTs are considerably more common than nongranular and also are much less likely to contain high-grade dysplasia or invasive cancer compared with nongranular LSTs.

SPECTRUM OF DISEASE

The modern colonoscopist should understand the molecular basis of colorectal cancer as it relates to the spectrum of precancerous lesions that must be detected and removed during colonoscopy. It is often said that the molecular profiles of any 2 colorectal cancers are never identical. However, 3 broad categories of molecular pathways have been described (**Table 1**) and have clinical implications for the colonoscopist.

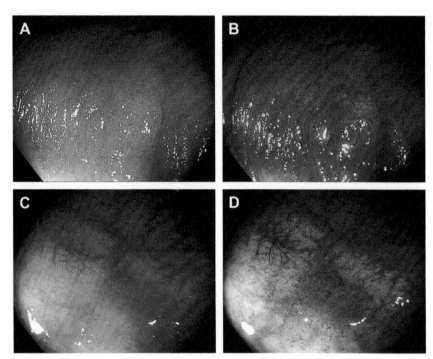

Fig. 2. (*A–D*) Examples of flat conventional adenomas in the proximal colon: (*A*) first lesion in white light, (*B*) first lesion in narrow band imaging, (*C*) second lesion in white light, (*D*) second lesion in narrow band imaging.

The most common molecular pathway is the chromosomal instability (CIN) pathway, in which cancers arise through the conventional adenomatous polyp. Adenomas carry point mutations in tumor suppressor genes and oncogenes, which commonly include the adenomatous polyposis coli gene, the *k-ras* oncogene, and the p53 tumor suppressor gene (see **Table 1**). Conventional adenomas are classified as tubular, tubulovillous, or villous, and the tubulovillous and villous adenomas are said to contain "villous elements." Adenomas with villous elements have a greater chance of having high-grade dysplasia or invasive cancer compared with tubular adenomas. All

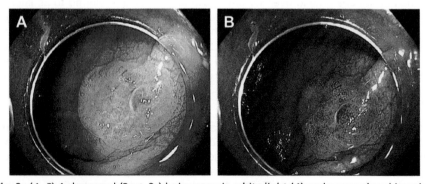

Fig. 3. (*A, B*) A depressed (2a + 2c) lesion seen in white light (*A*) and narrow band imaging (*B*). This lesion had invasive adenocarcinoma at pathology.

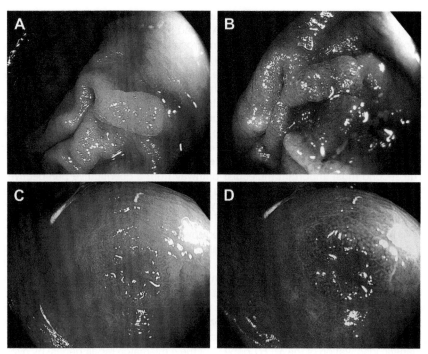

Fig. 4. (*A–D*) Examples of 2a lesions with pseudodepressions. (*A*) First lesion in white light, (*B*) first lesion in narrow band imaging, (*C*) second lesion in white light, (*D*) second lesion in narrow band imaging.

conventional adenomas by definition are dysplastic, which should be classified as low grade or high grade. In the CIN pathway, the passage of an adenoma from low-grade to high-grade dysplasia and then to invasive cancer is believed to typically require 10 to 20 years, although the process may occur more quickly in elderly patients whose adenomas may have accumulated more mutations.[9] However, because the dwell time of small tubular adenomas is typically decades, the consequences of missing a small (6–9 mm) or diminutive (1–5 mm) tubular conventional adenoma are almost always minimal.

The least common of the molecular pathways is the Lynch syndrome, in which patients are born with inherited germline mutations in 1 of the 4 mismatch repair genes

Table 1					
Colorectal cancer – molecular basis					
Pathway	Frequency	Genes	MSI	Precursor	Speed
CIN	65%–70%	APC K-ras p53	No	Adenoma	Slow
Lynch	3%	MLH1 MLH2 MLH6 PMS2	Yes	Adenoma	Fast
CIMP	30%–35%	BRAF	Sometimes	Serrated	Can be fast

(*MLH1, MSH2, MSH6, PMS2*). Patients carrying these mutations are prone to deletions in short repeating sequences of DNA called microsatellites. When these errors are not repaired, the result is referred to as microsatellite instability. Tumor suppressor genes and oncogenes with microsatellites in their coding regions are susceptible to mutation in patients with Lynch syndrome. Mutations normally occur at a relatively high rate but are repaired by the mismatch repair system; in Lynch syndrome, there is failure to repair these mutations, and patients can accumulate mutations in cancer genes faster than this process occurs in normal individuals. The result is the potential for even a small adenoma to transform into cancer in a few years. Therefore, the goal of detection in patients with Lynch syndrome is the complete clearing of all precancerous lesions, including tiny conventional adenomas.

The second most important molecular pathway from a quantitative perspective is also the most recent to be recognized. This pathway is often designated the "serrated pathway" or the "hypermethylation pathway" or "CIMP-high" pathway, referring to the CpG island methylator phenotype (CIMP).[10-13] These tumors account for about 30% of all colorectal cancers and are distributed toward the proximal colon. Rather than mutation in the *k-ras* oncogene, they typically carry mutations in the *BRAF* oncogene. *BRAF* is in the same signaling pathway as *k-ras,* and concomitant mutations in both *k-ras* and *BRAF* are distinctly uncommon in colorectal cancers, occurring in only 1% of tumors. *BRAF* mutation is almost synonymous with CIMP-high colorectal cancer. Approximately half of CIMP-high colorectal cancers are microsatellite unstable, and CIMP-high tumors account for about 80% of all microsatellite unstable colorectal cancers. The origin of microsatellite instability in CIMP-high tumors is epigenetic inactivation of the *MLH1* gene (1 of the 4 mismatch repair genes) by hypermethylation of its promoter region.

From the colonoscopist's perspective, the precursor of the hypermethylated tumors is not the conventional adenoma but rather a group of lesions called "serrated." The World Health Organization advises that serrated lesions be grouped into 3 major histologic categories (**Box 1**),[14] which includes hyperplastic polyps, sessile serrated polyps (synonymous with sessile serrated adenomas), and traditional serrated adenomas. The principle precursor of hypermethylated tumors is the sessile serrated polyp, which shares with hypermethylated tumors proximal colon location, hypermethylation, and *BRAF* mutation (see **Box 1**). Serrated lesions can be readily distinguished from conventional adenomas during endoscopy. They have a color similar to the surrounding mucosa, indistinct edges, no or few blood vessels on the surface, and their presence is often signaled by either a "mucus cap" or collection of debris, which often accumulates near the lesion edge (**Fig. 5**).[15]

Table 2 summarizes the full spectrum of precancerous lesions that must be detected by the advanced colonoscopist with regard to their histology, shape, location in the colon, and propensity to advanced histology. The modern colonoscopist

---

Box 1
World Health Organization recommended terminology for serrated lesions

Hyperplastic polyp

Sessile serrated polyp (same as sessile serrated adenoma)

    Without cytologic dysplasia

    With cytologic dysplasia

Traditional serrated adenoma

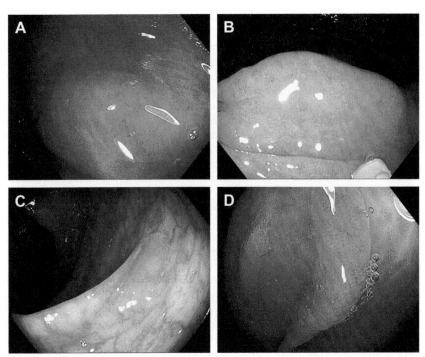

Fig. 5. (*A–D*) Examples of sessile serrated polyps (also called sessile serrated adenomas) from the proximal colon. Note the mucous caps on the lesions, areas of debris on the edges of some of the lesions, and poorly defined edges.

must acknowledge and understand this spectrum of disease, be fully familiar with the endoscopic appearance of each component, and be fully trained in techniques for effective resection of these lesions.

VARIABLE DETECTION OF CANCER

Why discuss routine withdrawal technique, which for decades was taken for granted as the simplest and most straightforward aspect of colonoscopy? The reason is accumulating evidence that significant percentages of colonoscopists are ineffective in

Table 2 Spectrum of precancerous lesions in the colorectum				
Lesion	Paris Shape	Distribution	Prevalence	Pathology
Traditional adenomatous polyps	1p 1s	Left Throughout	Low Common	Mostly LGD Mostly LGD
Flat adenomas (lesions)	2a	Greater to right	Common	Mostly LGD
Depressed adenomas (lesions)	2c 2a + 2c 2c + 2a	Greater to right	Rare	↑↑ HGD and invasive cancer
Sessile serrated adenoma (polyp)	1s or 2a	Greater to right	Common	Distinction from HP may not be reliable
TSA	1s or 1p	Left colon	Rare	Uncertain

detection and prevention of cancer. With regard to cancer prevention, at least 5 studies have demonstrated that gastroenterologists on average are more effective than nongastroenterologists in preventing colorectal cancer during colonoscopy.[16–20] The explanation for the differences may lie in training, but these remain unproved. Several studies have demonstrated that colonoscopists are generally more effective in preventing left-sided compared with right-sided cancer.[16,20–24] In 2 studies from Canada, where colonoscopy is performed largely by surgeons, colonoscopy provided no protection against right-sided cancer relative to cancer rates in the general population.[22,23] However, because patients undergoing colonoscopy were often symptomatic, they may have had higher prevalence rates of right-sided cancer than the general population, and lowering the right-sided incidence rate of cancer to that of the general population might represent an achievement for colonoscopy. In studies from Germany[24] and the United States,[20,25] where colonoscopy is performed largely by gastroenterologists, colonoscopy did provide protection against right-sided cancer, but the protection was less than achieved for left-sided cancer. Subsequent evaluation of the Canadian studies showed that when colonoscopy was performed in Canada by gastroenterologists, there was protection against right-sided cancer, but again with less protection than seen for left-sided cancer.[16,17]

Canadian studies also showed that colonoscopy performed by physicians with higher cecal intubation rates and higher polypectomy rates was associated with better protection against right-sided colon cancer.[17] In a screening colonoscopy study done in Poland, in which colonoscopy was performed by gastroenterologists, patients of doctors with adenoma detection rates less than 20% had hazard ratios for the development of interval cancer more than 10 times greater than patients colonoscoped by doctors with adenoma detection rates higher than the recommended target of 20% (for a mixed gender population).[26]

These data establish that variable detection is problematic, since low detection is associated with failure to prevent colorectal cancer.

VARIABLE DETECTION OF ADENOMAS

The best evidence for variable detection of adenomas comes from studies reporting the adenoma detection rates of members of the same gastroenterology group (**Table 3**).[3–6] These reports have consistently identified a 3-fold to 6-fold range for the adenoma detection rate (percentage of subjects aged ≥50 years undergoing

Table 3
Variable detection of adenomas among gastrointestinal doctors

	Number of Doctors	Lowest ADR	Highest ADR	Range
Barclay Illinois 2006	12	9.4%	32.7%	3.5
Chen Indiana 2007	9	15.5%	41.1%	2.7
Imperiale Indiana 2009	25	7%	44%	6.3
Shaukat Minnesota 2009	51	10%	39%	3.9

colonoscopy with one or more adenomas identified). Variable detection extends to identification of large adenomas[3,4] and patients who have multiple adenomas.[3,4] With detection expressed as adenomas per colonoscopy, rather than adenoma detection rate, the range of detection among members of the same gastroenterology group becomes magnified and can exceed 10-fold.[3] Under these circumstances, the lowest-level detectors are missing more than 90% of the adenomas in the colon and more than half of the large adenomas in a colon. The impact of variable adenoma detection becomes magnified when the results of individual colonoscopies are subjected to postpolypectomy surveillance follow-up recommendations. The postpolypectomy surveillance guidelines, which assume uniform performance of colonoscopy, recommend shorter-term follow-up when patients have any adenoma compared with no adenoma and even shorter follow-up when there are advanced adenomas, or 3 or more adenomas, compared with the low-risk patient with 1 or 2 small tubular adenomas. The result is a "double protection, double unprotection phenomenon" (**Box 2**). In this scenario, the high-level detector initially clears the colon better than the low-level detector and then paradoxically brings patients back at shorter intervals compared with the low-level detector. The low-level detector tells more patients that they are normal (when they are not) and these patients return at longer intervals.

VARIABLE DETECTION OF SERRATED LESIONS

Two recent studies have evaluated the range of detection of serrated lesions in the proximal colon among colonoscopists in the same gastroenterology groups. In this context, serrated refers to both sessile serrated polyp and hyperplastic polyp, primarily because this distinction is not reliable pathologically, even among gastrointestinal specialist pathologists.[27,28] The range of detection between the highest and the lowest detecting numbers of the groups was 7-fold to 18-fold, suggesting that serrated lesions are an even greater source of missed lesions than conventional adenomas. **Table 4** lists clinical factors that have been associated with interval cancers. Notice that these factors include hypermethylation, microsatellite instability, and proximal colon location, all factors associated with the CIMP-high pathway, again suggesting that missed serrated lesions are a major problem in colonoscopy detection.

WITHDRAWAL TECHNIQUE

In 1997, investigators at Indiana University reported the results of a tandem colonoscopy study in which 183 patients underwent 2 colonoscopies on the same day.[29]

Box 2
Factors associated with interval (post-colonoscopy cancers)
Proximal colon location
Microsateillite instability
CpG Island Methylator Phenotype
Colonoscopy by nongastroenterologists
Colonoscopy by doctors with low adenoma detection rates
Colonoscopy by doctors with low polypectomy rates
Colonoscopy by doctors with low cecal intubation rates
Baseline colonoscopy indication of positive fecal blood test versus screening

| Table 4
ADR-interval interaction	
High ADR: Patients Doubly Protected	**Low ADR: Patients Doubly Unprotected**
Colons are better cleared	Colons are poorly cleared
More patients come back at earlier intervals	More patients are told they are normal and can return at long intervals

The overall miss rate for adenomas was 27% but individual endoscopists demonstrated a range of miss rates from 17% to 48%. In 2000, a follow-up study in which 10 consecutive videotaped colonoscopy examinations performed by the endoscopist with the lowest miss rate and 10 examinations from the endoscopist with the highest miss rate were shown randomly to 4 gastroenterologists.[30] The video evaluations were blinded to who or how many endoscopists had performed the individual examinations and scored them for 4 quality parameters, including the time of inspection, the quality of examining the proximal sides of folds, the quality of cleaning residual fluid, and the adequacy of colonic distention. The endoscopist with the lower miss rate had a higher average withdrawal time and had substantially higher quality scores for each of the 4 quality parameters.[30] This became the first evidence associating colonoscopy withdrawal technique with adenoma detection. Subsequently, other studies have associated these same factors with detection but few additional associations have been made. Recently, investigators from the Mayo Clinic Jacksonville found that endoscopists with higher adenoma detection focus on the central portion of the video monitor compared with low-level detectors who focus more on the periphery.[31] Apparently, endoscopists can be trained to change their focus. Additional study is needed to determine whether high-level detectors bring more or all of the colonic mucosa into the central portion of the monitor by manipulation of the insertion tube. A variety of factors, including personality traits, have been suggested to account for variable withdrawal technique, because the principles of good withdrawal technique do not seem conceptually difficult to master. In support of this contention, a videotaping study reported that endoscopists consistently altered their withdrawal technique toward methods associated with better detection as soon as they became aware that their examinations were being video recorded.[32] Because no training was given in improved technique, the results suggest that endoscopists know how to perform careful technique but simply were not using careful technique in the absence of being observed.

Older barium enema studies[33] and more recent computed tomographic colonography studies[34] suggest that proximal sides of folds and flexures are hot spots for failed detection. Thus, colonoscopists should be alert to these areas, including the medial wall of the cecum, the medial wall of the distal ascending colon, and the proximal sides of rectal valves. Because colonoscopy is less effective at preventing right-sided colon cancer, consideration should be given to extra time and examination or performing a second examination of the right colon in certain circumstances. The greatest predictor of having missed a lesion is the number of lesions already detected.[35] Therefore, when one or more lesions are found in the right colon during an initial careful examination from the cecum to the hepatic flexure, consider a second examination. There is much discussion about the use of retroflexion in the right colon, but available evidence indicates that a second examination in the forward view is as effective as a second examination performed in retroflexion.[36] Retroflexion is more difficult when there is a substantial loop or bend in the scope but relatively easy when the insertion tube is short and straight.[35]

When a second examination of the right colon is performed, the instrument is readvanced to the cecum, which is fully reinspected in the forward view. My personal technique for retroflexion includes deflecting the bending section in the maximum up and left direction, and performing counterclockwise rotation of the insertion tube without advancement. Once retroflexion is achieved, the colonoscope is slowly withdrawn to the hepatic flexure or proximal transverse colon, and retroflexion is unwound in a relatively open space. Proximal colon retroflexion is performed with an adult or pediatric colonoscope but should not be performed in the descending or sigmoid colons with a colonoscope. The technique is important to master, because it often makes the difference in success in removing difficult-to-access polyps.[37,38]

After withdrawal to the dentate line, retroflexion should be performed in the rectum, unless the rectum is narrow and might not readily accommodate the diameter of the colonoscope bending section in the U-turn position. A narrow rectum is readily examined in the forward view. Retroflexion of the rectum was the source of 10% of colonic perforations in one series,[39] and neither deflection of the bending section nor advancement should occur against palpable resistance.

WITHDRAWAL TIME

In 2002, the US Multisociety Task Force on Colorectal Cancer made the first recommendation regarding withdrawal times for colonoscopy.[40] Based on limited evidence of average withdrawal times by endoscopists with low adenoma miss rates, the task force recommended that the withdrawal phase of colonoscopies in which no polypectomies or biopsies were performed should average 6 to 10 minutes.[40] In 2006, a gastroenterology group in Rockford, Illinois reported that colonoscopists with withdrawal times longer than 6 minutes had adenoma detection rates substantially higher than those with withdrawal times less than 6 minutes.[3] The same year, a joint task force of the American College of Gastroenterology and American Society for Gastrointestinal Endoscopy altered the recommendation to indicate that average withdrawal time should exceed 6 minutes in normal colonoscopies in which no polypectomies or biopsies were performed.[41]

Both quality recommendations indicated that the primary measure of the quality of mucosal inspection is not the withdrawal time but the adenoma detection rate, which should exceed 25% for men aged 50 years and older undergoing screening colonoscopy and 15% for women.[40,41] Despite these recommendations, withdrawal time was used by many colonoscopists as the sole measure of the quality of inspection, because it was easier to measure than the adenoma detection rate.

Retrospective studies have consistently shown a statistical association between withdrawal time and adenoma detection,[42] but the association may not hold for individual endoscopists.[43]

Although withdrawal time should be recorded in every examination, we consider that it has only marginal importance for endoscopists who have adequate adenoma detection rates. However, endoscopists with adenoma detection rates below the recommended thresholds must extend their withdrawal times to an average of 6 minutes and more. Although both guidelines recommended that the 6 minute withdrawal time not be applied to individual cases, the 6 minute benchmark has been applied in specific medical-legal cases, and from a medical-legal perspective it may be advisable for the withdrawal time to exceed 6 minutes in every patient with a fully intact colon.

CORRECTION OF LOW-LEVEL DETECTION

Correcting low-level detection has generally proved to be difficult. An excellent review of this topic found that most approaches reported have been unsuccessful.[42] Of particular interest, mandating withdrawal times of a certain length has been generally unsuccessful,[42] suggesting that endoscopists must actually use the time to perform an effective withdrawal examination.

Two approaches have thus far proved successful. Both of them involved an educational component. In the first, members of the Rockford, Illinois gastroenterology group reviewed techniques associated with high-level detection and then utilized a timer, which sounded every 2 minutes once withdrawal had begun and targeted a total examination time of at least 8 minutes.[44] Endoscopists were encouraged to have examined each quarter of the colon's length for at least 2 minutes. The program resulted in improvements in adenoma detection across the board. More recently, the Mayo Clinic Jacksonville reported the value of the EQUIP Program, in which a didactic session was presented to review the spectrum of precancerous lesions in the colon, followed by an emphasis on examination technique. In a randomized controlled trial, endoscopists participating in the EQUIP Program improved their adenoma detection rates, but controls did not.[45]

SUMMARY

Advanced colonoscopy skill must be demonstrated by measurement of the adenoma detection rate. High-level detection is associated with white-light examination technique that involves adequate time; meticulous probing of the proximal sides of folds, flexures, and valves; adequate colonic distention; and effort to clean up residual debris. Careful white-light examination technique, as well as other potential but as yet undiscovered characteristics of high-level detectors, has a greater influence on detection than ancillary imaging developments, including chromoendoscopy, electronic chromoendoscopy, and inspection aids for the proximal sides of folds such as cap-fitted colonoscopy and the Third Eye Retroscope. Much work remains to achieve the goal of effectively reducing or eliminating variable detection during colonoscopy. This includes widespread education of colonoscopists during and after training in the spectrum of precancerous lesions in the colorectum and their endoscopic appearances, in effective examination technique, and in mandating quality measurements, particularly the adenoma detection rate. New approaches to reducing variable detection, including the use of systematic videorecording of examinations, correction of visual gaze patterns, and development of insights into personality and behavioral factors that influence detection, warrant aggressive investigation.

REFERENCES

1. Rex DK. Maximizing detection of adenomas and cancers during colonoscopy. Am J Gastroenterol 2006;101:2866–77.
2. Rex DK. Update on colonoscopic imaging and projections for the future. Clin Gastroenterol Hepatol 2010;8:318–21.
3. Barclay RL, Vicari JJ, Doughty AS, et al. Colonoscopic withdrawal times and adenoma detection during screening colonoscopy. N Engl J Med 2006;355: 2533–41.
4. Chen SC, Rex DK. Endoscopist can be more powerful than age and male gender in predicting adenoma detection at colonoscopy. Am J Gastroenterol 2007;102: 856–61.
5. Imperiale TF, Glowinski EA, Juliar BE, et al. Variation in polyp detection rates at screening colonoscopy. Gastrointest Endosc 2009;69:1288–95.
6. Shaukat A, Oancea C, Bond JH, et al. Variation in detection of adenomas and polyps by colonoscopy and change over time with a performance improvement program. Clin Gastroenterol Hepatol 2009;7:1335–40.

7. The Paris endoscopic classification of superficial neoplastic lesions: esophagus, stomach, and colon: November 30 to December 1, 2002. Gastrointest Endosc 2003;58:S3–43.

8. Rex DK. Narrow-band imaging without optical magnification for histologic analysis of colorectal polyps. Gastroenterology 2009;136:1174–81.

9. Brenner H, Hoffmeister M, Stegmaier C, et al. Risk of progression of advanced adenomas to colorectal cancer by age and sex: estimates based on 840,149 screening colonoscopies. Gut 2007;56:1585–9.

10. Rex DK, Ahnen DJ, Baron JA, et al. Serrated lesions of the colorectum: review and recommendations from an expert panel. Am J Gastroenterol 2012. http://dx.doi.org/10.1038/ajg.2012.161.

11. Leggett B, Whitehall V. Role of the serrated pathway in colorectal cancer pathogenesis. Gastroenterology 2010;138:2088–100.

12. Snover DC. Update on the serrated pathway to colorectal carcinoma. Hum Pathol 2011;42:1–10.

13. Huang CS, Farraye FA, Yang S, et al. The clinical significance of serrated polyps. Am J Gastroenterol 2011;106:229–40.

14. Snover D, Ahnen DJ, Burt RW, et al. Serrated polyps of the colon and rectum and serrated ("hyperplastic") polyposis. In: Bozman FT, Carneiro F, Hruban RH, et al, editors. WHO classification of tumours. Pathology and genetics. Tumours of the digestive system. 4th edition. Berlin: Springer-Verlag; 2010.

15. Tadepalli US, Feihel D, Miller KM, et al. A morphologic analysis of sessile serrated polyps observed during routine colonoscopy (with video). Gastrointest Endosc 2011;74:1360–8.

16. Singh H, Nugent Z, Demers AA, et al. The reduction in colorectal cancer mortality after colonoscopy varies by site of the cancer. Gastroenterology 2010;139:1128–37.

17. Baxter N, Sutradhar R, Forbes DD, et al. Analysis of administrative data finds endoscopist quality measures asociated with post-colonoscopy colorectal cancer. Gastroenterology 2011;140:65–72.

18. Rabeneck L, Paszat LF, Saskin R. Endoscopist specialty is associated with incident colorectal cancer after a negative colonoscopy. Clin Gastroenterol Hepatol 2010;8:275–9.

19. Rex DK, Rahmani EY, Haseman JH, et al. Relative sensitivity of colonoscopy and barium enema for detection of colorectal cancer in clinical practice. Gastroenterology 1997;112:17–23.

20. Baxter NN, Warren JL, Barrett MJ, et al. Association between colonoscopy and colorectal cancer mortality in a US cohort according to site of cancer and colonoscopist specialty. J Clin Oncol 2012. http://dx.doi.org/10.1200/JCO.2011.40.4772.

21. Lakoff J, Paszat LF, Saskin R, et al. Risk of developing proximal versus distal colorectal cancer after a negative colonoscopy: a population-based study. Clin Gastroenterol Hepatol 2008;6:1117–21.

22. Singh H, Nugent Z, Mahmud SM, et al. Predictors of colorectal cancer after negative colonoscopy: a population-based study. Am J Gastroenterol 2010;105:663–73.

23. Baxter NN, Goldwasser MA, Paszat LF, et al. Association of colonoscopy and death from colorectal cancer. Ann Intern Med 2009;150:1–8.

24. Brenner H, Chang-Claude J, Seiler CM, et al. Does a negative screening colonoscopy ever need to be repeated? Gut 2006;55:1145–50.

25. Singh G, Gerson LB, Wang H, et al. Screening colonoscopy, colorectal cancer and gender: an unfair deal for the fair sex? Gastrointest Endosc 2007;65:AB100.

26. Kaminski MF, Regula J, Kraszewska E, et al. Quality indicators for colonoscopy and the risk of interval cancer. N Engl J Med 2010;362:1795–803.

27. Hetzel J, Huang CS, Coukos JA, et al. Variation in the detection of serrated polyps in an average risk colorectal cancer screening cohort. Am J Gastroenterol 2010; 105:2656–64.
28. Kahi CJ, Hewett DG, Norton DL, et al. Prevalence and variable detection of proximal colon serrated polyps during screening colonoscopy. Clin Gastroenterol Hepatol 2011;9:42–6.
29. Rex DK, Cutler CS, Lemmel GT, et al. Colonoscopic miss rates of adenomas determined by back-to-back colonoscopies. Gastroenterology 1997;112:24–8.
30. Rex DK. Colonoscopic withdrawal technique is associated with adenoma miss rates. Gastrointest Endosc 2000;51:33–6.
31. Almansa C, Shahid MW, Heckman MG, et al. Association between visual gaze patterns and adenoma detection rate during colonoscopy: a preliminary investigation. Am J Gastroenterol 2011;106:1070–4.
32. Rex DK, Hewett DG, Raghavendra M, et al. The impact of videorecording on the quality of colonoscopy performance: a pilot study. Am J Gastroenterol 2010;105: 2312–7.
33. Miller RE, Lehman G. Polypoid colonic lesions undetected by endoscopy. Radiology 1978;129:295–7.
34. Pickhardt PJ, Nugent PA, Mysliwiec PA, et al. Location of adenomas missed by optical colonoscopy. Ann Intern Med 2004;141:352–9.
35. Hewett DG, Rex DK. Miss rate of right-sided colon examination during colonoscopy defined by retroflexion: an observational study. Gastrointest Endosc 2011; 74:246–52.
36. Harrison M, Singh N, Rex DK. Impact of proximal colon retroflexion on adenoma miss rates. Am J Gastroenterol 2004;99:519–22.
37. Rex DK, Khashab M. Colonoscopic polypectomy in retroflexion. Gastrointest Endosc 2006;63:144–8.
38. Pishvaian AC, Al-Kawas FH. Retroflexion in the colon: a useful and safe technique in the evaluation and resection of sessile polyps during colonoscopy. Am J Gastroenterol 2006;101:1479–83.
39. Quallick MR, Brown WR. Rectal perforation during colonoscopic retroflexion: a large, prospective experience in an academic center. Gastrointest Endosc 2009;69:960–3.
40. Rex DK, Bond JH, Winawer S, et al. Quality in the technical performance of colonoscopy and the continuous quality improvement process for colonoscopy: recommendations of the U.S. Multi-Society Task Force on Colorectal Cancer. Am J Gastroenterol 2002;97:1296–308.
41. Rex DK, Petrini JL, Baron TH, et al. Quality indicators for colonoscopy. Gastrointest Endosc 2006;63:S16–28.
42. Corley DA, Jensen CD, Marks AR. Can we improve adenoma detection rates? A systematic review of intervention studies. Gastrointest Endosc 2011;74: 656–65.
43. Fatima H, Rex DK, Rothstein R, et al. Cecal insertion and withdrawal times with wide-angle versus standard colonoscopes: a randomized controlled trial. Clin Gastroenterol Hepatol 2008;6:109–14.
44. Barclay RL, Vicari JJ, Greenlaw RL. Effect of a time-dependent colonoscopic withdrawal protocol on adenoma detection during screening colonoscopy. Clin Gastroenterol Hepatol 2008;6:1091–8.
45. Ussui V, Coe SG, Ngamruengphong S, et al. Long term increases in adenoma detection at colonoscopy. Follow up of a randomized controlled clinical trial. Gastrointest Endosc 2012;75:AB300.

Colonoscopic Polypectomy
Current Techniques and Controversies

David G. Hewett, MBBS, MSc, PhD, FRACP

KEYWORDS

- Colonoscopy • Polypectomy • Adenoma • Colorectal cancer • Cold snare
- Electrocautery • Anticoagulation

KEY POINTS

- Colonoscopic polypectomy is fundamental to effective colonoscopy.
- Operator variability influences the quality of colonoscopy for both detection and resection.
- Multiple questions remain about best practice techniques for colonoscopic polypectomy. Cold snaring seems to offer safe, effective, and efficient resection for small and diminutive polyps.
- Further research is urgently needed to investigate the apparent variation in polypectomy outcomes, and establish an evidence base for effective polypectomy.

 Video demonstrating cold snare polypectomy technique in small and diminutive polyps accompanies this article at http://www.gastro.theclinics.com/

INTRODUCTION

Polypectomy is fundamental to the practice of colonoscopy. The importance of polypectomy derives from the natural history of colorectal cancer (CRC) and its disruptive impact on the polyp-cancer sequence. By removing cancer precursors, polypectomy reduces CRC incidence and mortality.[1,2] Data on the therapeutic benefit of colonoscopic polypectomy are derived from indirect evidence and longitudinal observational studies. Indirect evidence includes a population-level reduction in overall CRC incidence, likely due to CRC screening.[3] Longitudinal evidence includes the adenoma-cohort studies in which long-term follow-up after adenoma removal in the National Polyp Study and other international cohort studies demonstrated a reduction in CRC incidence[1,4] and mortality.[2,5]

School of Medicine, The University of Queensland, Mayne Medical Building, Herston Road, Herston, Brisbane, Queensland 4006, Australia
E-mail address: d.hewett@uq.edu.au

Gastroenterol Clin N Am 42 (2013) 443–458
http://dx.doi.org/10.1016/j.gtc.2013.05.015
0889-8553/13/$ – see front matter © 2013 Elsevier Inc. All rights reserved.

VARIATION IN COLONOSCOPY AND POLYPECTOMY EFFECTIVENESS

Despite this potential, colonoscopy is not perfect.[6] It is now clear that colonoscopy does not offer complete protection against CRC, particularly in the proximal colon.[7,8] Interval (postcolonoscopy) cancers are clearly associated with the quality of colonoscopy performance.[9–11] The factors contributing to this variation in effectiveness are multiple, including inadequate bowel preparation, incomplete insertion, and tumor biology, including the serrated pathway of neoplasia.[12]

However, individual operator factors are likely the most important contributor.[12,13] Studies show wide variation in levels of adenoma detection[14,15] and serrated polyp detection[16,17] between endoscopists and a clear relationship between adenoma detection and rates of interval cancer.[9–11] Also, interval cancers are more commonly due to missed, than new lesions.[18]

Emerging data extend this issue of operator variation to the effectiveness of polypectomy. It has been estimated that up to 27% of interval cancers may be due to incomplete endoscopic resection.[19–22] The recent Complete Adenoma Resection (CARE) study has cast substantial doubt on the effectiveness of routine polypectomy techniques for complete histologic eradication.[23] It showed high rates (over 10%) of incomplete hot snare resection of nonpedunculated neoplastic polyps (5–20 mm) and, importantly, rates of incomplete resection that varied significantly between endoscopists (6.5%–22.7%). Serrated polyps were a particular problem because they were almost four times more likely to be incompletely resected than adenomas (relative risk 3.74, 95% CI 2.04–6.84), with an incomplete resection rate approaching 50% for large serrated lesions. Other studies have questioned the effectiveness of resection with a biopsy forceps, with incomplete adenoma resection rates of up to 38%.[24,25]

GENERAL PRINCIPLES OF POLYPECTOMY

This variation in polypectomy outcomes indicates that some techniques are more effective than others are. It also highlights the relative lack of research attention and training on polypectomy techniques.[26,27] As a result, recommendations regarding polypectomy technique are limited by a lack of evidence and are based on expert opinion and uncontrolled observational studies.[26,28–30] Few clinical trial data have been available on the effectiveness and safety of specific techniques,[31] and most have focused on postpolypectomy bleeding.[32–34] Only recently have animal and clinical trials begun to define an evidence-base for basic polypectomy technique.[35–40]

Most endoscopists, therefore, perform polypectomy as they were taught in fellowship or from expert commentary at postgraduate training courses.[41] A 2004 survey of US gastroenterologists demonstrated substantial variation in polypectomy practices for lesions less than 10 mm.[42] For example, for resection of polyps 4 to 6 mm, hot snare was used by 59%, cold snare by 15%, cold biopsy forceps by 19%, and hot biopsy forceps (HBF) by 21%.

The goals of colonoscopic polypectomy are the effective, safe, and efficient resection and retrieval of precancerous lesions. Techniques to accomplish these goals must completely eradicate pathologic tissue while minimizing the risk of complications, specifically perforation and hemorrhage. Most complications from colonoscopy (with experienced operators) are related to polypectomy.[43] Further, because of the prevalence of small polyps, most polypectomy complications result from their removal.[44,45] Polypectomy complications are also more likely with an increasing number and size of resected polyps[44,46,47] and proximal location.[48]

Polypectomy is difficult to learn, requiring skills in instrument handling including the ability to precisely and efficiently control the instrument tip and therapeutic devices. It is an important element of the overall task of colonoscopy, yet colonoscopy competency assessment has tended to focus on insertion skills and measurement of completion or intubation rates.[49,50] It is likely that polypectomy skills require a baseline level of competence at instrument handling and tip control, although this has not been clarified. Specific polypectomy competencies have been defined only recently.[51,52]

Within the limits of the current evidence base and lack of formal recommendations,[26] this article describes current techniques and discusses controversies for basic colonoscopic polypectomy.

TECHNIQUES FOR RESECTION OF SMALL AND DIMINUTIVE POLYPS

Small polyps are very common. Most (>90%) colorectal polyps are less than 10 mm.[53,54] High-level adenoma detectors are now able to consistently achieve adenoma prevalence rates of approximately 40% to 50% in patients who have index screening colonoscopies.[55–58] Therefore, effective techniques to remove these lesions must be optimized.

Cold forceps are readily applied to diminutive polyps, 3 mm or less, and are virtually without risk. However, cold forceps removal is associated with high rates of incomplete resection, particularly with increasing polyp size when multiple bites are more likely required.[24,59] Piecemeal forceps resection limits visualization of any remaining adenomatous tissue due to blood contamination of the biopsy defect, which makes complete resection much less likely. The use of large capacity forceps that allow the polyp to be completed engulfed by the forceps and removed in a single piece may mitigate this risk. However, it seems that even jumbo forceps are associated with high rates (18%) of residual adenoma on postresection biopsy sampling.[37]

The addition of electrocautery to forceps removal is intended to ensure tissue destruction. However, in practice, this benefit is not realized. In particular, HBF are not effective, with high rates of incomplete resection (up to 30%), even for polyps less than 5 mm.[60–62] Also, HBF are associated with unacceptable rates of complications, notably uncontrolled, asymmetric, and transmural thermal injury to the colonic wall, resulting in perforation and rates of delayed postpolypectomy hemorrhage.[40,63–67] HBF should certainly not be used for polyps greater than 5 mm because of the risk of residual adenoma[68] and, in the author's view, cannot be recommended at all.

I never use HBF, I use cold forceps sparingly, and I aim to avoid piecemeal cold forceps resection. It is my practice to use large-capacity cold forceps for only the most tiny, diminutive of polyps (1–2 mm) that can be removed in a single bite, often by only partly opening the forceps to facilitate polyp entrapment. They seem most useful when the polyp is relatively inaccessible for efficient snaring; for example, located in the left field of endoscopic view and/or cannot be easily repositioned for snare placement (because of instrument looping or specific location at a flexure).

Cold snaring is the preferred technique for virtually all small (<10 mm) and most diminutive (≤5 mm) polyps. It is now well established as a safe and efficient technique for lesions less than 10 mm.[29,62,69] Cold snaring allows efficient resection of polyp tissue in a single piece, with a margin of normal tissue to ensure complete eradication. It is readily applied to most polyps less than 10 mm. Occasionally, polyps less than 10 mm are narrow-based and bulky or pedunculated. In these occasional situations, hot snare resection may be warranted because of the higher risk of immediate bleeding with a more vascular pedicle.

Like cold forceps, cold snaring is essentially without risk.[70] Bleeding is typically minor, immediate, and insignificant.[38] The advantage of cold techniques is the capacity to visualize immediately any significant bleeding from injury to submucosal vessels (which is the usual cause of delayed bleeding). As a result, cold snaring can be regarded as safe in patients taking antiplatelet agents or therapeutic anticoagulation.[28] A large Italian observational study of 1015 consecutive polyps confirmed the safety of cold techniques for polyps less than 10 mm, showing a low rate of immediate bleeding (1.8%), and no delayed bleeding or perforation.[71] Antiplatelet agents (aspirin, ticlopidine) predicted bleeding, although patients taking clopidogrel were excluded. Other small studies suggest that cold snaring may be more efficient than hot snaring.[38,39]

The effectiveness of cold snaring for polyp resection has not been well studied. Observational data suggest it may be more effective than forceps techniques,[62,72] yet its effectiveness compared with hot snaring has not been evaluated in prospective randomized studies. The recent CARE study[23] casts doubt on the effectiveness of hot snare polypectomy, which is unresolved for cold snaring. Studies comparing the completeness of polyp resection for cold versus hot snaring are required.

Cold Snaring

The technique of cold snaring is fundamentally different from snaring with electrocautery (**Fig. 1**, **Table 1**, Video 1). With hot snaring, capturing excess tissue around the polyp should be avoided and, once snared, the lesion should be lifted into the lumen by tenting the sheath away from the colon wall, to avoid electrocautery injury to the colon wall. With cold snaring, the goal is to capture and resect a 1 to 2 mm margin of normal tissue around the polyp. To achieve this, and to prevent the polyp specimen from flying away, the snare sheath should remain embedded within the

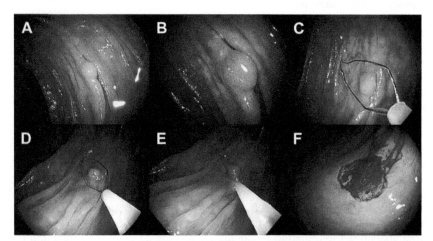

Fig. 1. The technique of cold snaring. (*A*) A diminutive polyp in the transverse colon. (*B*) Image enhancement (narrow-band imaging) shows an adenoma (*brown color, brown vessels, oval and tubular surface pattern*). (*C*) The polyp is aligned with the instrument channel at 5 o'clock and the snare opened (Exacto, US Endoscopy, Mentor, OH, USA). (*D*) The snare is advanced distal to the lesion, and the instrument tip angled down and right into the colon wall. (*E*) The snare is closed while the snare sheath is kept angled into the colon wall, capturing a complete rim of normal tissue around the lesion. (*F*) The resection defect shows minor bleeding after suctioning of polyp tissue.

Table 1
Differences in technique between hot and cold snaring

	Cold Snaring	Hot Snaring
Margin of normal tissue	Yes: at least 1–2 mm	Minimal
Tenting of lesion	No: snare sheath should remain pressed against colon wall	Yes: for application of electrocautery
Snare closure	Continuous until polyp guillotined	Snare closure stopped once resistance detected (or mark on snare handle reached)
Air aspiration	Not essential (can help snare to grasp polyp)	Yes
Electrocautery	No	Yes

colon wall during snare closure. The endoscopist should advance the sheath to at least 2 mm of the distal edge of the polyp and keep the sheath in this position while the snare is full closed around the polyp and the tissue guillotined. This may require gentle forward pressure on the snare sheath (or instrument) or angulation of the instrument tip into the wall (typically downward and right tip angulation) during snare closure. Suction can help the snare to capture the polyp and surrounding tissue. Next, the snare is gradually and completely closed in a single, continuous movement to guillotine the tissue. Once the tissue has been transected, the polyp tissue typically remains within or adjacent to the polypectomy defect, if the sheath has not been lifted during snare closure. The polyp can then be readily suctioned and retrieved.[70]

Precise and efficient manipulation of the snare sheath and wire requires skill in tip control. For additional control of the instrument tip, particularly for simultaneous movement of the snare, angulation controls, and insertion tube (forward or back), consider stabilizing the insertion tube between the fourth and fifth fingers of the left hand (the left-hand scope grip).[73] This frees the right hand to manipulate the snare sheath within the instrument channel, or the right or left angulation control for additional tip control.

Snare choice has an impact on the ease and efficiency of cold snaring, although evidence is lacking. Most experts use diminutive minisnares (9–15 mm), including snare shapes that facilitate capturing a rim of normal tissue around the lesion. The diameter (thickness) of the wire is also relevant because it affects the ease of cold transection. For snare closure, some endoscopists advocate marking the snare handle to assist in estimating the amount of tissue ensnared.[74] This is typically not required with cold snaring because there is no requirement to pause once the snare is closed around the polyp. Rather, after the polyp is encircled, the snare is gradually and completely closed and the polyp is guillotined in a single, continuous, and controlled movement of the snare handle. This is distinct from hot snaring in which inadvertent guillotining of the polyp before the application of electrocautery must be avoided.[74]

Occasionally, the snare may fail to cut through and guillotine the tissue. If this occurs, it is likely that the snare has captured some submucosa, which is preventing complete transection (**Fig. 2**). Failure to cold transect may occur more often with broader based polyps (approaching 10 mm), although can occur when excess normal tissue has been captured adjacent to a small polyp. In my experience, it does seem to happen less often with thin wire mini snares or dedicated cold snares. At this point, it is best to avoid application of electrocautery because of the risk of thermal injury to

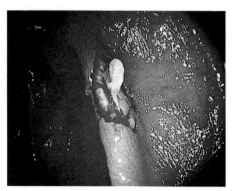

Fig. 2. A protruding remnant of submucosa in the base of a polypectomy defect, which initially prevented snare transection during cold snaring of a diminutive polyp.

submucosal vessels and delayed bleeding. My approach is to keep the snare tightly closed and wait a few seconds because the snare will often slowly transect the tissue. If not, with the snare tightly closed, cautiously lift the snare away from the colon wall, attempting to encourage release of the entrapped submucosa. Sometimes, this may require slight relaxation of the snare wire, although it is best to avoid fully reopening the snare because the margin of normal mucosa may be lost or the polyp may be resected piecemeal.

Cold snaring allows rapid and immediate visualization of the polypectomy defect after resection. The margins of the defect can be quickly inspected to confirm complete resection. There is typically minor capillary bleeding after cold resection, which is trivial and not clinically significant. Very occasionally, there is more prominent bleeding streaming from the base of the defect, usually in patients with coagulopathy or therapeutic anticoagulation. The benefit of cold snaring is the immediate visualization of any significant bleeding, which can be readily treated with clips.

Pedunculated Polyps

Pedunculated polyps require a different technique, more typical of traditional hot snare polypectomy. The snare should be carefully positioned around the stalk approximately one-half to one-third the distance between the polyp head and the colon wall, allowing sufficient resection margin in case of malignancy within the polyp head and leaving sufficient stalk tissue to regrasp in the event of bleeding. Access to the lesion should be optimized, and it is advisable to consider repositioning the patient so that the stalk attachment is not in a dependent segment of the colon. This allows ready visualization and access to the stalk in the event of immediate postresection bleeding. Once snared, the lesion should be lifted away from the colonic wall, being careful to minimize contact with the opposing colonic wall to avoid contralateral electrocautery injury. For large pedunculated lesions, ancillary strategies to prevent postpolypectomy bleeding should be considered (see the article by Sanchez-Yague and colleagues elsewhere in this issue).

UNCERTAINTIES AND CONTROVERSIES
The Use of Electrocautery

Traditionally, electrosurgical current (electrocautery) has been used in combination with mechanical transection for resection of all polyps with either snare or biopsy techniques. Electrocautery simultaneously ensures acute hemostasis while providing thermal fulguration of the polypectomy margins to ensure obliteration of pathologic tissue. The snare prevents blood flow by mechanically coapting blood vessel walls while heat seals the vessels closed.

However, the optimal choice of electrosurgical current is unresolved. There are few data to guide decisions regarding current or other electrosurgical settings, and power outputs between electrosurgical generators are not easily compared.[74] Many experts have advocated pure low-power coagulation, which provides good immediate hemostasis, but likely a higher chance of transmural thermal injury and a higher rate of delayed bleeding.[75] Blended current achieves effective transection with a lower depth of thermal injury and delayed bleeding, although rates of immediate bleeding are higher. Improvements in technology have seen the introduction of more sophisticated electrosurgical generators in which power output is microprocessor-controlled and responsive to tissue impedance. Output power is adjusted automatically and applied cyclically, alternating between cutting and coagulation current to minimize depth and spread of thermal injury. Many endoscopists have begun to use these systems for complex polypectomy.[76] The contribution of type of electrosurgical current to variable polypectomy effectiveness is unknown.

However, electrocautery is responsible for virtually all of the complications associated with polypectomy.[46] The risk of complications increases with the number of polypectomies performed with electrocautery.[47] As a result, cold mechanical techniques have become the preferred strategy for small and diminutive polyps.[27–29,45,71]

Resection of Serrated Polyps

Serrated polyps (specifically, sessile serrated adenoma or polyp [SSA/P]) pose a particular problem for colonoscopy and polypectomy.[77] They are likely significant contributors to postcolonoscopy interval CRC[78,79] due to failures in detection,[16,17] but also failures in resection as highlighted by the CARE study.[23] SSA/P are typically flat subtle lesions draped over or thickening folds, with a yellow-brown mucus cap.[77] They have characteristically indistinct margins that blend imperceptibly with normal mucosa (**Fig. 3**), particularly when their mucus cap is removed.

Optimal and effective techniques for resection of serrated polyps have not been established. Cold snaring is suitable for smaller lesions less than 10 mm. However, the CARE study showed overall rates of incomplete resection for SSA/P of 31% (and 47.6% for 10–20 mm lesions). These data emphasize the need to delineate carefully the margin of the lesion before resection, to avoid recurrence (**Fig. 4**). Image-enhancement techniques may have a role in this regard. For example, preresection

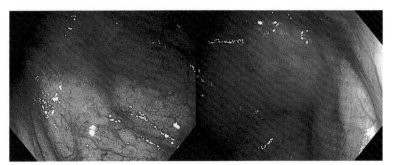

Fig. 3. Two sessile serrated adenomas in the ascending colon. The lesions are very flat with a minimal mucus cap and indistinct margins.

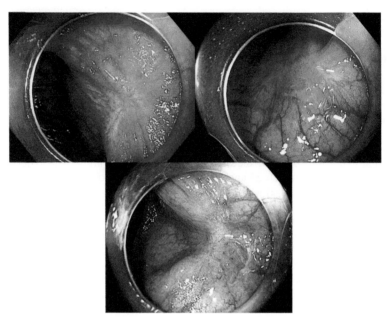

Fig. 4. Three examples of residual sessile serrated adenoma within polypectomy scars, after previous incomplete resection.

marking of the lesion margins after topical dye spray application or visualization with narrow-band imaging. Submucosal injection of dilute indigo carmine or methylene blue seems helpful in defining the lesion for subsequent resection. These techniques need further research.

Confirming Complete Resection

After endoscopic resection, the margins of the polypectomy defect should be carefully inspected to ensure complete removal of all visible pathologic tissue. Methods to assess and document complete resection at the time of polypectomy have not been determined. There are no data to support a role for endoscopic image-enhancement technologies, although they warrant further evaluation, particularly given the variable outcomes seen in the CARE study.[23]

Management of Anticoagulation or Antiplatelet Therapy

Recommendations from the American Society for Gastrointestinal Endoscopy (ASGE) provide guidance on the management of anticoagulation and antiplatelet agents for patients undergoing colonoscopy with polypectomy.[80] This is an important and common scenario given the prevalence of cardiovascular disease and related therapies in patients having colonoscopy. The ASGE has developed categories of procedural bleeding risk and patient thromboembolic risk (**Box 1**). Diagnostic colonoscopy without polypectomy but including mucosal biopsy is regarded as low risk for bleeding,[81] and the ASGE recommends that antiplatelet and anticoagulation therapy can be continued. The ASGE guidelines regard polypectomy as a high-risk procedure for bleeding, although they do not distinguish between polypectomy with and without the use of electrocautery. Mucosal biopsy is not regarded as high risk, and some endoscopists extend mucosal biopsy to include cold snare resection of polyps.[45]

Box 1

ASGE categories of risk for thromboembolic complications of endoscopy

Higher risk conditions	Atrial fibrillation with valvular heart disease, prosthetic valve, active congestive heart failure, left ventricular ejection fraction <35%, history of thromboembolism, hypertension, diabetes, or age >75 years
	Mechanical valve in mitral position
	Mechanical valve with previous thromboembolism
	Acute coronary syndrome
	Coronary stent (within 1 year)
	Nonstented percutaneous coronary intervention after myocardial infarction
Low-risk conditions	Uncomplicated atrial fibrillation without valvular disease
	Bioprosthetic valve
	Mechanical valves in aortic position
	Deep vein thrombosis
Higher risk procedures	Colonoscopy with polypectomy
	Colonoscopy with dilation
	Colonoscopy with tumor ablation
Low-risk procedures	Colonoscopy with biopsy (cold)

Adapted from ASGE Standards of Practice Committee. Management of antithrombotic agents for endoscopic procedures. Gastrointest Endosc 2009;70:1063; with permission.

For high-risk procedures, the guidelines suggest aspirin and NSAIDs may be continued, although they allow clinicians to stop therapy for 5 to 7 days depending on the underlying indication for treatment. Data on aspirin show only a small risk of bleeding,[82–85] although this is likely higher with resection of large polyps.[86] The ASGE recommends that clopidogrel be stopped 7 to 10 days before the procedure. Clopidogrel does seem to be associated with a small but higher rate of postpolypectomy bleeding.[87] To reduce the risk of withdrawing clopidogrel, it is suggested that aspirin be continued (or substituted).

Decisions about the management of warfarin are guided by the indication for anticoagulation and procedural risk. Like aspirin and clopidogrel, warfarin may be continued for colonoscopy with mucosal biopsy. For polypectomy, the guidelines advise warfarin withdrawal. For patients with low thromboembolic risk, warfarin can be stopped 3 to 5 days before the procedure. Bridging therapy with outpatient low molecular weight heparin (LMWH), or inpatient unfractionated heparin, is recommended for high-risk patients periprocedurally, although LMWH should be withheld 24 hours before the scheduled procedure time.[88]

The ASGE guidelines recommend that decisions on reinstitution of anticoagulation and antiplatelet agents should be individualized. Considerations include procedure risk (polypectomy, use of electrocautery, size of defect) and indications for antithrombotic therapy. For example, it is my practice to try to delay reinstitution of clopidogrel, LMWH, or warfarin for as long as possible after hot snare polypectomy, particularly for large lesions. Resumption of bridging therapy or early reinstitution of warfarin is associated higher rates of postprocedural bleeding after polypectomy.[89,90] Obviously, this has to be balanced with the risk of a thrombotic event; hence, communication and coordination of care with the patient's other health care providers are very important.

Several areas of uncertainty remain (**Box 2**). For example, what is the safety of cold snare polypectomy in patients on antiplatelet or anticoagulant therapy? This approach

---

Box 2
Uncertainties about basic polypectomy technique

Which technique is most effective and safe, and for what type of lesion?

What is the incomplete resection rate for cold snaring?

Which factors explain incomplete resection?

- Specific tools and techniques (high-definition instrument, type or shape of snare, margin of normal tissue, piecemeal resection)
- Type of electrosurgical current (pure coagulation vs microprocessor-controlled alternating current)
- Use of image-enhancement techniques to define margins of lesion (before) and defect (after)
- Use of adjunctive thermal therapy (argon plasma coagulation)

Is piecemeal cold snaring effective. If so, for what type of lesion?

Which specific techniques are effective and safe for resection of serrated lesions?

Which outcome measure should be used for studying effectiveness of polypectomy?

How can completeness of polypectomy be best assessed at the time of resection?

What techniques ensure safety of polypectomy in patients on antiplatelet or anticoagulant therapy (cold snaring, clip closure of defect)?

Adapted from Kahi CJ, Rex DK. Why we should CARE about polypectomy technique. Gastroenterology 2013;144:17; with permission.

---

theoretically allows visualization and treatment of immediate bleeding at the time of resection, yet needs further study. In addition, what is the role of clip closure of polypectomy defects to prevent bleeding in patients remaining on or resuming antiplatelet or anticoagulant therapy? Endoscopic clips have been used to prophylactically close hot snare polypectomy defects in anticoagulated patients[91] and to reduce the risk of bleeding after resection of large polyps.[92]

Surveillance After Polypectomy

Updated surveillance guidelines have recently been published by the US Multi-Society Task Force on Colorectal Cancer.[93] These guidelines now incorporate recommendations about serrated polyp surveillance and advise surveillance intervals based on both the most recent colonoscopy and a previous examination showing neoplasia. Recommendations require risk stratification of patients into three groups on findings at baseline colonoscopy: no adenomas or polyps, low-risk adenomas (LRA; 1–2 tubular adenomas <10 mm), and high-risk adenomas (HRA; adenoma with high-grade dysplasia, villous histology, or size ≥10 mm or number ≥3). All recommendations regarding surveillance interval presume a high-quality baseline examination in terms of extent of examination, intensity of mucosal inspection, and bowel preparation.

Recommendations for the timing of the first surveillance examination are summarized in **Box 3**. In general, the timing is as follows:

- Patients with no adenomas or small distal hyperplastic polyps should have surveillance colonoscopy in 10 years
- Patients with LRA should have a surveillance interval of between 5 and 10 years
- Patients with HRA should have surveillance at 3 years.

Box 3
Recommended screening and polyp surveillance intervals for individuals with baseline average risk

After findings at baseline examination	
No adenomas or polyps	10 years
Small (<10 mm) hyperplastic polyps in rectum or sigmoid	10 years
LRA	
1–2 small (<10 mm) tubular adenomas	5–10 years
Sessile serrated polyps <10 mm without cytologic dysplasia	5 years
HRA	
3 to 10 adenomas	3 years
>10 adenomas	Within 3 years
≥1 adenomas ≥10 mm or with villous histology or with high-grade dysplasia	3 years
Sessile serrated polyps ≥10 mm or with cytologic dysplasia	3 years
Traditional serrated adenoma	3 years
After findings at surveillance examination	
No adenoma (and LRA on baseline colonoscopy)	10 years
No adenoma (and HRA on baseline colonoscopy)	5 years
LRA	5 years
HRA	3 years

Adapted from Lieberman DA, Rex DK, Winawer SJ, et al. Guidelines for colonoscopy surveillance after screening and polypectomy: a consensus update by the US Multi-Society Task Force on Colorectal Cancer. Gastroenterology 2012;143:844–57; with permission.

Recommendations for subsequent surveillance are derived from baseline and first surveillance findings. Notably, patients with LRA at baseline and a negative first surveillance examination can have colonoscopy in 10 years. Patients with HRA at baseline or surveillance colonoscopy should continue to have a 3-year surveillance interval.

The guidelines now incorporate surveillance for serrated polyps, although this remains controversial because of a lack of evidence from prospective studies.[77,93] Current recommendations, based on low-quality evidence, suggest categorizing large (≥10 mm) sessile serrated polyps or those with cytologic dysplasia as HRA; conversely, small (<10 mm) sessile serrated polyps with no cytologic dysplasia can be managed as LRA.

SUMMARY

Colonoscopic polypectomy is fundamental to effective colonoscopy. However, operator variability influences the quality of colonoscopy for both detection and resection. Multiple questions remain about best practice techniques for colonoscopic polypectomy. Cold snaring seems to offer safe, effective, and efficient resection for small and diminutive polyps. Further research is urgently needed to investigate the apparent variation in polypectomy outcomes and to establish an evidence base for effective polypectomy.

SUPPLEMENTARY DATA

Supplementary data related to this article can be found online at http://dx.doi.org/10.1016/j.gtc.2013.05.015.

REFERENCES

1. Winawer SJ, Zauber AG, Ho MN, et al. Prevention of colorectal cancer by colonoscopic polypectomy. N Engl J Med 1993;329:1977–81.
2. Zauber AG, Winawer SJ, O'Brien MJ, et al. Colonoscopic polypectomy and long-term prevention of colorectal-cancer deaths. N Engl J Med 2012;366: 687–96.
3. Sedjo RL, Byers T, Barrera E Jr, et al. A midpoint assessment of the American Cancer Society challenge goal to decrease cancer incidence by 25% between 1992 and 2015. CA Cancer J Clin 2007;57:326–40.
4. Citarda F, Tomaselli G, Capocaccia R, et al. Efficacy in standard clinical practice of colonoscopic polypectomy in reducing colorectal cancer incidence. Gut 2001;48:812–5.
5. Jorgensen OD, Kronborg O, Fenger C. The Funen Adenoma Follow-up Study. Incidence and death from colorectal carcinoma in an adenoma surveillance program. Scand J Gastroenterol 1993;28:869–74.
6. Hewett DG, Kahi CJ, Rex DK. Does colonoscopy work? J Natl Compr Canc Netw 2010;8:67–77.
7. Baxter NN, Goldwasser MA, Paszat LF, et al. Association of colonoscopy and death from colorectal cancer. Ann Intern Med 2009;150:1–8.
8. Brenner H, Chang-Claude J, Seiler CM, et al. Protection from colorectal cancer after colonoscopy: a population-based, case-control study. Ann Intern Med 2011;154:22–30.
9. Kaminski MF, Regula J, Kraszewska E, et al. Quality indicators for colonoscopy and the risk of interval cancer. N Engl J Med 2010;362:1795–803.
10. Baxter NN, Sutradhar R, Forbes SS, et al. Analysis of administrative data finds endoscopist quality measures associated with postcolonoscopy colorectal cancer. Gastroenterology 2011;140:65–72.
11. Rogal SS, Pinsky PF, Schoen RE. Relationship between detection of adenomas by flexible sigmoidoscopy and interval distal colorectal cancer. Clin Gastroenterol Hepatol 2013;11:73–8.
12. Hewett DG, Kahi CJ, Rex DK. Efficacy and effectiveness of colonoscopy: how do we bridge the gap? Gastrointest Endosc Clin N Am 2010;20:673–84.
13. Adler A, Wegscheider K, Lieberman D, et al. Factors determining the quality of screening colonoscopy: a prospective study on adenoma detection rates, from 12 134 examinations (Berlin colonoscopy project 3, BECOP-3). Gut 2013;62: 236–41.
14. Barclay RL, Vicari JJ, Doughty AS, et al. Colonoscopic withdrawal times and adenoma detection during screening colonoscopy. N Engl J Med 2006;355: 2533–41.
15. Chen SC, Rex DK. Endoscopist can be more powerful than age and male gender in predicting adenoma detection at colonoscopy. Am J Gastroenterol 2007;102:856–61.
16. Hetzel JT, Huang CS, Coukos JA, et al. Variation in the detection of serrated polyps in an average risk colorectal cancer screening cohort. Am J Gastroenterol 2010;105:2656–64.
17. Kahi CJ, Hewett DG, Norton DL, et al. Prevalence and variable detection of proximal colon serrated polyps during screening colonoscopy. Clin Gastroenterol Hepatol 2011;9:42–6.
18. Pohl H, Robertson DJ. Colorectal cancers detected after colonoscopy frequently result from missed lesions. Clin Gastroenterol Hepatol 2010;8:858–64.

19. Pabby A, Schoen RE, Weissfeld JL, et al. Analysis of colorectal cancer occurrence during surveillance colonoscopy in the Dietary Polyp Prevention Trial. Gastrointest Endosc 2005;61:385–91.
20. Farrar WD, Sawhney MS, Nelson DB, et al. Colorectal cancers found after a complete colonoscopy. Clin Gastroenterol Hepatol 2006;4:1259–64.
21. Martinez ME, Baron JA, Lieberman DA, et al. A pooled analysis of advanced colorectal neoplasia diagnoses after colonoscopic polypectomy. Gastroenterology 2009;136:832–41.
22. Leung K, Pinsky P, Laiyemo AO, et al. Ongoing colorectal cancer risk despite surveillance colonoscopy: the Polyp Prevention Trial Continued Follow-up Study. Gastrointest Endosc 2010;71:111–7.
23. Pohl H, Srivastava A, Bensen SP, et al. Incomplete polyp resection during colonoscopy: results of the Complete Adenoma Resection (CARE) study. Gastroenterology 2013;144:74–80.e1.
24. Efthymiou M, Taylor AC, Desmond PV, et al. Biopsy forceps is inadequate for the resection of diminutive polyps. Endoscopy 2011;43:312–6.
25. Liu S, Ho SB, Krinsky ML. Quality of polyp resection during colonoscopy: are we achieving polyp clearance? Dig Dis Sci 2012;57:1786–91.
26. Rex DK. Have we defined best colonoscopic polypectomy practice in the United States? Clin Gastroenterol Hepatol 2007;5:674–7.
27. Kahi CJ, Rex DK. Why we should CARE about polypectomy technique. Gastroenterology 2013;144:16–8.
28. Hewett DG, Rex DK. Colonoscopy and diminutive polyps: hot or cold biopsy or snare? Do I send to pathology? Clin Gastroenterol Hepatol 2011;9:102–5.
29. Tappero G, Gaia E, De Giuli P, et al. Cold snare excision of small colorectal polyps. Gastrointest Endosc 1992;38:310–3.
30. Pattullo V, Bourke MJ, Tran KL, et al. The suction pseudopolyp technique: a novel method for the removal of small flat nonpolypoid lesions of the colon and rectum. Endoscopy 2009;41:1032–7.
31. Brooker JC, Saunders BP, Shah SG, et al. Treatment with argon plasma coagulation reduces recurrence after piecemeal resection of large sessile colonic polyps: a randomized trial and recommendations. Gastrointest Endosc 2002;55:371–5.
32. Shioji K, Suzuki Y, Kobayashi M, et al. Prophylactic clip application does not decrease delayed bleeding after colonoscopic polypectomy. Gastrointest Endosc 2003;57:691–4.
33. Di Giorgio P, De Luca L, Calcagno G, et al. Detachable snare versus epinephrine injection in the prevention of postpolypectomy bleeding: a randomized and controlled study. Endoscopy 2004;36:860–3.
34. Paspatis GA, Paraskeva K, Theodoropoulou A, et al. A prospective, randomized comparison of adrenaline injection in combination with detachable snare versus adrenaline injection alone in the prevention of postpolypectomy bleeding in large colonic polyps. Am J Gastroenterol 2006;101:2805–9.
35. Moss A, Bourke MJ, Kwan V, et al. Succinylated gelatin substantially increases en bloc resection size in colonic EMR: a randomized, blinded trial in a porcine model. Gastrointest Endosc 2010;71:589–95.
36. Moss A, Bourke MJ, Metz AJ. A randomized, double-blind trial of succinylated gelatin submucosal injection for endoscopic resection of large sessile polyps of the colon. Am J Gastroenterol 2010;105:2375–82.
37. Draganov PV, Chang MN, Lieb J, et al. Randomized controlled trial of two types of biopsy forceps for polypectomy of small sessile colorectal polyps. Gastrointest Endosc 2010;71:AB194.

38. Paspatis GA, Tribonias G, Konstantinidis K, et al. A prospective randomized comparison of cold vs hot snare polypectomy in the occurrence of postpolypectomy bleeding in small colonic polyps. Colorectal Dis 2011;13:e345–8.

39. Ichise Y, Horiuchi A, Nakayama Y, et al. Prospective randomized comparison of cold snare polypectomy and conventional polypectomy for small colorectal polyps. Digestion 2011;84:78–81.

40. Metz AJ, Moss A, McLeod D, et al. A blinded comparison of the safety and efficacy of hot biopsy forceps electrocauterization and conventional snare polypectomy for diminutive colonic polypectomy in a porcine model. Gastrointest Endosc 2013;77(3):484–90.

41. Rex DK. Colonoscopic polypectomy. Rev Gastroenterol Disord 2005;5:115–25.

42. Singh N, Harrison M, Rex DK. A survey of colonoscopic polypectomy practices among clinical gastroenterologists. Gastrointest Endosc 2004;99:414–8.

43. Rabeneck L, Paszat LF, Hilsden RJ, et al. Bleeding and perforation after outpatient colonoscopy and their risk factors in usual clinical practice. Gastroenterology 2008;135:1899–906, 1906.e1.

44. Levin TR, Zhao W, Conell C, et al. Complications of colonoscopy in an integrated health care delivery system. Ann Intern Med 2006;145:880–6.

45. Tolliver KA, Rex DK. Colonoscopic polypectomy. Gastroenterol Clin North Am 2008;37:229–51, ix.

46. Ko CW, Dominitz JA. Complications of colonoscopy: magnitude and management. Gastrointest Endosc Clin N Am 2010;20:659–71.

47. Ko CW, Riffle S, Michaels L, et al. Serious complications within 30 days of screening and surveillance colonoscopy are uncommon. Clin Gastroenterol Hepatol 2010;8:166–73.

48. Heldwein W, Dollhopf M, Rosch T, et al. The Munich Polypectomy Study (MUPS): prospective analysis of complications and risk factors in 4000 colonic snare polypectomies. Endoscopy 2005;37:1116–22.

49. Cass OW, Freeman ML, Peine CJ, et al. Objective evaluation of endoscopy skills during training. Ann Intern Med 1993;118:40–4.

50. Sedlack RE. Training to competency in colonoscopy: assessing and defining competency standards. Gastrointest Endosc 2011;74:355–66.e1–2.

51. Gupta S, Anderson J, Bhandari P, et al. Development and validation of a novel method for assessing competency in polypectomy: direct observation of polypectomy skills. Gastrointest Endosc 2011;73:1232–9.e2.

52. Gupta S, Bassett P, Man R, et al. Validation of a novel method for assessing competency in polypectomy. Gastrointest Endosc 2012;75:568–75.

53. Regula J, Rupinski M, Kraszewska E, et al. Colonoscopy in colorectal-cancer screening for detection of advanced neoplasia. N Engl J Med 2006;355:1863–72.

54. Lieberman D, Moravec M, Holub J, et al. Polyp size and advanced histology in patients undergoing colonoscopy screening: implications for CT colonography. Gastroenterology 2008;135:1100–5.

55. Rex DK, Helbig CC. High yields of small and flat adenomas with high-definition colonoscopes using either white light or narrow band imaging. Gastroenterology 2007;133:42–7.

56. Hewett DG, Rex DK. Cap-fitted colonoscopy: a randomized, tandem colonoscopy study of adenoma miss rates. Gastrointest Endosc 2010;72:775–81. http://dx.doi.org/10.1016/j.gie.2010.04.030.

57. Kahi CJ, Anderson JC, Waxman I, et al. High-definition chromocolonoscopy vs. high-definition white light colonoscopy for average-risk colorectal cancer screening. Am J Gastroenterol 2010;105:1301–7. http://dx.doi.org/10.1038/ajg.2010.51.

58. Hewett DG, Rex DK. Inspection on instrument insertion during colonoscopy: a randomized controlled trial. Gastrointest Endosc 2012;76:381–7.

59. Woods A, Sanowski R, Wadas D, et al. Eradication of diminutive polyps: a prospective evaluation of bipolar coagulation versus conventional biopsy removal. Gastrointest Endosc 1989;35:536–40.

60. Vanagunas A, Jacob P, Vakil N. Adequacy of "hot biopsy" for the treatment of diminutive polyps: a prospective randomized trial. Am J Gastroenterol 1989; 84:383–5.

61. Peluso F, Goldner F. Follow-up of hot biopsy forceps treatment of diminutive colonic polyps. Gastrointest Endosc 1991;37:604–6.

62. Ellis K, Shiel M, Marquis S, et al. Efficacy of hot biopsy forceps, cold microsnare, and microsnare with cautery techniques in the removal of diminutive colonic polyps [abstract]. Gastrointest Endosc 1997;45:AB107.

63. Wadas DD, Sanowski RA. Complications of the hot biopsy forceps technique. Gastrointest Endosc 1988;34:32–7.

64. Quigley EM, Donovan JP, Linder J, et al. Delayed, massive hemorrhage following electrocoagulating biopsy ("hot biopsy") of a diminutive colonic polyp. Gastrointest Endosc 1989;35:559–63.

65. Dyer WS, Quigley EM, Noel SM, et al. Major colonic hemorrhage following electrocoagulating (hot) biopsy of diminutive colonic polyps: relationship to colonic location and low-dose aspirin therapy. Gastrointest Endosc 1991;37:361–4.

66. Weston AP, Campbell DR. Diminutive colonic polyps: histopathology, spatial distribution, concomitant significant lesions, and treatment complications. Am J Gastroenterol 1995;90:24–8.

67. Chino A, Karasawa T, Uragami N, et al. A comparison of depth of tissue injury caused by different modes of electrosurgical current in a pig colon model. Gastrointest Endosc 2004;59:374–9.

68. Gilbert DA, DiMarino AJ, Jensen DM, et al. Status evaluation: hot biopsy forceps. American Society for Gastrointestinal Endoscopy. Technology Assessment Committee. Gastrointest Endosc 1992;38:753–6.

69. McAfee J, Katon R. Tiny snares prove safe and effective for removal of diminutive colorectal polyps. Gastrointest Endosc 1994;40:301–3.

70. Deenadayalu VP, Rex DK. Colon polyp retrieval after cold snaring. Gastrointest Endosc 2005;62:253–6.

71. Repici A, Hassan C, Vitetta E, et al. Safety of cold polypectomy for <10 mm polyps at colonoscopy: a prospective multicenter study. Endoscopy 2012;44: 27–31.

72. Urquhart P, Brown G. The effectiveness of cold snare polypectomy for the removal of small sessile colonic polyps [abstract]. Gastrointest Endosc 2012; 75:AB328.

73. Rex DK. Maximizing control of tip deflection with sound ergonomics: the "left hand shaft grip". Gastrointest Endosc 2007;65:950–1 [author reply: 951].

74. Waye JD. Polypectomy: basic principles. In: Waye JD, Rex DK, Williams CB, editors. Colonoscopy: principles and practice. 2nd edition. Hoboken (NJ): Blackwell; 2009. p. 572–81.

75. Van Gossum A, Cozzoli A, Adler M, et al. Colonoscopic snare polypectomy: analysis of 1485 resections comparing two types of current. Gastrointest Endosc 1992;38:472–5.

76. Holt BA, Bourke MJ. Wide field endoscopic resection for advanced colonic mucosal neoplasia: current status and future directions. Clin Gastroenterol Hepatol 2012;10:969–79.

77. Rosty C, Hewett DG, Brown IS, et al. Serrated polyps of the large intestine: current understanding of diagnosis, pathogenesis, and clinical management. J Gastroenterol 2013;48(3):287–302.
78. Sawhney MS, Farrar WD, Gudiseva S, et al. Microsatellite instability in interval colon cancers. Gastroenterology 2006;131:1700–5.
79. Arain MA, Sawhney M, Sheikh S, et al. CIMP status of interval colon cancers: another piece to the puzzle. Am J Gastroenterol 2010;105:1189–95.
80. ASGE Standards of Practice Committee. Management of antithrombotic agents for endoscopic procedures. Gastrointest Endosc 2009;70:1060–70.
81. Gerson LB, Gage BF, Owens DK, et al. Effect and outcomes of the ASGE guidelines on the periendoscopic management of patients who take anticoagulants. Am J Gastroenterol 2000;95:1717–24.
82. Shiffman ML, Farrel MT, Yee YS. Risk of bleeding after endoscopic biopsy or polypectomy in patients taking aspirin or other NSAIDS. Gastrointest Endosc 1994;40:458–62.
83. Hui AJ, Wong RM, Ching JY, et al. Risk of colonoscopic polypectomy bleeding with anticoagulants and antiplatelet agents: analysis of 1657 cases. Gastrointest Endosc 2004;59:44–8.
84. Yousfi M, Gostout CJ, Baron TH, et al. Postpolypectomy lower gastrointestinal bleeding: potential role of aspirin. Am J Gastroenterol 2004;99:1785–9.
85. Sawhney MS, Salfiti N, Nelson DB, et al. Risk factors for severe delayed postpolypectomy bleeding. Endoscopy 2008;40:115–9.
86. Moss A, Bourke MJ, Williams SJ, et al. Endoscopic mucosal resection outcomes and prediction of submucosal cancer from advanced colonic mucosal neoplasia. Gastroenterology 2011;140:1909–18.
87. Singh M, Mehta N, Murthy UK, et al. Postpolypectomy bleeding in patients undergoing colonoscopy on uninterrupted clopidogrel therapy. Gastrointest Endosc 2010;71:998–1005.
88. O'Donnell MJ, Kearon C, Johnson J, et al. Brief communication: preoperative anticoagulant activity after bridging low-molecular-weight heparin for temporary interruption of warfarin. Ann Intern Med 2007;146:184–7.
89. Witt DM, Delate T, McCool KH, et al. Incidence and predictors of bleeding or thrombosis after polypectomy in patients receiving and not receiving anticoagulation therapy. J Thromb Haemost 2009;7:1982–9.
90. Gerson LB, Michaels L, Ullah N, et al. Adverse events associated with anticoagulation therapy in the periendoscopic period. Gastrointest Endosc 2010;71:1211–7.e2.
91. Friedland S, Soetikno R. Colonoscopy with polypectomy in anticoagulated patients. Gastrointest Endosc 2006;64:98–100.
92. Liaquat H, Rohn E, Rex DK. Prophylactic clip closure reduced the risk of delayed postpolypectomy hemorrhage: experience in 277 clipped large sessile or flat colorectal lesions and 247 control lesions. Gastrointest Endosc 2013;77(3):401–7.
93. Lieberman DA, Rex DK, Winawer SJ, et al. Guidelines for colonoscopy surveillance after screening and polypectomy: a consensus update by the US Multi-Society Task Force on Colorectal Cancer. Gastroenterology 2012;143:844–57.

Advanced Endoscopic Resection of Colorectal Lesions

Andres Sanchez-Yague, MD[a,b], Tonya Kaltenbach, MD, MS[a], Gottumukkala Raju, MD[c], Roy Soetikno, MD[a,*]

KEYWORDS

- Colonoscopy • Advanced endoscopic resection • Endoscopic mucosal resection
- Endoscopic submucosal dissection • Colorectal cancer

KEY POINTS

- Advanced endoscopic resection techniques represent the most cost-effective option for the management of difficult colorectal lesions.
- Proficiency in optical diagnosis, techniques to prevent complications and to resect are key to the management of complex colorectal lesions.
- All the team members should fully understanding the techniques and equipment needed to perform them.

INTRODUCTION

Recent advances in endoscopic imaging and resection allow clinicians to identify and determine lesions that are amenable to curative resection and apply techniques that ensure their complete and safe resection,[1] while referring cancer-harboring lesions to surgery. However, these developments occurred after many clinicians finished training in an era in which lesions were described as either pedunculated or sessile and treated with a hot snare, without the benefit of image enhancement, resection, hemostatic, and closure techniques that developed in the last decade. Current therapeutic colonoscopists should be able to make an optical diagnosis of the lesion and apply the most appropriate technique to remove the lesion completely and safely. Based on our practice, this article shares our views on advanced endoscopic resection of colorectal lesions (**Box 1**). It focuses on the resection of the nonpolypoid colorectal neoplasm (NP-CRN) because of its importance and because its resection often requires advanced techniques.

[a] Endoscopy Unit, Veterans Affairs Palo Alto and Stanford University, 3801 Miranda Avenue, Palo Alto, CA 93404, USA; [b] Endoscopy Unit, Hospital Costa del Sol, Autovia A-7, Km 187, Marbella 29603, Spain; [c] Department of Gastroenterology, Hepatology and Nutrition, The University of Texas MD Anderson Cancer Center, 1515 Holcombe Boulevard, Unit 1466, Houston, TX 77030, USA
* Corresponding author.
E-mail address: giendo@me.com

Gastroenterol Clin N Am 42 (2013) 459–477
http://dx.doi.org/10.1016/j.gtc.2013.05.012
0889-8553/13/$ – see front matter © 2013 Elsevier Inc. All rights reserved.

gastro.theclinics.com

Box 1
Indications for advanced endoscopic resection in the colon

Nonpolypoid colorectal neoplasms

Lesions greater than 2 cm

Difficult locations

    Dentate line

    Ileocecal valve

    Appendiceal orifice

    Folds

Lesions over scars

Lesions in chronic inflammatory bowel disease

Large pedunculated lesions

Rectal carcinoids

Large lipomas

Patients with impaired coagulation

    Anticoagulation medication

    Antiplatelet medication

    Thrombocytopenia

RESECTION OF NP-CRN
Characterization of NP-CRN

Endoscopic characterization of the colorectal lesion is the first step in the assessment of whether a lesion is a candidate for curative endoscopic resection. This characterization can be undertaken using the shape of the lesion (macroscopic characterization) as well as the mucosal surface pit pattern and vascular pattern (microscopic characterization). Lesions amenable for curative resection are those limited to the mucosa and, perhaps, superficial submucosa, whereas those extending to deep submucosa are not candidates for endoscopic resection.[2]

Macroscopic characterization

Macroscopic characterization of a lesion provides information about its endoscopic appearance, its malignant potential, and the skill level required for its resection.[2] There are 2 macroscopic types: (1) type 0, the superficial lesions; and (2) types 1 to 5, the advanced cancers (**Box 2**). Type 0 includes the colorectal polyps, herein called lesions because the term polyp connotes abnormal growth of tissue projecting from mucous membrane. Type 0 can be classified into protruding or polypoid, and nonprotruding or nonpolypoid. Polypoid lesions are further subtyped into pedunculated (0–Ip) and sessile (0–Is). Nonpolypoid lesions can be subtyped into the superficial elevated (0–IIa), flat (0–IIb), and depressed (0–IIc) types. In the colon and rectum, the superficial elevated types are commonly classified together with flat lesions because of their shapes being tabletop flat, and because the true colorectal flat (0–IIb) lesions are rare. Flat colorectal neoplasms equal to or larger than 10 mm are called lateral spreading tumors (LSTs). LSTs are differentiated into granular LST (LST-G) and nongranular LST (LST-NG).[3]

Box 2
Paris/Japanese classification

Type 0: lesions with superficial appearance

    0 to I: Protruding

        0 to Is: Sessile

        0 to Ip: Pedunculated

    0 to II: Nonprotruding and nonexcavated

        0 to IIa: Slightly elevated

        0 to IIb: Flat

        0 to IIc: Slightly depressed

        0 to IIa + IIc, 0 to IIc + IIa: Elevated and depressed

    0 to III: Excavated

Type 1 to 5: lesions with muscularis propria involvement

Macroscopic characterization provides superior information about the risk of early cancer compared with size of the lesion. NP-CRNs have higher risk of early cancer than the polypoid-CRNs, irrespective of size.[3] The observation that the larger the polypoid neoplasms the higher the risk of deeper submucosal invasion does not apply for NP-CRNs. In NP-CRNs, the difference in the size of lesions with superficial and deep submucosal invasion is not pronounced. LST-Gs with even-sized nodules have a low risk (<2%) of submucosal invasion, irrespective of size, whereas LST-Gs with mixed-sized nodules have a higher risk of submucosal invasion (7.1% for lesions <20 mm and 38% for lesions >30 mm),[3] with the point of invasion usually located under the largest nodule.[4] The LST-NGs, particularly those that have a thinner center (LST-NG with pseudodepression) also have a high risk of submucosal invasion: 12.5% for lesions less than 20 mm to 83.3% for lesions more than 30 mm.[3] In such lesions the points of invasion are typically multifocal.[4] Although depressed lesions are uncommon (1%–6% of NP-CRNs), their risks of submucosal invasion are the highest: the overall risks are reported to be 27% to 35.9% compared with 0.7% to 2.4% in the flat lesions.[3]

In addition to the macroscopic classification, there are several other important clues to submucosal invasion in NP-CRN, including fold convergence, expansion appearance, and ulceration (**Box 3**).[5,6]

Microscopic characterization (optical diagnosis)
Optical diagnosis is a real-time, in vivo microscopic characterization of a lesion at the tissue level during endoscopy that is based on objective criteria[7] and is reproducible.[8] Objectivity based on standardized and reproducible criteria is important to bring the validity of the optical diagnosis to the same level as pathologic diagnosis. Both electronic and dye-based image-enhanced endoscopy techniques are conceptually similar to the application of the various stains in pathology and can delineate the neoplastic borders. They can enhance optical diagnosis and provide information on the depth of invasion.[9]

In practice, we routinely use image-enhanced endoscopy to make an optical diagnosis. Following a detailed high-definition white light inspection of the lesion, we perform image-enhanced endoscopy using narrow band imaging (NBI) to systematically characterize the lesion color and mucosal surface and microvascular patterns. We apply the Narrow Band Imaging International Colorectal Endoscopic (NICE)

Box 3
Findings that suggest submucosal deep invasion

Macroscopic signs:

    Expansive appearance

    Deep depression in surface

    Irregular bottom of a depression

    Fold convergence

    Tumor size

    Presence of white spots (chicken-skin appearance)

    Redness

    Firm consistency

NBI NICE type 3

Pit pattern type V invasive

Nonlifting sign positive[a]

[a] False positive can occur due to desmoplastic reaction, scarring from prior biopsies or incomplete EMR, India ink tattooing or chronic inflammatory disease.

---

classification to make an optical diagnosis (type 1, hyperplastic; type 2, adenomatous or superficial invasive carcinoma [<1000 μm]; or type 3, deep submucosal invasive cancer) (**Fig. 1**).[7,10] Lesions that are a good match with the criteria are considered to have high confidence. We spray diluted indigo carmine (0.2%) to confirm the diagnosis of a depressed lesion, which is characterized by dye pooling into the depressed area. The indigo carmine solution can also help delineate the borders of the lesion before and during resection. We do not routinely apply the Kudo classification, although it can be useful to confirm the optical diagnosis. We use the clinical classification: hyperplastic, adenoma, and deeply invasive, as proposed by Matsuda and colleagues.[6]

Optical diagnosis is vital to the management of complex colorectal lesions. All of the lesions shown in this article were optically diagnosed before resection. Deep submucosal invasive lesions are generally not resected by endoscopy because their resections are associated with increased risks of complications, and they have a high risk of metastasis.

The nonlifting sign

The nonlifting sign, which is assessed during the submucosal injection, provides further opportunity to assess for the possibility of submucosal invasion. The nonlifting sign has shown a predictive positive value of 80%, negative predictive value of 96%, and an overall accuracy of 94.8%.[11] It can be falsely positive because of submucosal fibrosis (secondary to prior biopsies, incomplete resection, or cauterization), desmoplastic reaction under the lesion, prior India ink tattooing, or presence of ulceration.

RESECTION TECHNIQUES

Resection techniques to treat difficult colorectal lesions include the inject-and-cut endoscopic mucosal resection (EMR), EMR with specialized cap (EMR-C), EMR with band ligation (EMR-L), underwater EMR, endoscopic submucosal dissection (ESD), and specialized polypectomy techniques (**Box 4**).

NBI International Colorectal Endoscopic (NICE) Classification *

	Type 1	Type 2	Type 3
Color	Same or lighter than background	Browner relative to background (verify color arises from vessels)	Brown to dark brown relative to background; sometimes patchy whiter areas
Vessels	None, or isolated lacy vessels coursing across the lesion	Brown vessels surrounding white structures**	Has area(s) of disrupted or missing vessels
Surface Pattern	Dark or white spots of uniform size, or homogeneous absence of pattern	Oval, tubular or branched white structures** surrounded by brown vessels	Amorphous or absent surface pattern
Most likely pathology	Hyperplastic	Adenoma***	Deep submucosal invasive cancer
Pic samples	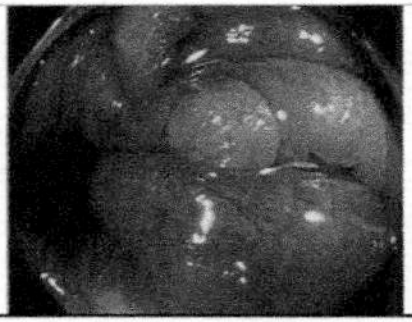	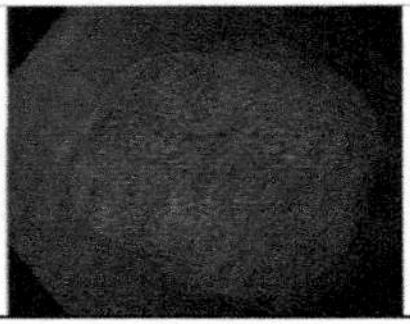	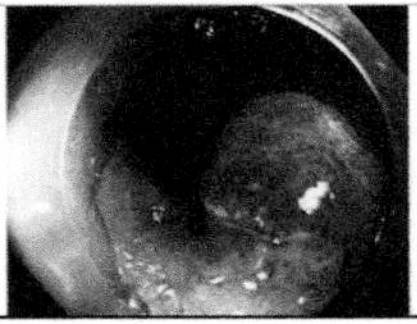

* Can be applied using colonoscopes with or without optical (zoom) magnification

** These structures (regular or irregular) may represent the pits and the epithelium of the crypt opening.

*** Type 2 consists of Vienna classification types 3, 4 and superficial 5 (all adenomas with either low or high grade dysplasia, or with superficial submucosal carcinoma). The presence of high grade dysplasia or superficial submucosal carcinoma may be suggested by an irregular vessel or surface pattern, and is often associated with atypical morphology (e.g., depressed area).

Fig. 1. NICE classification.

Box 4
Advanced resection techniques
Inject-and-cut EMR
EMR-C[a]
Underwater EMR
ESD
ESD-universal
Ligate and let go (for colonic lipomas)
EMR of rectal carcinoid using band ligation[a]
[a] Unsafe in the colon due to high risk of muscularis propria entrapment.

General Recommendations

Personnel
Personnel who are proficient in the use of the range of equipment and the intricacies of the technical procedure details, and who remain calm to manage complications are critical assets in performing advanced resections.

Equipment
We use high-definition adult colonoscopes with a water jet channel. We often use the therapeutic upper endoscopes when the lesion is located in the left colon. Pediatric colonoscopes featuring a smaller diameter may be useful to retroflex in the right colon to manage lesions extending over folds. Distal attachments can be helpful to improve visualization behind folds and stabilize the endoscope tip.[12] We use CO_2 insufflation because it has been shown to improve patient comfort during and after the procedure, and it decreases the risk of tension pneumoperitoneum if a perforation were to occur. The accessories that we routinely use are shown in **Box 5**.

Choice of sedation
The ideal sedation is conscious (moderate sedation). Deep sedation with propofol may result in labored breathing, which makes the colon move significantly and interferes with the EMR. Furthermore, patient repositioning, which is often required in order to optimize the procedure, may be difficult in obese patients.

Injection
Injection solutions Saline is commonly used worldwide. Glyceol, which is composed of glycerin, fructose, and NaCl solution, is commonly used in Japan. Hyaluronic acid solutions have shown longer duration of mucosal elevation compared with saline,[13] independently of the concentration used (0.4%, 0.2%, or 0.13%). However, it does not cause a significantly higher elevation of the mucosa compared with saline.[14] Other solutions have been described in search of a solution that stays longer, but none is commonly used.

Injection techniques We use a dynamic submucosal injection technique[15] (**Fig. 2**) that is designed to create a generous bulge under the lesion. In this technique, after puncturing the mucosa and inserting the needle into the submucosa, a small amount of saline is injected to confirm insertion into the submucosal layer, followed by rapid large-volume injection. Unlike the variceal injection technique, in which the needle is kept stationary during the injection (static injection technique), dynamic submucosal

---

Box 5
Standard equipment and accessories used for advanced endoscopic resection

1. High-definition endoscope with water jet

    Colonoscope

    Pediatric colonoscope

    Therapeutic upper endoscope

2. Carbon dioxide regulator

3. Water irrigator with pedal activator

4. Distal attachments compatible with selected endoscope

5. Indigo carmine in a 60-mL syringe

6. Injection needle (25 gauge)

7. Electrosurgical generator

8. Injectant (10-mL syringes of indigo carmine and saline; tattoo agent)

9. Stiff snares (small and large)

10. ESD knife (dual knife)

11. Biopsy forceps (standard and jumbo cold forceps)

12. Endoscopic clips (if using resolution, we take the sheath off)

13. Endoscopic loop

14. Band ligator

15. Argon plasma coagulator with straight catheter

16. Coagulation forceps (Coagrasper, hot biopsy forceps)

17. Retrieval net

18. Multichannel suction trap

19. Pins and Styrofoam

---

injection involves moving the needle within the submucosa by slowly deflecting the tip of the endoscope or gently pulling the catheter back to create the desired mound of submucosal fluid cushion with injection. At the same time, air is suctioned out of the lumen. In essence, the submucosal bulge is sculpted.

It is important to appreciate the difference between the dynamic and static injection techniques. In the static technique, after inserting the needle into the submucosa, the needle is kept stationary until an adequate amount of fluid is slowly infused. In this technique the lumen is maintained insufflated to allow visualization of the lesion during injection. A common disappointment after the static injection technique has been inadequate thickness of the submucosal cushion, which is unsatisfactory for successful resection, because the injected saline spreads thinly throughout the area rather than collecting as a mound under the lesion.

EMR

The inject-and-cut EMR
The inject-and-cut EMR is a simple technique that is widely used for removal of large flat or sessile lesions. Lesions larger than 20 mm cannot be removed in a single piece (en bloc resection), and in such cases piecemeal resection is required.[3]

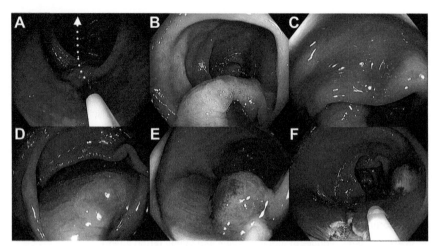

Fig. 2. The dynamic injection technique. The dotted arrow shows the planned path of the needle that was to be followed during injection (*A*). Diluted indigo carmine solution in saline was injected rapidly while lifting the tip of the endoscope and suctioning the lumen (*B*). Further injection (*C*). After 8 to 10 mL of injection, there was a large submucosal cushion (*D*). A stiff 10-mm snare was used to capture the lesion and surrounding normal tissue (*E*). After resection (*F*).

We use a stiff snare for EMR after dynamic submucosal injection. If an LST-G mixed lesion with a large nodule is encountered, it is important to resect the large nodule in a single piece and submit it in a separate bottle of formalin after fixing it because of the likelihood of advanced features or invasive carcinoma underneath such a lesion.[4] Our preference is to resect LST-NGs en bloc if they are less than 20 mm.

After capturing the lesion with a snare, the lumen is insufflated with air to stretch the wall, and the snare is lifted up while the snare is slightly loosened to release any entrapped muscularis propria. The lesion is then strangled and transected using blended current: 35 W in the left and 40 W in the right side of the colon. In large lesions requiring piecemeal resection, successive resections should be performed using the free resection margin from prior resection as an anchor point. Additional submucosal injections can be performed through the already-visible submucosa to create a cushion if necessary for safe resection. It is important to keep the snare parallel to the wall during piecemeal resection to avoid entrapping muscle when a snare is deployed at an angle.

Prevention of recurrence using argon plasma coagulation

A major drawback of piecemeal resection is the risk of leaving residual tissue at the end of resection, which can ensure recurrence in 100% of cases. We resect all visible neoplastic tissue. Application of argon plasma coagulation (APC) to the borders and bridges of the resected area may burn microscopic residual tissue to reduce the risk of recurrence.[16]

EMR-C

EMR-C with a prepositioned snare in the colon has been regarded as unsafe because of the theoretic risk of entrapment of thin colon wall during suction of the lesion into the cap resulting in perforation, although this technique is widely used in the resection of lesions of the rectum where the wall is thick.[17,18]

Underwater EMR

Binmoeller and colleagues[19] observed that the muscularis propria of the colon and rectum that are filled with water stay circular during endoscopic ultrasonography. Thus, he proposed to use water immersion to eliminate the need for submucosal injection during mucosal resection. To perform this technique once the lesion is identified, the air is suctioned and 500 mL to 1 L of water are infused until complete filling of the lumen is achieved. Once underwater, the margins of the lesion are marked using APC. The resection is performed using a 15-mm duckbill snare with blended current. To maximize tissue capture a torque-and-crimp technique is used. APC can be delivered underwater as well. Note that the lesions are resected in piecemeal fashion.

ESD

En bloc resection is recommended for lesions that are deemed to have high risk of harboring high-grade dysplasia or superficial submucosal invasion, or lesions that may be difficult to remove using the other available techniques. The indications for ESD recommended by the Japan Colorectal ESD Standardization Implementation Working Group include lesions difficult to remove en bloc (including LST-NG, especially of the pseudodepressed type; lesions showing a Vi pit pattern; or lesions 0–I with suspicion of adenocarcinoma); lesions with underlying fibrosis; sporadic localized lesions in ulcerative colitis; or local residual lesions after prior EMR (**Box 6**).[20,21]

A recent systematic review[22] comprising 22 studies and 2841 treated lesions reported en bloc resection rate of 96% with an R0 rate of 88%. Surgery was necessary in a few cases (2% of lesions) mainly because of incomplete resection or complications (1%). Intramucosal cancer was present in 44%, and submucosal cancer was found in 11% of specimens.

The ESD technique comprises several steps (**Fig. 3**). First, the lesion is delineated, although marking the borders in the colon and rectum is usually not necessary. After submucosal injection of fluid, a circumferential incision is first performed, beginning at the proximal border. Half of the circumference is incised and submucosal dissection is performed in this half of the circumference. In some cases retroflexion may be necessary to complete this step. Then circumferential incision is completed and the submucosa is completely dissected from the distal side. During resection any bleeding vessels should be coagulated before continuing resection. Any possible perforations should be closed using endoclips.

Box 6
Indication of ESD for colorectal tumor

Large (>20 mm in diameter) lesions that are indicated for endoscopic, rather than surgical, resection and in which en bloc resection using inject-and-cut EMR is difficult

  LST-NG, particularly of the pseudodepressed type

  Lesions showing V invasive type pit pattern

  Carcinoma with submucosal infiltration

  Large depressed-type lesion

  Large elevated lesion suspected to be a cancer

Mucosal lesions with fibrosis

Local residual early carcinoma after endoscopic resection

Sporadic localized tumors in chronic inflammation

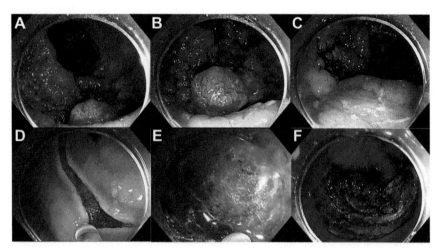

Fig. 3. ESD for a large, granular, lateral spreading tumor with a prominent nodule located in the rectum (*A*). We studied the nodule in detail (*B*). The submucosa around the lesion is injected using diluted indigo carmine in saline (*C*). Circumferential incision is performed using a dual knife (*D*). After circumferential incision, the submucosa is slowly dissected using the dual knife. Multiple submucosal injections are necessary to elevate the submucosa and continue the dissection (*E*). Result after resection. The specimen was 8 cm in diameter (*F*).

The ESD-universal

Although colonic ESD has been performed in Japan for years, standardization of the technique remains difficult and adoption of the technique is slow.[23] Thus, additional techniques to allow en bloc resection need to be adopted. ESD-universal is a concept of ESD that reflects the goal of an en bloc resection. The concept involves performing a circumferential incision and partial dissection to free the lesion, followed by en bloc snare resection of the lesion (**Fig. 4**) or, in some cases, a complete submucosal dissection. This technique has been used with LSTs up to 40 mm with good results.[24]

ADVANCED RESECTION IN CERTAIN LOCATIONS

Lesions located proximal to the dentate line, ileocecal (IC) valve, appendiceal orifice, and lesions behind a fold or folds may require additional techniques.

Dentate Line

The dentate line separates the rectum from the anoderm, an area highly sensitive to pain. To prevent pain during resection, injection of diluted lidocaine 1% via a standard sclerotherapy needle can be useful.[25,26] We inject the lidocaine solution above the dentate line first, which is painless, and, when the bleb reaches the dentate line, we inject further above and distal to the bleb (**Fig. 5**). The use of distal attachment cap that is 3 to 4 mm away from the tip of the endoscope (band ligation cap after deploying the bands) can be useful to keep the anal canal open and the endoscope in a stable position. Thus, the lesion can be well visualized and the lesion can be removed uneventfully. Larger lesions may also require removal while the endoscope is in the retroflex position.

IC Valve

Lesions at the IC valve represent a challenge for endoscopic resection. Although the risk of perforation should not be higher given the presence of fatty tissue in the

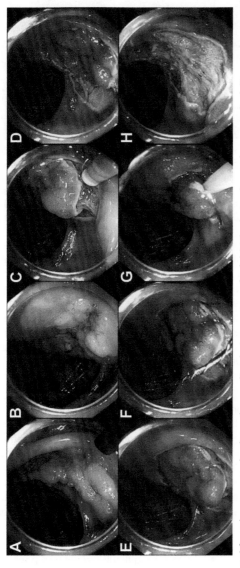

Fig. 4. ESD-universal for a large, granular, lateral spreading lesion on top of a fold. The lesion has to be precisely delineated, especially the area behind the fold. A cap is useful in this case to improve visualization (*A*). Although a generous submucosal bulge is formed, a pseudodepressed area can be identified at the lesion center (*B*). Circumferential incision was performed using a dual knife and completed in 12 minutes, which is the first step of the ESD-universal technique (*C*). Lesion overview after completion of the circumferential incision (*D*). Injection directly into the exposed submucosa allows elevation of the pseudodepressed area (*E*). Snaring is performed using a 20-mm stiff snare, which represents the second step of the ESD-universal technique (*F*). Once the snare is maneuvered around the lesion, it is tightened, catching the lesion in 1 piece (*G*). Lesion site after en bloc resection performed in 15 minutes (*H*).

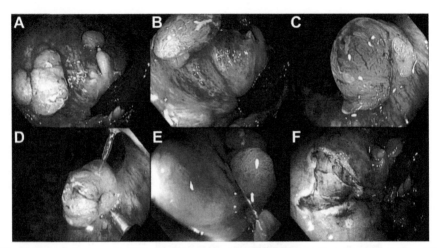

Fig. 5. Retroflex view of a 20-mm rectal sessile lesion (*left*) contacting the dentate line (*A*). Detail of the lesion contacting the dentate line (*retroflex view*) (*B*). The lesion seen on forward view (*C*). Injection of lidocaine 1% under the lesion (*D*). Once the bleb reaches the dentate line, further injections are performed below it (not shown). A stiff snare is closed around the lesion. The maneuver is performed in retroflex view (*E*). Ulcer after lesion resection (*retroflex view*) (*F*). The patient did not complain of pain during or after the procedure.

submucosa at this area, these lesions are especially difficult to resect because of poor access and inadequate visualization, especially if they extend into the ileum or down into the cecum, with a higher risk of recurrence.[27] To remove polyps affecting the IC valve, we prefer to use a short cap attached to the distal tip of the endoscope. The cap allows pushing of the IC valve folds and maintains a more stable position to optimize visualization of the lesion. Submucosal injection is often used to provide additional cushioning. Complete delineation of the lesion may require a combination of forward and retroflex views, along with insertion of the endoscope into the terminal ileum and slow removal to determine the internal margin of the lesion.

Appendiceal Orifice

Polyps arising from the appendix are rare, although endoscopic resection of adenomatous polyps, typically pedunculated, have been reported using snares.[28] Polyps located adjacent to the appendiceal orifice, although not arising from the appendix itself, represent a challenge for endoscopic resection, especially those that are nonpolypoid. The concerns in these cases include the thin cecal wall and the potential for an appendiceal inflammation caused by injection close to the appendix. However, we are not aware of reports describing appendicitis from submucosal injection into the periappendiceal area. Lesions that extend into the appendix require surgery.

Behind Fold(s)

The resection of a lesion behind a fold may be difficult because of poor visualization of the border and/or inability to place the accessories to permit injection or snaring. Several systematic steps can be performed. The first step is to delineate the border to determine the amount of polyp hidden behind the fold, or folds. The fold(s) can be pushed using a biopsy forceps or a snare. The distal attachment cap can be useful because it can be used to push the fold down or sideways, thus allowing visualization and subsequent treatment. With or without a cap, submucosal injection technique can be used to lift the lesion above the level of the fold(s). As an alternative, if the lesion is located in the cecum, ascending colon, distal sigmoid, and rectum, retroflexion can be performed and the lesion can be treated with the endoscope in the retroflexion view.

Lesions Over Scars

Resection of lesions over scars can be difficult because the submucosal injection can be ineffective, often resulting in a superficial mucosal bleb instead of a submucosal bleb; the lesion can be difficult to snare because of slippage of snare during its closure; the muscularis propria under the lesion may be inadvertently snared and result in perforation; and the lesion is typically resected in piecemeal fashion, making the pathology interpretation difficult. The procedure typically lasts a long time because some areas of polyp tethered to the wall may require the use of a biopsy forceps to remove them in pieces. Resection of a colorectal neoplasm over a scarred area poses risks to all parties involved: the patient who is left with a risk of high complications and recurrence, the endoscopists for assuming the increased risk of the procedure, the pathologist for potential misinterpretation of the piecemeal resection, and society for wasted resources when the lesion could be resected completely by an expert clinician.

Scarring of the submucosa and tethering of the polyp can result from prior treatment (cold or hot biopsy; polypectomy snaring, including partial, EMR, India ink injection, or coagulation) or chronic inflammation from inflammatory bowel disease.

Scarring prevents the submucosa from expanding during injection, which is observed as the nonlifting sign. In addition to the difficulty in resecting nonlifted lesion, the nonlifting sign is also observed in submucosally invasive cancers, which leads to difficulty in assessing the malignant potential of the lesion (discussed later).

Endoscopic techniques for resection of a nonlifted benign lesion with tethering of the lesion caused by fibrosis from prior intervention include repeat mucosal resection, ESD, ablation using APC, or repeated biopsy followed by APC ablation. The difficulty is that repeat resection often necessitates referral to an experienced endoscopist. In our practice, we try to inject with saline and remove as much visible neoplasm as possible using a small (10 mm) stiff snare. We reserve the use of APC for when there is minimal, if any, visible lesion. The base of the lesion requires coagulation.

ADVANCED RESECTION IN CHRONIC INFLAMMATORY BOWEL DISEASE

The EMR of nonpolypoid or sessile lesions in patients with chronic inflammatory bowel disease present a special challenge because of increased risk of colorectal cancer, suppressed immune system from use of immunomodulators and steroids, difficulty in delineating the border of the lesion, and significant difficulty in capturing the lesion using a snare because of underlying fibrosis. In addition, descriptions of the technique and efficacy of endoscopic resection in patients with inflammatory bowel disease are sparse. In our limited experience, submucosal injection usually produces partial, if any, lifting. The resection then requires small cuts, which is not ideal. The application of ESD-U in such patients is an attractive endoscopic technique.[29]

ENDOSCOPIC RESECTIONS OF LARGE PEDUNCULATED LESIONS

Large pedunculated lesions in the colon and rectum include polyps arising from the mucosa and those arising from the submucosa (lipoma). These lesions can easily be differentiated by examining the mucosal pattern of the head of the polyp, which is abnormal for the mucosal lesions and normal for the lipomas. Prevention of complications is critical in the resection of both types of lesions.

Resection of Large Pedunculated Mucosal Lesions

Large pedunculated polyps are fed by multiple large vessels, which increase the risk of bleeding after resection. Strategies to reduce the risk of bleeding include the use of an Endoloop, endoscopic clips, and epinephrine injection.

Endoscopic looping technique

The Endoloop has been conclusively shown in several clinical studies to significantly reduce the risk of bleeding after polypectomy of large pedunculated polyps. In one study, the risk of bleeding in polyps greater than or equal to 2 cm decreased significantly from approximately 15% to 2.7% ($P<.05$).[30] In another study of polyps larger than 1 cm, the risk decreased from 12% to nil ($P<.05$).[31] The injection of epinephrine before looping expectantly leads to improper loop placement because the loop tends to become loose after the epinephrine has been absorbed. However, the Endoloop can be difficult to deploy; knowledge of its proper placement is required.

In order to use the Endoloop safely and efficaciously, several steps must be followed, as shown in **Box 7**.

Endoscopic clipping technique

Some investigators have advocated the use of endoclips to strangulate the stalk before resection, thus preventing postpolypectomy bleeding (**Fig. 6**). Up to 3 clips might be needed even though bleeding has been observed in 5.9% of cases, probably caused by insufficient compression of the feeding vessel.[32,33] Clips are successful in polyps with thin stalks, whereas those with thick stalks require a loop.

The steps for precise clip application are shown in **Box 8**.

Volume reduction technique

To ease snaring of the head, large snares can be used, although it is still technically challenging, or the head size can be decreased by injecting epinephrine solution into it and waiting for size reduction. Between 4 and 8 mL of 1:10,000 epinephrine should typically be injected into the head of the polyp at 2 to 4 sites, which results in an immediate blanching of the head. This step is followed by additional injections of 2 to 4 mL of epinephrine into the stalk in 2 or more sites. In about 5 minutes, the

---

Box 7
Technique to deploy the Endoloop

1. The patient is position such that the polyp attaches from 12 o'clock position.

2. The endoscope is then rotated so that the stalk of the polyp is at the 6 o'clock position.

3. The loop is opened from the proximal or lateral aspect of its head.

4. The loop is positioned by repeated movements of closing and opening its sheath, until the loop is positioned closest to the wall.

5. The loop is then tightened, while the sheath is simultaneously opened.

6. It takes time for the loop to fully tighten. Thus, repeated motion to tighten it is required.

7. Snare resection is accomplished by closing the snare as tightly as possible, otherwise the burn will occur at the site of the loop placement.

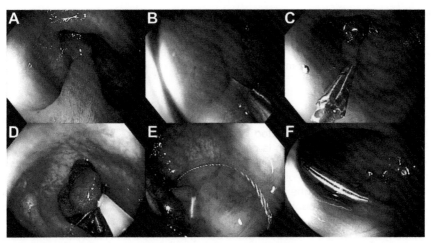

Fig. 6. Clipping the stalk of a pedunculated polyp before polypectomy to prevent bleeding. The polyp was located in the sigmoid colon (*A*). The clip has to be adjusted to the area closest to the colonic wall (*B*). Complete closure around the stalk needs to be assessed. Once the clip is placed, the polyp head turns dark red (*C*). The snare has to be maneuvered over the head and closed between the head and the clip. It has to be positioned away from the head so that there is enough resected pedicle for a proper histopathology study and also enough distance from the clip to prevent dislodgment after resection, thus defeating the purpose of clipping (*D*, *E*). Pedicle with the clip in place after lesion resection (*F*).

polyp shrinks to permit snare resection. The colonoscopy could be completed before resecting large lesions in the left colon.[34]

Removal of Large Colorectal Lipomas

Resection of large colorectal lipomas used to be associated with a significant risk of perforation, because a large amount of cautery was applied in order to overcome the poor conduction of fatty tissue. However, large colorectal lipomas are almost always benign. Thus, their removal is best accomplished by the ligate-and-let-go technique, which we have previously described.[35] In short, the best method to remove large colorectal lipomas is to place an Endoloop (following steps 1 to 6 in **Box 7**) and then leave it for resection through slow transection.

Box 8
Technique to deploy the endoscope clip before polypectomy of pedunculated polyps

1. The patient is positioned such that the polyp attaches from the 12 o'clock position.

2. The endoscope is then rotated so that the stalk of the polyp is at 6 o'clock position.

3. The clip needs to be adjusted to the base of the stalk close to the colonic wall.

4. Some endoclips allow rotation and multiple opening/closing maneuvers.

5. Once deployed, the presence of ischemic signs indicates that the polyp has been adequately strangulated.

6. If the polyp has a broad stalk, application of several clips may be necessary.

EMR OF RECTAL CARCINOIDS USING BAND LIGATION

Band ligation for endoscopic resection of adenomas has been performed in the rectum with good results.[36,37] Because of the thinness of the colon wall, the use of band ligation has been deemed unsafe.

COMPLICATIONS

The main complications are bleeding and perforation. Bleeding should be arrested when it occurs, using a dedicated hot coagulation forceps, hot biopsy forceps, or APC for minor bleeding. When large vessels are present or the bleeding cannot be arrested using coagulation, we use endoscopic clips to ligate the bleeding vessels. Perforations occur in 0.1% of therapeutic colonoscopies. Precautions to avoid perforations include applying the snare on the stalk away from the wall in pedunculated polyps, using dynamic submucosal injection technique in sessile and flat lesions to separate the lesion from muscularis propria with an adequate submucosal cushion, accurately identifying the resection plane during piecemeal EMR and ESD, and taking preventive measures if a deep resection is undertaken.[38] It is important to be able to identify deep cuts or perforations because these need to be closed immediately with the clips during the same endoscopy session.

FOLLOW-UP
Repeat Colonoscopy

Follow-up colonoscopy should be performed 3 to 6 months after piecemeal EMR to assess resection completeness and remove any residual or recurrent lesion.[39] High-definition endoscopes are preferred. We look for the scar of prior resection, which can be recognized by the mucosal changes or the presence of a tattoo. The area should be studied under white light and image-enhanced endoscopy techniques as previously detailed. If the area shows no signs of local macroscopic recurrence, then targeted pathology biopsies of the scar area should be taken. If a residual or recurrent lesion is recognized, either EMR or ESD should be performed.

Referral to Surgery After EMR or ESD

In some cases the pathologic analysis of the specimen may reveal the presence of adenocarcinoma. If the lesion is limited to the mucosa, which in the United States is called high-grade dysplasia, the available studies have shown no risk of lymph node metastasis.[40,41] In contrast, adenocarcinomas with invasion into the submucosa harbor a 6% to 12% risk of lymph node metastasis.[42–44] Further studies have shown that well-differentiated adenocarcinomas with submucosal invasion less than 1000 μm and lesions without lymphatic or vascular involvement have small, if not nil, risk of lymph node metastasis.[27,45] Thus, in Japan, endoscopic resections are indicated for NP-CRN with these features, whereas in Western countries endoscopic resections are limited to NP-CRN with high-grade dysplasia or intramucosal carcinoma. Polypoid-CRNs are typically classified according to the method described by Haggit and colleagures.[46] Submucosal invasion into the submucosa beyond the neck of the pedunculated polyp, or into the submucosa of sessile, poor differentiation, and lymphovascular invasion necessitates surgery.

SUMMARY

Advanced endoscopic resection techniques allow curative treatment of difficult colonic lesions and avoid the need for surgery in certain cases. If endoscopic resection is indicated, the choice of the most appropriate resection technique depends on lesion characteristics and endoscopist expertise.

REFERENCES

1. Soetikno R, Gotoda T. Con: colonoscopic resection of large neoplastic lesions is appropriate and safe. Am J Gastroenterol 2009;104(2):272–5.
2. The Paris endoscopic classification of superficial neoplastic lesions: esophagus, stomach and colon. Gastrointest Endosc 2003;58(Suppl 6):S3–43.
3. Kudo S, Lambert R, Allen JI, et al. Nonpolypoid neoplastic lesions of the colorectal mucosa. Gastrointest Endosc 2008;68(Suppl 4):S3–47.
4. Uraoka T, Saito Y, Matsuda T, et al. Endoscopic indications for endoscopic mucosal resection of laterally spreading tumours in the colorectum. Gut 2006; 55(11):1592–7.
5. Saitoh Y, Obara T, Watari J, et al. Invasion depth diagnosis of depressed type early colorectal cancers by combined use of videoendoscopy and chromoendoscopy. Gastrointest Endosc 1998;48(4):362–70.
6. Matsuda T, Parra-Blanco A, Saito Y, et al. Assessment of likelihood of submucosal invasion in non-polypoid colorectal neoplasms. Gastrointest Endosc Clin N Am 2010;20(3):487–96.
7. Hewett DG, Kaltenbach T, Sano Y, et al. Validation of a simple classification system for endoscopic diagnosis of small colorectal polyps using narrow-band imaging. Gastroenterology 2012;143(3):599–607.e1.
8. McGill S, Evangelou E, Ionnidis J, et al. Narrow band imaging to differentiate neoplastic and non-neoplastic colorectal polyps in real time: a meta-analysis of diagnostic operating characteristics. Gut, in press.
9. Kaltenbach T, Sano Y, Friedland S, et al. American Gastroenterological Association (AGA) Institute technology assessment on image-enhanced endoscopy. Gastroenterology 2008;134(1):327–40.
10. Hayashi N, Tanaka S, Hewett DG, et al. Endoscopic prediction of deep submucosal invasive carcinoma: validation of the Narrow Band Imaging (NBI) International Colorectal Endoscopic (NICE) classification. Gastrointest Endosc, in press.
11. Kobayashi N, Saito Y, Sano Y, et al. Determining the treatment strategy for colorectal neoplastic lesions: endoscopic assessment or the non-lifting sign for diagnosing invasion depth? Endoscopy 2007;39(8):701–5.
12. Sanchez-Yague A, Kaltenbach T, Yamamoto H, et al. The endoscopic cap that can (with videos). Gastrointest Endosc 2012;76(1):169–78.e1–2.
13. Yoshida N, Naito Y, Kugai M, et al. Efficacy of hyaluronic acid in endoscopic mucosal resection of colorectal tumors. J Gastroenterol Hepatol 2011;26(2): 286–91.
14. Fujishiro M, Yahagi N, Kashimura K, et al. Comparison of various submucosal injection solutions for maintaining mucosal elevation during endoscopic mucosal resection. Endoscopy 2004;36(7):579–83.
15. Soetikno R, Kaltenbach T. Dynamic submucosal injection technique. Gastrointest Endosc Clin N Am 2010;20(3):497–502.
16. Zlatanic J, Waye JD, Kim PS, et al. Large sessile colonic adenomas: use of argon plasma coagulator to supplement piecemeal snare polypectomy. Gastrointest Endosc 1999;49(6):731–5.
17. Inoue H, Kawano T, Tani M, et al. Endoscopic mucosal resection using a cap: techniques for use and preventing perforation. Can J Gastroenterol 1999;13(6): 477–80.

18. Soetikno RM, Inoue H, Chang KJ. Endoscopic mucosal resection - current concepts. Gastrointest Endosc Clin N Am 2000;10(4):595–617.
19. Binmoeller KF, Weilert F, Shah J, et al. "Underwater" EMR without submucosal injection for large sessile colorectal polyps (with video). Gastrointest Endosc 2012; 75(5):1086–91.
20. Tanaka S, Oka S, Chayama K. Colorectal endoscopic submucosal dissection: present status and future perspective, including its differentiation from endoscopic mucosal resection. J Gastroenterol 2008;43(9):641–51.
21. Tanaka S, Oka S, Kaneko I, et al. Endoscopic submucosal dissection for colorectal neoplasia: possibility of standardization. Gastrointest Endosc 2007;66(1): 100–7.
22. Repici A, Hassan C, De Paula Pessoa D, et al. Efficacy and safety of endoscopic submucosal dissection for colorectal neoplasia: a systematic review. Endoscopy 2012;44(2):137–50.
23. Tanaka S, Terasaki M, Kanao H, et al. Current status and future perspectives of endoscopic submucosal dissection for colorectal tumors. Dig Endosc 2012; 24(Suppl 1):73–9.
24. Terasaki M, Tanaka S, Oka S, et al. Clinical outcomes of endoscopic submucosal dissection and endoscopic mucosal resection for laterally spreading tumors larger than 20 mm. J Gastroenterol Hepatol 2012;27(4):734–40.
25. Sanchez-Yague A, Yamaguchi Y, Takao T, et al. Endoscopic submucosal dissection of a lower rectal polyp proximal to the dentate line by using local lidocaine injection. Gastrointest Endosc 2011;73(2):405–7.
26. Nakadoi K, Tanaka S, Hayashi N, et al. Clinical outcomes of endoscopic submucosal dissection for rectal tumor close to the dentate line. Gastrointest Endosc 2012;76(2):444–50.
27. Kitajima K, Fujimori T, Fujii S, et al. Correlations between lymph node metastasis and depth of submucosal invasion in submucosal invasive colorectal carcinoma: a Japanese collaborative study. J Gastroenterol 2004;39(6):534–43.
28. Khawaja FI. Colonoscopic removal of an appendiceal polyp. Saudi J Gastroenterol 2002;8(3):93–5.
29. Kaltenbach T, Soetikno R. Endoscopic resection of large colon polyps. Gastrointest Endosc Clin N Am 2013;23(1):137–52.
30. Di Giorgio P, De Luca L, Calcagno G, et al. Detachable snare versus adrenalin stalk injection in the prevention of post-polypectomy bleeding. A controlled randomized study. Endoscopy 2004;36(10):860–3.
31. Iishi H, Tatsuta M, Narahara H, et al. Endoscopic resection of large pedunculated colorectal polyps using a detachable snare. Gastrointest Endosc 1996; 44:594–7.
32. Boo SJ, Byeon JS, Park SY, et al. Clipping for the prevention of immediate bleeding after polypectomy of pedunculated polyps: a pilot study. Clin Endosc 2012;45(1):84–8.
33. Luigiano C, Ferrara F, Ghersi S, et al. Endoclip-assisted resection of large pedunculated colorectal polyps: technical aspects and outcome. Dig Dis Sci 2010; 55(6):1726–31.
34. Hogan RB, Hogan RB 3rd. Epinephrine volume reduction of giant colon polyps facilitates endoscopic assessment and removal. Gastrointest Endosc 2007; 66(5):1018–22.
35. Kaltenbach T, Milkes D, Friedland S, et al. Safe endoscopic treatment of large colonic lipomas using endoscopic looping technique. Dig Liver Dis 2008; 40(12):958–61.

36. Van Os EC, Gostout CJ, Geller A, et al. Band ligation-assisted endoscopic resection of a flat rectal adenoma containing infiltrating adenocarcinoma. Gastrointest Endosc 1997;45(3):322–4.
37. Ono A, Fujii T, Saito Y, et al. Endoscopic submucosal resection of rectal carcinoid tumors with a ligation device. Gastrointest Endosc 2003;57(4):583–7.
38. Raju GS, Saito Y, Matsuda T, et al. Endoscopic management of colonoscopic perforations (with videos). Gastrointest Endosc 2011;74(6):1380–8.
39. Rex DK, Kahi CJ, Levin B, et al. Guidelines for colonoscopy surveillance after cancer resection: a consensus update by the American Cancer Society and US Multi-Society Task Force on Colorectal Cancer. CA Cancer J Clin 2006; 56(3):160–7 [quiz: 185–6].
40. Morson BC, Whiteway JE, Jones EA, et al. Histopathology and prognosis of malignant colorectal polyps treated by endoscopic polypectomy. Gut 1984; 25(5):437–44.
41. Fujimori T, Kawamata H, Kashida H. Precancerous lesions of the colorectum. J Gastroenterol 2001;36(9):587–94.
42. Kyzer S, Begin LR, Gordon PH, et al. The care of patients with colorectal polyps that contain invasive adenocarcinoma. Endoscopic polypectomy or colectomy? Cancer 1992;70(8):2044–50.
43. Minamoto T, Mai M, Ogino T, et al. Early invasive colorectal carcinomas metastatic to the lymph node with attention to their nonpolypoid development. Am J Gastroenterol 1993;88(7):1035–9.
44. Cooper HS. Surgical pathology of endoscopically removed malignant polyps of the colon and rectum. Am J Surg Pathol 1983;7(7):613–23.
45. Mou S, Soetikno R, Shimoda T, et al. Pathologic predictive factors for lymph node metastasis in submucosal invasive (T1) colorectal cancer: a systematic review and meta-analysis. Surg Endosc, in press.
46. Haggitt RC, Glotzbach RE, Soffer EE, et al. Prognostic factors in colorectal carcinomas arising in adenomas: implications for lesions removed by endoscopic polypectomy. Gastroenterology 1985;89(2):328–36.

Cap-Assisted Colonoscopy

Amit Rastogi, MD

KEYWORDS

- Cap-assisted colonoscopy • Polyp detection rate • Adenoma detection rate
- Cecal intubate rate • Cecal intubation time

KEY POINTS

- Cap-assisted colonoscopy is a simple, practical, and inexpensive technique that serves several useful purposes in enhancing the performance of colonoscopy.
- It helps improve polyp detection by its ability to visualize the otherwise blind mucosal areas on the proximal aspects of folds and flexures, although its effect on adenoma detection has been inconsistent.
- By helping navigate the colon more efficiently, it facilitates intubation of the cecum faster and with lesser patient discomfort.
- Cap-assisted colonoscopy can be tried as a salvage procedure in cases of failed cecal intubation with regular colonoscopy.
- Cap-assisted colonoscopy also is of assistance during polypectomy, especially for polyps located on the proximal aspects of folds.
- In cases of diverticular bleeding, use of cap helps localize the bleeding diverticulum and in the treatment of the bleeding stigmata.

INTRODUCTION

Colonoscopy is considered the preferred method for colorectal cancer screening, especially in the United States.[1] With the recent US Multi-Society Task Force guidelines[2] emphasizing that the goal of screening should be the prevention of colorectal cancer, the role of colonoscopy has assumed even greater significance. The central premise by which colonoscopy prevents colon cancer is the detection and removal of precursor lesions, such as adenomas. Colonoscopy remains an imperfect tool, however, for the prevention of colorectal cancer. One of the major reasons for this is that adenomas can be missed during colonoscopy, even when the procedure is performed by expert endoscopists using meticulous technique.[3] Adenoma detection rate is considered an important quality indicator of colonoscopy performance and its clinical relevance was highlighted in a recent study showing that the adenoma detection rate of endoscopists is independently associated with interval colorectal cancer.[4]

Conflict of Interest: Received research grant support from Olympus America Inc.
Kansas City VA Medical Center, University of Kansas, 4801 Linwood Boulevard, Kansas City, MO 64128, USA
E-mail address: amitr68@hotmail.com

Gastroenterol Clin N Am 42 (2013) 479–489
http://dx.doi.org/10.1016/j.gtc.2013.05.008
0889-8553/13/$ – see front matter Published by Elsevier Inc.

gastro.theclinics.com

Therefore, efforts to improve and optimize adenoma detection rates continue to be an active area of research in the field of colonoscopy.

REASONS FOR MISSING ADENOMAS

Several reasons have been attributed for missing adenomas during colonoscopy. These include inadequate bowel preparation,[5,6] suboptimal technique,[7] shorter withdrawal time,[8] presence of flat/depressed/subtle lesions evading detection, and the inability to visualize the proximal sides of haustral folds, flexures, rectal valves, and ileocecal valve. Incomplete visualization continues to be a vexing problem for endoscopists with a wide range of experience. The haustral folds in the colon are of varying dimensions and can shield significant amount of mucosal surface area from the view of the endoscopist. One of the elements of good inspection technique during the withdrawal phase of colonoscopy is to inspect between folds by torquing the colonoscope and/or deflecting its tip. But this maneuver is limited by the extent of tip deflection and angle of view of the lens at the colonoscope tip as well as the loss of visualization when the colonoscope tip closely approximates the mucosa, leading to a red out. The fact that lesions located on the proximal aspects of colonic folds are prone to be missed during colonoscopy was highlighted in a study that used CT colonography as the reference standard.[9] This study showed that majority of clinically significant adenomas that are missed during colonoscopy are located on the proximal sides of folds. There are 3 methods that aid in inspecting these blind mucosal areas, which include cap-assisted colonoscopy, third eye colonoscopy,[10] and retroflexion of the colonoscope.[11] This review discusses the different aspects of cap-assisted colonoscopy.

CAP-ASSISTED COLONOSCOPY
Mechanism of Action of Cap

Cap-assisted colonoscopy is a simple technique using a small transparent cap attached to the tip of the colonoscope (**Figs. 1–3**). The cap is shaped like a hollow cylinder and, depending on its length, a portion of it protrudes for a variable distance beyond the tip of the colonoscope. This portion of the cap helps depress the colonic folds while keeping an appropriate distance between the mucosa and the lens at the tip of colonoscope, thus preventing loss of visualization and facilitating the inspection of the mucosal areas on the proximal aspects of folds, flexures, and valves

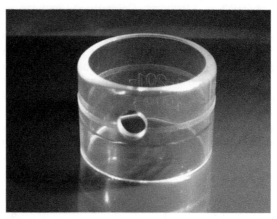

Fig. 1. Cap with a side hole.

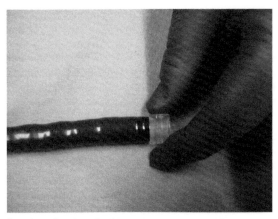

Fig. 2. Cap being fitted to the tip of colonoscope.

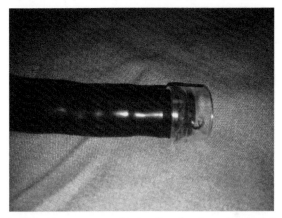

Fig. 3. Cap fitted to the colonoscope and extending for 4 mm beyond the tip.

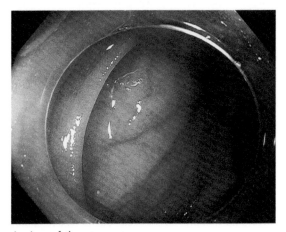

Fig. 4. Colonoscopic view of the cap.

(**Fig. 4**).[12–15] Furthermore, the cap can improve mucosal inspection by stretching or splaying colonic mucosa that might have otherwise folded over and obscured small lesions from the view of the endoscopist.[13] The cap can also be of assistance during insertion of the colonoscope by pushing away folds and helping with luminal orientation and better visualization at bends.[12,16,17] This helps the endoscopist insert the colonoscope with less air insufflation. Finally, the cap can be used to hook colonic folds at acute bends and help reduce loops in the colonoscope.[18]

Type of Caps

Caps are of varying lengths, ranging from 2 mm to 10 mm. The most commonly used one protrudes for approximately 4 mm beyond the tip of colonoscope after being tightly secured (see **Fig. 4**). Caps come in different diameters that fit snugly on colonoscopes of various sizes (adult colonoscope, pediatric colonoscope, and magnification colonoscope). The distal end of the cap is horizontal and the edges are rounded to minimize mucosal trauma. The newer version of the cap has a side hole for drainage of fluid and fecal material that might get entrapped within the interior confines of the cap and can, therefore, obscure the view. Another variation of the cap used in one study[19] is the retractable cap (**Fig. 5**). This cap extends to the desired length beyond the tip of colonoscope by the injection of air with a 10-mL syringe and retracts by aspiration of the air. The maximum extension possible is 7 mm. Various synonyms used for cap in

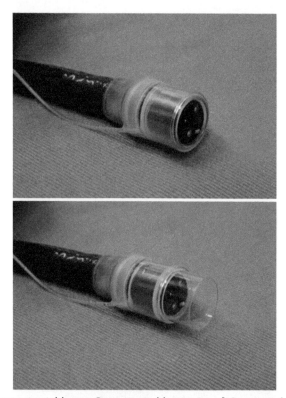

Fig. 5. Transparent retractable cap. Cap retracted (*upper panel*) Cap extended (*lower panel*). (*From* Horiuchi A, Nakayama Y. Improved colorectal adenoma detection with a transparent retractable extension device. Am J Gastroenterol 2008;103:341–5; with permission.)

the literature include hood, transparent hood, transparent extension device, and distal attachment.

Cap-assisted colonoscopy has been studied for a variety of endpoints that include adenoma or polyp detection rates, cecal intubation rates, cecal intubation time, patient discomfort during colonoscopy, and efficiency in colonoscopy. The literature pertinent to each of these endpoints is reviewed.

CAP-ASSISTED COLONOSCOPY FOR ADENOMA/POLYP DETECTION

Cap-assisted colonoscopy has been tested for improving adenoma/polyp detection since the late 1990s. The majority of earlier studies, including randomized controlled trials (RCTs) comparing cap-assisted colonoscopy to standard colonoscopy, were conducted in Asia[12,14,16,17,19–23] and have shown mixed results. More recently, this technique has been evaluated in Western countries. The first RCT on cap-assisted colonoscopy conducted in United States was by Hewett and Rex.[15] This was a tandem design study with 100 subjects, of whom 52 were randomized to undergo cap-assisted colonoscopy and 48 to regular high-definition colonoscopy as the first procedure, followed by a second colonoscopy by the alternate method. Patients undergoing cap-assisted colonoscopy first had a significantly lower adenoma miss rate compared with those who underwent a regular colonoscopy as the first procedure (21% vs 33%; $P = .039$). The difference in the miss rate was, however, seen only for diminutive (≤ 5 mm) adenomas (22% vs 35%; $P = .037$). In another RCT by Rastogi and colleagues,[13] conducted at a tertiary-care veterans hospital, 420 subjects were randomized to either cap-assisted colonoscopy or regular high-definition colonoscopy. The proportion of subjects with at least 1 adenoma was higher with cap-assisted colonoscopy (69% vs 56%; $P = .009$). Cap-assisted colonoscopy also detected a significantly higher number of adenomas per subject compared with regular colonoscopy (2.3 vs 1.4; $P<.001$). Therefore, cap-assisted colonoscopy detected a 13% higher number of subjects with at 1 one adenoma and 59% higher adenomas per subject. A higher number of subjects with right-sided adenomas and total number of right-sided adenomas were also detected by the cap-assisted procedures. A majority of the subjects enrolled in this study were male veterans and more than 90% had an excellent or good bowel preparation, thereby limiting the generalizability of the results. Contrary to the results of these 2 studies, an RCT from the Netherlands[24] did not find an increment in adenoma detection with cap-assisted colonoscopy. This study was conducted at 2 centers by 5 endoscopists, and randomly allocated 1380 participants to cap-assisted colonoscopy or regular colonoscopy. The proportion of subjects with at least 1 adenoma was similar in the 2 groups (28% vs 28%; relative risk [RR] 0.98; 95% CI, 0.82–1.16). The mean number of adenomas per subject was also similar (0.50 vs 0.49; $P = .91$). A large RCT from Hong Kong[16] involving 1000 subjects showed lower adenoma detection rates with cap-assisted colonoscopy. The adenoma detection rate was 30.5% in the cap-assisted group compared with 37.5% in the regular colonoscopy group ($P = .018$). Similarly, the number of adenomas per subject was also lower in the cap-assisted group (0.63 vs 0.96; $P = .023$). This study, however, had limitations because there was less satisfactory bowel preparation and shorter withdrawal time in the cap-assisted group, factors that could have had a negative impact on the adenoma detection rates. The type of cap used in all these studies had a length of 4 mm protruding beyond the tip of colonoscope. Horiuchi and Nakayama[19] used a specially designed cap, called a retractable transparent hood, and found that although the proportion of patients with adenomas was similar compared with colonoscopy without the device (29% vs 24%; $P = .11$), the total number of adenomas detected was significantly higher (205 vs 150; $P = .04$).

Other RCTs have compared cap-assisted colonoscopy with regular colonoscopy but have reported polyp detection rates without information on polyp histopathology. Kondo and colleagues[12] found that the polyp detection rate was significantly higher with the cap (49% versus 39%; $P = .04$). In another study by Harada and colleagues,[17] the detection rates of polyps was similar with and without the cap (43% vs 42%; $P = .86$). Similarly, Tee and colleagues[23] reported no difference in the polyp detection rates between colonoscopies performed with and without the cap (33% vs 31%; $P = .75$).

An exhaustive meta-analysis of the RCTs comparing cap-assisted colonoscopy with regular colonoscopy was recently published.[25] A total of 16 RCTs were included with 8991 subjects, of whom 4501 underwent cap-assisted colonoscopy and 4490 standard colonoscopy. Twelve trials were identified for comparison of polyp detection rates. Cap-assisted colonoscopy detected a significantly higher proportion of subjects with polyps compared with regular colonoscopy (52.5% vs 47.5%, RR 1.08; 95% CI, 1.00–1.17). Number-needed-to-treat analysis showed that 27 patients would need to undergo cap-assisted colonoscopy for 1 additional patient detected with polyps. For adenoma detection rates, 6 trials were identified and no significant difference was seen between cap-assisted colonoscopy and regular colonoscopy (46.8% vs 45.3%; RR 1.04; 95% CI, 0.90–1.19).

CAP-ASSISTED COLONOSCOPY FOR CECAL INTUBATION RATE AND CECAL INTUBATION TIME

Several studies have compared cap-assisted colonoscopy with regular colonoscopy for cecal intubation rate and cecal intubation time. A recent meta-analysis of RCTs on cap-assisted colonoscopy[25] included 10 studies that included cecal intubation rates and found no significant difference between cap-assisted colonoscopy and regular colonoscopy (96.4% vs 95.6%; RR 1.00; 95% CI, 0.90–1.02). There was, however, statistical heterogeneity among these trials. Although it seems that cap-assisted colonoscopy does not confer any significant benefit over regular colonoscopy for cecal intubation, there is evidence to suggest that it may be useful in difficult cases. Lee and colleagues[16] compared cap-assisted with regular colonoscopy for success as rescue procedures. In their study, patients in whom the cecum could not be reached during the initial procedure by cap or the regular method underwent a second colonoscopy by the alternate method. Cap-assisted colonoscopy achieved a higher rescue rate in cecal intubation compared with regular colonoscopy (67% vs 21%; $P = .003$). An earlier study by the same group[18] had evaluated cap-assisted colonoscopy for consecutive patients with difficult regular colonoscopy defined as failure to pass through the sigmoid colon after 20 minutes of examination or failure to reach the cecum at the end of the procedure. For these patients, the procedure was repeated with the cap. Of the 100 patients in whom the cecum could not be reached by regular colonoscopy, success was achieved with the cap in 94 patients. Therefore, cap-assisted colonoscopy can be considered a rescue method when regular colonoscopy fails to intubate the cecum. My personal experience has been that cap-assisted colonoscopy is effective as a back-up procedure in difficult cases. The potential benefit of using the cap is that it helps in luminal orientation at bends by keeping the colonic mucosa away from the lens at the colonoscope tip. This assists in negotiating sharp turns by better anticipation of the direction[17] and also allows for insertion of the colonoscope with less air insufflation. As a result, there is less chance of looping of the colonoscope during insertion, with greater likelihood of reaching the cecum. Another potential mechanism for improved cecal intubation is the ability to hook the folds, especially at turns, with the tip of the colonoscope augmented by the cap. This helps reduce loops, thereby straightening the colonoscope and facilitating insertion.

As far as time to insert to the cecum is concerned, cap-assisted colonoscopy has been shown superior to regular colonoscopy in multiple trials.[12,13,16,17,19,21,24] Harada and colleagues[17] conducted a prospective randomized study with the primary aim of comparing the cecal intubation time between cap-assisted colonoscopy and regular colonoscopy. The mean cecal intubation time with the cap was 10.2 ± 12.5 minutes, which was significantly shorter than that with regular colonoscopy (13.4 ± 15.8 min; $P = .024$). The impact of cap on cecal intubation time was more prominent in the expert endoscopist (≥ 5000 colonoscopies) group compared with those with moderate experience (≤ 3000 colonoscopies). In the randomized trial by Lee and colleagues,[16] the mean cecal intubation time was 1.2 minutes shorter in the cap-assisted procedures. In the study by Rastogi and colleagues,[13] the mean time to reach the cecum was 3.29 minutes with the cap-assisted method compared with 3.98 minutes with regular colonoscopy ($P<.001$). In another recently published large RCT by de Wijkerslooth and colleagues,[24] the cecal intubation time was also significantly lower with cap-assisted colonoscopy compared with regular colonoscopy (7.7 ± 5.0 min vs 8.9 ± 6.2 min; $P<.001$). Kondo and colleagues[12] showed that cap-assisted colonoscopy shortened the cecal intubation time and, in a stratified subanalysis, the effect was strongest in the subgroups of women and older patients. Ten RCTs comparing cecal intubation times between cap-assisted colonoscopy and regular colonoscopy were included in the meta-analysis by Ng and colleagues.[25] Of these, 7 showed lower cecal intubation time with cap-assisted colonoscopy. Although there was significant statistical heterogeneity, the mean cecal intubation time in the cap-assisted group was significantly lower compared with regular colonoscopy (mean difference = -0.64 min; 95% CI, -1.19 to -0.10). No RCT has shown a longer cecal intubation time with the cap method.

CAP-ASSISTED COLONOSCOPY AND PATIENT DISCOMFORT

Cap-assisted colonoscopy has been compared with regular colonoscopy for patient discomfort and pain during the procedure. Two studies showed no significant differences.[16,20] Harada and colleagues,[17] however, showed that the level of patient discomfort was significantly lower with the cap. In this study, all procedures were started without sedation, and intravenous midazolam was only when a patient requested it or complained of intolerable pain. The frequency of use of sedative was similar in the 2 groups. The patients who did not get sedation were asked to complete a questionnaire regarding the level of discomfort experienced by using a visual analog scale graded into 3 categories: comfortable, acceptable, and intolerable. The proportion of subjects who were comfortable was significantly higher in the cap-assisted group (36% vs 28%; $P = .04$) and those who answered intolerable were significantly lower compared with the regular colonoscopy group (18% vs 25%; $P = .04$). In another study,[26] assessment of pain experienced by patients was assessed postprocedure on a modified 100-mm visual analog scale, on which 0 was defined as pain-free and 100 as extremely painful. Patients undergoing cap-assisted colonoscopy reported lower levels of procedural pain—visual analog scale of pain 29 versus 43 for regular colonoscopy ($P = .01$). In the more recent study by the Amsterdam group,[24] discomfort during colonoscopy was scored using the 5-point Gloucester Comfort

Score, which ranges from no discomfort to extreme discomfort. The overall score was lower in the cap-assisted group compared with the regular colonoscopy group (2.0 vs 2.2; $P = .03$). There is no study showing a higher level of patient discomfort with cap-assisted colonoscopy compared with regular colonoscopy.

CAP-ASSISTED COLONOSCOPY AND POLYPECTOMY

Caps have been used to assist in removal of lesions in the gastrointestinal tract for the past 2 decades, since the report by Inoue and colleagues.[27] Most often this involves sucking the lesion into the compartment between the edge of the cap and the tip of colonoscope, followed by snaring the lesion or applying a band around it, followed by snaring. In the colon, however, this technique has not been embraced routinely. The cap affords, however, a mechanical advantage for endoscopic mucosal resection of polyps, especially those located on the proximal aspects of folds. Because the cap depresses the folds to expose their proximal aspects, it helps in better visualization of the entire polyp located in these areas. The cap also helps stabilize the tip of colonoscope and, therefore, keeps the polyp relatively stationary at an appropriate distance for its removal. These factors help achieve a more complete and efficient polypectomy for polyps in these locations. Park and colleagues[28] conducted a prospective controlled trial in which 329 patients undergoing endoscopic mucosal resection of colon polyps were randomized to either cap-assisted colonoscopy or regular colonoscopy. The mean size of polyps detected was similar in the 2 groups (11.65 mm vs 12.16 mm). The mean time ($\pm$SD) required for endoscopic mucosal resection of 1 polyp, however, was shorter in the cap-assisted group compared with the regular colonoscopy group (3.5 ± 4.5 min vs 4.2 ± 5.1 min; $P = .01$). Subgroup analysis showed that although there was no difference in the time taken to resect pedunculated polyps, there was a significant difference in the resection of nonpedunculated polyps (cap: 3.4 ± 5.0 min vs regular: 3.9 ± 4.7 min; $P = .018$).

CAP-ASSISTED COLONOSCOPY FOR DIVERTICULAR BLEEDING

Cap-assisted colonoscopy also is a useful accessory in the management of diverticular bleeding. It helps in examining diverticuli present between folds that may evade detection and complete visualization during regular colonoscopy. Once the bleeding stigmata within a diverticulum is found, the cap then helps align the target for therapy (ie, a visible vessel or clot within the diverticulum) with the axis of the colonoscope[29] and also stabilizes the colonoscope in relation to the diverticulum for precise application of hemostatic therapy, such as clips or thermal cautery. If the bleeding stigmata within the diverticulum is not visible, then the cap can be used to evert the diverticulum and allow for inspection of the entire mucosal lining of the diverticulum dome.[30] The rim of the cap also provides some tamponade effect prior to hemostatic therapy by pressure at the neck or slight suction of the dome of the diverticulum.[30] Although these are practical observations made by connoisseurs of cap-assisted colonoscopy, there as yet is no RCT comparing the cap method with regular colonoscopy in patients with suspected diverticular bleeding.

CAP-ASSISTED COLONOSCOPY FOR TRAINEES AND LESS-EXPERIENCED ENDOSCOPISTS

Studies have also evaluated the performance of trainees and less-experienced endoscopists with cap-assisted colonoscopy. In one study,[31] 6 trainees, with experience of fewer than 10 colonoscopies each, were randomly assigned to perform the procedure with or without the cap under the supervision of an attending colonoscopist. Success-ful cecal intubation was defined as reaching the cecum within 20 minutes without the assistance of the supervising attending. There were 300 procedures performed in each group. The cecal intubation rate was significantly higher in the cap-assisted group (81% vs 63%; $P<.001$) and the average cecal intubation time was significantly shorter in the cap-assisted group (13.7 min vs 18.7 min; $P<.001$). In another study,[22] one experienced (>5 years experience) and one inexperienced (<1 year experience) endoscopist performed both cap-assisted and regular colonoscopy. The time taken to reach the cecum for the experienced endoscopist was similar with or without the cap. In contrast, for the inexperienced endoscopist, the time taken to reach the cecum was significantly shorter with the cap (9.5 min vs 12.5 min; $P<.05$). The visual analog scale scores of abdominal pain and distension felt by the subjects were also signifi-cantly lower in the cap-assisted group for the inexperienced endoscopist. Caps can, therefore, serve as a useful accessory in assisting novice endoscopists in the performance of more efficient colonoscopy.

COMPLICATIONS

There have been no major complications reported due to the use of cap during colo-noscopy. In one study,[19] the investigators reported mild local submucosal petechial lesions in the rectal mucosa in 9% of subjects undergoing colonoscopy with the trans-parent retractable device that extends for a maximum of 7 mm beyond the tip of co-lonoscope. Retroflexion in the rectum or intubation of the terminal ileum is not hampered by the cap. The potential drawback of cap-assisted colonoscopy is the additional cost burden associated with the cap (approximately $30).

SUMMARY

Cap-assisted colonoscopy is a simple, practical, and inexpensive technique that serves several useful purposes in enhancing the performance of colonoscopy. It helps improve polyp detection by its ability to visualize the otherwise blind mucosal areas on the proximal aspects of folds and flexures, although its effect on adenoma detection has been inconsistent. By helping navigate the colon more efficiently, it facilitates intu-bation of the cecum faster and with lesser patient discomfort. Cap-assisted colonos-copy can be tried as a salvage procedure in cases of failed cecal intubation with regular colonoscopy. Cap can also be of assistance during polypectomy, especially for polyps located on the proximal aspects of folds. Finally, in cases of diverticular bleeding, use of the cap can help in localizing the bleeding diverticulum and in the treatment of the bleeding stigmata.

REFERENCES

1. Lieberman DA. Clinical practice. Screening for colorectal cancer. N Engl J Med 2009;361:1179–87.
2. Levin B, Lieberman DA, McFarland B, et al. Screening and surveillance for the early detection of colorectal cancer and adenomatous polyps, 2008: a joint guideline from the American Cancer Society, the US Multi-Society Task Force on Colorectal Cancer, and the American College of Radiology. Gastroenterology 2008;134:1570–95.
3. Rex DK, Cutler CS, Lemmel GT, et al. Colonoscopic miss rates of adenomas determined by back-to-back colonoscopies. Gastroenterology 1997;112:24–8.

4. Kaminski MF, Regula J, Kraszewska E, et al. Quality indicators for colonoscopy and the risk of interval cancer. N Engl J Med 2010;362:1795–803.

5. Froehlich F, Wietlisbach V, Gonvers JJ, et al. Impact of colonic cleansing on quality and diagnostic yield of colonoscopy: the European Panel of Appropriateness of Gastrointestinal Endoscopy European multicenter study. Gastrointest Endosc 2005;61:378–84.

6. Harewood GC, Sharma VK, de Garmo P. Impact of colonoscopy preparation quality on detection of suspected colonic neoplasia. Gastrointest Endosc 2003; 58:76–9.

7. Rex DK. Colonoscopic withdrawal technique is associated with adenoma miss rates. Gastrointest Endosc 2000;51:33–6.

8. Barclay RL, Vicari JJ, Doughty AS, et al. Colonoscopic withdrawal times and adenoma detection during screening colonoscopy. N Engl J Med 2006;355: 2533–41.

9. Pickhardt PJ, Nugent PA, Mysliwiec PA, et al. Location of adenomas missed by optical colonoscopy. Ann Intern Med 2004;141:352–9.

10. Leufkens AM, DeMarco DC, Rastogi A, et al. Effect of a retrograde-viewing device on adenoma detection rate during colonoscopy: the TERRACE study. Gastrointest Endosc 2011;73:480–9.

11. Hewett DG, Rex DK. Miss rate of right-sided colon examination during colonoscopy defined by retroflexion: an observational study. Gastrointest Endosc 2011; 74:246–52.

12. Kondo S, Yamaji Y, Watabe H, et al. A randomized controlled trial evaluating the usefulness of a transparent hood attached to the tip of the colonoscope. Am J Gastroenterol 2007;102:75–81.

13. Rastogi A, Bansal A, Rao DS, et al. Higher adenoma detection rates with cap-assisted colonoscopy: a randomised controlled trial. Gut 2012;61:402–8.

14. Dafnis GM. Technical considerations and patient comfort in total colonoscopy with and without a transparent cap: initial experiences from a pilot study. Endoscopy 2000;32:381–4.

15. Hewett DG, Rex DK. Cap-fitted colonoscopy: a randomized, tandem colonoscopy study of adenoma miss rates. Gastrointest Endosc 2010;72:775–81.

16. Lee YT, Lai LH, Hui AJ, et al. Efficacy of cap-assisted colonoscopy in comparison with regular colonoscopy: a randomized controlled trial. Am J Gastroenterol 2009;104:41–6.

17. Harada Y, Hirasawa D, Fujita N, et al. Impact of a transparent hood on the performance of total colonoscopy: a randomized controlled trial. Gastrointest Endosc 2009;69:637–44.

18. Lee YT, Hui AJ, Wong VW, et al. Improved colonoscopy success rate with a distally attached mucosectomy cap. Endoscopy 2006;38:739–42.

19. Horiuchi A, Nakayama Y. Improved colorectal adenoma detection with a transparent retractable extension device. Am J Gastroenterol 2008;103:341–5.

20. Tada M, Inoue H, Yabata E, et al. Feasibility of the transparent cap-fitted colonoscope for screening and mucosal resection. Dis Colon Rectum 1997;40:618–21.

21. Matsushita M, Hajiro K, Okazaki K, et al. Efficacy of total colonoscopy with a transparent cap in comparison with colonoscopy without the cap. Endoscopy 1998;30:444–7.

22. Dai J, Feng N, Lu H, et al. Transparent cap improves patients' tolerance of colonoscopy and shortens examination time by inexperienced endoscopists. J Dig Dis 2010;11:364–8.

23. Tee HP, Corte C, Al-Ghamdi H, et al. Prospective randomized controlled trial evaluating cap-assisted colonoscopy vs standard colonoscopy. World J Gastroenterol 2010;16:3905–10.
24. de Wijkerslooth TR, Stoop EM, Bossuyt PM, et al. Adenoma detection with cap-assisted colonoscopy versus regular colonoscopy: a randomised controlled trial. Gut 2012;61:1426–34.
25. Ng SC, Tsoi KK, Hirai HW, et al. The efficacy of cap-assisted colonoscopy in polyp detection and cecal intubation: a meta-analysis of randomized controlled trials. Am J Gastroenterol 2012;107:1165–73.
26. Shida T, Katsuura Y, Teramoto O, et al. Transparent hood attached to the colonoscope: does it really work for all types of colonoscopes? Surg Endosc 2008;22:2654–8.
27. Inoue H, Takeshita K, Hori H, et al. Endoscopic mucosal resection with a cap-fitted panendoscope for esophagus, stomach, and colon mucosal lesions. Gastrointest Endosc 1993;39:58–62.
28. Park SY, Kim HS, Yoon KW, et al. Usefulness of cap-assisted colonoscopy during colonoscopic EMR: a randomized, controlled trial. Gastrointest Endosc 2011;74:869–75.
29. Sanchez-Yague A, Kaltenbach T, Yamamoto H, et al. The endoscopic cap that can (with videos). Gastrointest Endosc 2012;76:169–78.e1–2.
30. Kaltenbach T, Watson R, Shah J, et al. Colonoscopy with clipping is useful in the diagnosis and treatment of diverticular bleeding. Clin Gastroenterol Hepatol 2012;10:131–7.
31. Park SM, Lee SH, Shin KY, et al. The cap-assisted technique enhances colonoscopy training: prospective randomized study of six trainees. Surg Endosc 2012;26:2939–43.

Retroview Colonoscopy

Jerome D. Waye, MD

KEYWORDS

- Retroview • Retroflexion • Colonoscopy • Missed lesions • Third Eye Retroscope

KEY POINTS

- Lesions in the right colon are often missed.
- Missed lesions may be hidden from view by standard colonoscopy techniques.
- Instruments that look behind folds in the colon will find hidden lesions.
- Retroview in the colon can discover many polyps and adenomas.
- Dedicated instruments are being developed to enhance right colon observations.

Videos of removal of a colon polyp during retroflexion in the right colon and retroview of a polyp accompany this article at http://www.gastro.theclinics.com/

INTRODUCTION

Most endoscopists perform retroview during colonoscopy. Most often, this is a retroflexion in the rectum to observe the rectal ampulla and to view the areas near the anus directly and up close. This maneuver is accomplished by performing a turn-around or U-turn maneuver in the capacious rectal ampulla, but retroflexion can also be performed in the proximal colon in a similar fashion. Because of the narrowing and multiple twists in the sigmoid colon, it is often difficult to perform retroflexion with a colonoscope in the left colon or sigmoid colon.

RECTAL RETROFLEXION

When colonoscopy was introduced as an alternative to the barium enema, rectal retroflexion was often performed inadvertently as the deflected tip turned around as the shaft was pushed forward. It did not take long for endoscopists to realize the value and the relative ease with which the colonoscope could be retroflexed in the rectum. This technique became widely used as a standard of the effectiveness of

No conflicts of interest.

Medicine, Icahn School of Medicine at Mount Sinai, Mount Sinai Hospital, 1 Gustave Levy Place, New York, NY 10029, USA

E-mail address: Jdwaye@aol.com

Gastroenterol Clin N Am 42 (2013) 491–505
http://dx.doi.org/10.1016/j.gtc.2013.05.013
0889-8553/13/$ – see front matter © 2013 Elsevier Inc. All rights reserved.

colonoscopy. In the retroflexion mode, the dentate line can be readily seen, usually in a 360° circumferential view; the mucosal junction between columnar mucosa and cuboidal mucosa of the anal canal is easily discernible; and at times, stratified squamous epithelium (external skin) can also be seen.

Over the years, rectal retroflexion became an integral feature of colonoscopy **(Fig. 1)**. Only recently has there been any investigation into its usefulness in discovering intrarectal pathologic conditions. This matter is of some controversy because some reports find that it has no additional pathologic findings, and others laud the benefits of this relatively simple maneuver.

As expected, it has been reported that rectal retroflexion is useful for the evaluation of hemorrhoids. However, 2 reports concluded that retroflexion in the rectum is a procedure with very little yield for perianal neoplasia. Saad and Rex[1] successfully performed rectal retroflexion in 94% of 1502 patients and discovered only one small tubular adenoma not seen on forward examination. A previous article by Cutler and Pop[2] inspected the rectal vault during scope withdrawal. They successfully performed the rectal retroflexion maneuver in 445 of 453 patients; they reported that this procedure yielded very little additional information because it revealed further findings in only 9 patients with 3 inflammatory pseudopolyps, 5 hyperplastic polyps, and one case of erosions.

In contrast, Varadarajulu and Ramsey[3] found that more than 50% of the lesions in the rectal vault were identified only on retroflexion, with 30 out of 60 patients having significant additional information discovered by rectal retroflexion. There are several other similar reports and case studies espousing the value of rectal retroflexion.[4,5]

TECHNIQUE FOR RECTAL RETROFLEXION

The technique of retroflexion has been described[3]: "The rectum was first thoroughly examined on direct view upon withdrawal of the instrument up to the anal verge. The endoscope was then re-advanced into the rectum and the shaft of the instrument

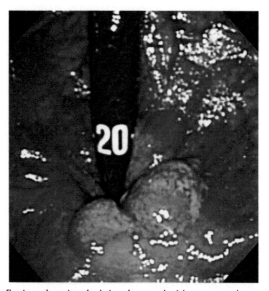

Fig. 1. Rectal retroflexion showing bulging hemorrhoids near anal verge. The white areas on hemorrhoids are caused by chronic prolapse.

was rotated clockwise while both control knobs were fully angulated to invert the tip of the endoscope for a close view of the perianal rectal ampulla."[3] The maneuver was considered successful if a complete 360° visualization of the distal rectum was obtained. In this report, retroflexion was successful in 590 of 600 consecutive patients (98.3%). Because of a contracted vault, 10 patients could not have their retroflexion performed. It is interesting that endoscope-induced trauma was not encountered in any of the patients, although 9 patients who had successful retroflexion complained of rectal pain during the procedure.

The author's technique is to carefully inspect the rectal mucosa down to the anal verge and then advance the colonoscope, placing the tip against a flat area of the mucosa at the level of the first rectal valve. The tip is then maximally deflected upward and gently advanced into the rectum. If resistance is encountered and the tip does not slide freely across the mucosa, the attempt is abandoned and another site is chosen for the retroflexion maneuver. The retroflexion attempt should be discontinued if patients complain of pain during the maneuver. It should not be attempted in the presence of a contracted small rectum such as occurs after radiotherapy or in inflammatory bowel disease. If the tip slides across mucosa easily (although a view of the lumen cannot be seen), the small outer dial control is then maximally deflected to the right and locked. The right hand, which moved and locked the small dial control, then grasps the instrument, and the scope is torqued markedly clockwise and withdrawn. This technique frees the tip from mucosal contact and affords a view of the shaft as it traverses the anal canal. The perianal area can be easily visualized by torque and withdrawal. It is not usually possible to retroflex the scope in the rectum by sole use of the dial controls, although these are effective to turn the tip into a retroflex position when the scope is outside of patients in a demonstration mode. The inability to freely retroflex in the rectum is caused by the radius of the tip deflection being greater than the spatial capacity of the rectal ampulla so that the tip is constrained and catches the wall, impairing free movement.

COMPLICATIONS WITH RECTAL RETROFLEXION

Perforations related to rectal retroflexion have been reported[6–12] that are generally caused by a contracted rectal vault or advancing the instrument against resistance. Saad and Rex[1] made a point that this maneuver should not be attempted if the rectum seems narrow. There are 2 specific instances when rectal retroflexion should be avoided, and these are ulcerative colitis and after radiation treatment of prostate cancer when the rectal vault may be contracted.

PROXIMAL COLON RETROFLEXION

A more thorough evaluation of the right colon has been popularized primarily because of recent reports showing that colon cancer can occur shortly following a negative colonoscopic examination and that colonoscopy may not protect against the development of right colon cancers.[13–15]

Hewett and Rex[16] were able to perform retroflexion in the right colon in almost 95% of patients in whom it was attempted, and an additional 10% of polyps were seen in addition to those discovered on forward view colonoscopy. Even with meticulous examination in the forward view, they missed 12% of large adenomas (≥1 cm) that were found on retroflexion.

In another study, a prototype tapered colonoscope with the distal 25 cm being similar to a pediatric-sized diameter tapering to a standard adult-sized colonoscope was compared with a standard pediatric variable-stiffness colonoscope.[17]

A retroflexion could be performed 98% of the time with the tapered scope as compared with 78% with the pediatric variable-stiffness colonoscope.

Two prototype instruments, one with a shorter bending section and the other with a tighter radius of tip deflection, showed a significantly higher rate of successful retroflexion compared with the standard pediatric colonoscope; there was no difference between them in the success rate of cecal retroflexion. The success of retroflexion in the cecum was 57% for the standard pediatric colonoscope and 91% and 94% for the prototype instruments.

Another study[17] was performed with similar instruments but using adult-diameter colonoscopes.

The instrument with a shorter bending section could be retroflexed in the cecum more often than the other, but there were no other significant differences noted with either instrument.

An earlier report by the Indiana Group had shown disappointing results for additional adenoma detection from retroflexion in the right colon during screening colonoscopy.[18] Following an initial examination, the cecum was then reintubated and the patients were randomized to a second examination either using a forward-viewing technique or using a retroflexed mode. It was found that the standard adult colonoscope could only be retroflexed in the cecum approximately 40% of the time, and a standard pediatric colonoscope could be retroflexed in the cecum approximately one-third of the time when attempted (**Fig. 2**).

When the second examination was performed in the standard forward view, the miss rates for polyps and adenomas during the initial examination were 37% and 33%, respectively. When the second examination was performed with retroflexion, the rates of missed polyps and adenomas were 38% and 23%, respectively. Thus, the calculated miss rate on the second examination performed in retroflexion was numerically lower than when the second examination was performed in the forward view. The explanation proffered in this report was that the retroflexion does not expose

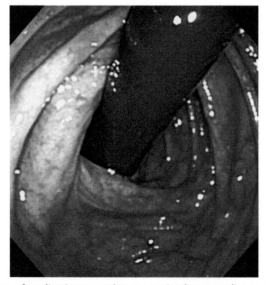

Fig. 2. Retroflexion of pediatric-type colonoscope in the ascending colon. The proximal aspects of folds can be seen.

the entire colon to view because the instrument may be difficult to maneuver during retroflexion or that polyps located in hidden positions on the proximal sides of folds are not the principal mechanism accounting for failure of detection during colonoscopy. Although no complications were seen during this randomized study, the investigators cautioned against routine retroflexion in the right colon because of the possibility of complications.

RETROFLEXION AND POLYPECTOMY

Two articles have discussed the removal of colon polyps during retroflexion with a colonoscope (Video 1).[19] Prototypes of the pediatric-type colonoscope (one with a shorter bending section and the other with a tighter tip deflection radius) were used in one of these studies.[20] Standard polypectomy procedures were used to remove 59 consecutive large sessile polyps proximal to the rectum.[20] Fourteen polyps were removed partially or completely in the retroflexion mode. There were no perforations and no complications related to retroflexion. The polyps removed in retroflexion could only barely be visualized in the forward view, and all could not have been removed except by using the retroflexion technique. A similar report[21] detailed 15 polypectomies with endoscopic retroflexion. All of the polyps were sessile and large (average size 38 mm, range 20–60 mm) and evenly distributed throughout the colon. The procedures were performed using a standard Pentax colonoscope (EC3831L, Pentax Precision Instrument Corporation, Orangeburg, NY).

The authors of both reports state that retroflexion attempts should be stopped if the endoscopist feels resistance when bending the tip or when trying to advance the scope. Oftentimes, the use of an upper endoscope may be a good alternative especially when retroflexing in the left colon.[21]

USE OF A GASTROSCOPE

A gastroscope, which has both a short nose and a short bending section, has been reported to be easily retroflexed in the right colon so that flat polyps can be removed in the retroflexion mode. In an article by Hurlstone and colleauges,[19] cecal intubation was achieved in 100% of cases using a gastroscope and all 76 patients had tumors that were situated on both sides of a fold, located on both the proximal and distal aspects. Endoscopic resection was possible in 61 patients who completed their protocol (8 were excluded by the endoscopic ultrasound criteria), with a 98% cure rate following endoscopic mucosal resection using a standard gastroscope. It is the opinion of the author of this article that although a gastroscope can often be passed to the cecum, it is not invariably the case because the length may be too short to allow advancement around several bends and folds of the colon, especially in tall or overweight patients.

TECHNIQUE FOR RETROFLEXION IN PROXIMAL COLON

This author's technique is to advance the instrument several haustral folds beyond the polyp. Loops are removed by withdrawing the scope to straighten the instrument as much as possible. The dial controls are pointed maximally up and to the right. The right/left control is locked, and the thumb maintains the large control wheel in an upward direction. The scope is then advanced a few centimeters to determine whether the tip will begin to slide across the mucosal surface or whether a loop forms in the shaft. If the tip slides freely, further advancement of the scope is performed to complete the retroflexion. If the scope shaft is pushed in but the tip does not move, then a loop is forming and the scope should be torqued in a clockwise fashion and withdrawn.

Once retroflexion view is obtained, the instrument tip can be controlled by torque around several folds of the ascending colon and may be withdrawn into the transverse colon by gentle manipulation of the shaft, torquing it to the right or to the left as necessary to insinuate the tip around acute angulations near the hepatic flexure.

The recent interest in the retroflexion view of the colon has been engendered by the reported miss rate of the colonoscope and of the inability of colonoscopy to prevent right-sided colon cancer.[13–15] Studies to measure the miss rate for colonoscopy have used several different methods.

TANDEM COLONOSCOPY

The concept of tandem colonoscopy is well suited for evaluation of missed lesions in the colon because polyps that are found are discrete, can be measured, are readily recognized, and are common. During tandem colonoscopy, the first examiner removes all polyps that are encountered so all polyps seen by the second endoscopy will represent overlooked lesions. One of the problems with tandem colonoscopy is that the endoscopists know they are part of a study and will pay special attention so as not to miss lesions. However, despite this heightened awareness from being part of a tandem colonoscopy experiment, trials that have evaluated the miss rate of polyps in the large bowel through performing a second-pass colonoscopy have revealed strikingly large numbers of polyps overlooked by the first examiner using the same standard colonoscopic equipment.

The first such study by Hixson and colleagues[22] found a 15% miss rate for adenomas less than 1 cm in size. Rex and colleagues,[23] in a study of 183 patients, reported a 27% miss rate for polyps smaller than 6 mm in diameter and only 6% for polyps larger than 9 mm. There was no significant difference in the miss rate of polyps in the right colon (27%) than in the left colon (21%). Although a substantial percentage (24%) of adenomas were missed, there was an inverse ratio between the miss rate and the size of the adenoma. In the summary of the report, the investigators recommended that technology be developed that may overcome the technical limitations of colonoscopy.

The more recent large multicenter European study[24] found miss rates of 28% for all polyps, 31% for hyperplastic polyps, and 21% for adenomas. However, the miss rate for all polyps 5 mm or larger was 12% and 9% for adenomas. Among the 14 polyps and 6 adenomas larger than 5 mm missed during the first examination, 5 polyps and 1 adenoma were sessile, and 9 polyps and 5 adenomas were flat. In all, 37 adenomas were overlooked in 286 patients, with the median size being 3 mm; however, the range of missed lesions was from 1 to 18 mm. This report also stated that 3 advanced adenomas were missed whose size varied from 15 to 18 mm. The investigators reported that there was a 27% rate of missed adenomas for lesions less than 5 mm in diameter, whereas the miss rate for lesions greater than 5 mm in diameter was 9%.

The most recent back-to-back colonoscopy study for missed lesions involved special effort to ensure a "quality examination."[25] This involved eliminating cases whereby the cecum was not intubated or when the bowel prep was poor. The examinations were performed by 2 experienced colonoscopists who have previously performed more than 3000 colonoscopies, and the withdrawal time was more than 6 minutes in every case. The second colonoscopy was performed immediately after conclusion of the first examination by the same examiner. A total of 149 patients completed all the criteria for enrollment in the study whereby all polyps were removed during the initial examination. The miss rates (polyps found on the second examination) for all polyps, all adenomas, adenomas 6 to 9 mm, and advanced adenomas were 16.8%, 17.0%, 7.2%, and 5.4%, respectively. The location of polyps in the right or left colon did not significantly affect the miss rate, which was positively correlated with the size of the polyp.

Despite the attention to quality in this study, the true adenoma miss rate is not known because the second colonoscopy was used as the gold standard. Their conclusion was that a significant number of adenomas (17.0%) and advanced adenomas (5.4%) were being missed during colonoscopy and that "development of new endoscopic techniques to overcome the technical limitations of the current colonoscopic examination is important."[25]

FOLLOW-UP COLONOSCOPY

Another method for estimating polyp miss rates is to evaluate results of colonoscopies performed at relatively brief intervals following an initial procedure with total polyp removal. In a retrospective analysis[26] of more than 15 000 colonoscopies, the polyp miss rate was evaluated by comparing findings on repeat colonoscopic examinations at 4 and 12 months after the initial colonoscopic examination. The miss rate was 17% for all polyps and 12% for neoplastic polyps, which is comparable with tandem colonoscopy studies.

The technique of the examination is critically important in the discovery of colon polyps. Flat neoplasms or sessile serrated polyps can elude detection by the casual or untrained observer,[27] even when they are in the field of view of the forward-viewing standard colonoscope.

However, a limitation of tandem examinations and studies involving a second colonoscopy at a later date is that a substantial proportion of polyps that are missed are located behind folds in the colon wall where they are hidden from the forward-viewing colonoscope. Thus, considering use of the same instrument a second time to be the gold standard ignores the fact that lesions behind folds are likely to be missed during both examinations. When studies are designed to compare standard colonoscopy with techniques capable of seeing behind folds, they generally find substantially higher adenoma miss rates compared with those determined in tandem studies.

COMPARISON WITH COMPUTERIZED TOMOGRAPHIC COLONOGRAPHY

Pickhardt and colleagues[28] did a computerized tomographic colonography (CTC) evaluation of more than 1200 people who had same-day CTC and colonoscopy. With segmental unblinding during a colonoscopic examination that followed the CTC, 10% of polyps were found only after the colonoscopist was told to review an area where a polyp was detected on the original CTC. Of the neoplasms originally missed but found on the second-look colonoscopy after segmental unblinding, 17 were tubular adenomas, 3 were tubulovillous adenomas, and 1 was a small adenocarcinoma (size range 6–17 mm). The miss rate for large adenomas (at least 1 cm) with colonoscopy was 12%. Most of the missed neoplasms were located on the edge or on the proximal aspect of a fold.[28]

In a separate study of 223 patients, Pickhardt's group[29] used CTC to demonstrate that 23.4% of the colonic surface is not visualized by direct straight end-on examinations from below and suggested this "may provide insight into potential limitations at optical colonoscopy."[29]

East and colleagues[30] used CTC modeling to simulate fields of view of 90°, 120°, 140°, and 170° to match the angle of view of various models of colonoscopes. They also simulated a 135° view with a retrograde-viewing auxiliary imaging device, which they described as equivalent to the image provided by the Third Eye Retroscope (TER) (Avantis Medical Systems, Sunnyvale, CA).

The percentage of visualized colonic surface increased with each increasing colonoscope angle-of-view increment. The total number of missed areas was approximately the same for fields of view of 90° to 140° but decreased when the field of view enlarged to 170°. Approximately only 85% of the colonic surface would have been visualized using a 140° angle of view, and this increased so that more of the surface would be seen when the examination was conducted using a 170° angle of view comparable with the Olympus 180 series colonoscopes (Olympus Medical Instruments, Tokyo, Japan).

With the simulation of optical colonoscopy by CTC software, using the commonly available 140° angle of view of most colonoscopes, approximately 13% of the colonic surface is unseen. Simulation of a colonoscope with a 170° field of view resulted in an almost 6% reduction in percentage of surface missed.

The simulated addition of a retrograde viewing auxiliary imaging device along with the 140° angle-of-view colonoscope led to an almost complete surface visualization with a 10-fold decrease in the area that was missed compared with that obtained using a wide-angle colonoscope with a 170° angle of view. When complemented by the 135° reverse view, both the 140° and the 170° angle-of-view colonoscopes provided essentially complete visualization of the colonic mucosa.

COLONOSCOPY AND PROTECTION AGAINST RIGHT COLON CANCER

The need to address hidden lesions has led to a series of trials, many of which involved an innovation in scope characteristics that would result in the ability to turn the tip of the colonoscope backward to see behind colon haustral folds and in the haustral pouches between folds. It has also led to the development of an auxiliary endoscope that permits visualization behind colon folds. Retroview in the right colon may become the new standard for colonoscopy, especially in view of current literature that lesions located there may be missed.

Currently there are 3 types of instruments that provide a retroview of the colon. These instruments are (1) the standard colonoscope, either pediatric or adult size; (2) a short tip-bending colonoscope (not commercially available); and (3) a pass-through mini-scope that automatically retroflexes to allow simultaneous forward and backward views of the colon.

THE TER

The only instrument that can allow viewing both the proximal and distal aspect of folds simultaneously during a colonoscopic examination is the TER, a fully developed mini-endoscope that is slim enough to fit through the biopsy channel of a standard or pediatric-type colonoscope (**Fig. 3**). When its tip emerges from the distal end of the channel, it automatically reverses direction 180°, so its video camera is aiming in the retrograde direction. Because the outside dimension of its U-shaped tip is only 7.5 mm, it can be pulled along with the colonoscope through even the most acute bends in the sigmoid colon. This technique is not possible with any other instruments currently manufactured.

When the TER is positioned beyond the tip of the colonoscope, it permits a retrograde view of the colon. Although the standard colonoscope provides an image of

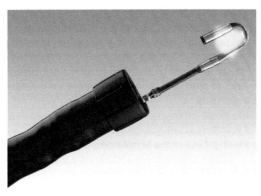

Fig. 3. The TER exits the biopsy channel of a pediatric colonoscope, and the tip turns to face the lens of the colonoscope. The light source is at the apex of the bend. (*Courtesy of* Avantis Medical Systems, Inc, Sunnyvale, CA; with permission.)

the colon in a forward direction, the TER looks backward toward and beyond the faceplate of the colonoscope, visualizing the proximal aspect of folds as the colonoscope simultaneously views their distal surfaces. The disposable TER has an integrated light-emitting diode (LED) light source and uses a dedicated video processor. Its retrograde video image is displayed side by side with the forward view of the colonoscope on a wide-screen monitor. The shaft of the device is 2.0 mm in diameter, and its 3.1-mm viewing portion is comprised of 2 segments with a camera at the tip. The fixed but flexible segments have a built-in angulation that, when exiting the accessory channel of the colonoscope, causes the tip to bend 180° so that the imaging chip is directed toward the faceplate of the colonoscope.

The outside distance across the 2 limbs of the U-turned TER tip is 7.5 mm, and the length of the camera-carrying segment is 12 mm. The 2-part bending portion, each with a 90° angulation, creates a U shape with an LED light that shines toward the colonoscope to illuminate the area behind it so that the area that is usually dark (behind the tip of the colonoscope) is bathed in a brilliant light illuminating several centimeters of distal bowel.

Torquing the retroscope with a knob outside the biopsy port changes the orientation of the Retroscope's tip so that it can be placed in a position to be washed by the water jet from the colonoscope whenever debris tends to obscure excellent vision. A locking mechanism keeps the TER in whichever position is optimal for distal visualization.

Ordinarily, the bright light from the Retroscope's LED would fool the sensor mechanism of the colonoscope into registering too much light, causing the colonoscope's light source to be dimmed. However, this effect has been minimized by synchronizing the flashes of the LED with the frame rate of the colonoscope's camera and can be further alleviated by switching the light source setting from *auto* to *manual*.

A greater challenge results from the fact that the Retroscope's camera is looking directly at the colonoscope's multiple fiber-optic light guides. Without a mechanism to compensate for this, the Retroscope would be blinded by the intense light shining into its lens.

The solution involves placing a disposable plastic cap over the tip of the colonoscope before the procedure. The cap places polarizing filters over each of the colonoscope's light guides, and in combination with a similar polarizing filter that is built into the Retroscope camera's lens, the system eliminates the glare.

The cap has an aperture that is aligned with the instrument channel to allow passage of the Retroscope or, when necessary, a biopsy forceps or snare. Another larger opening assures that the colonoscope's camera and water jet are unimpeded.

The tip of the TER is routinely situated about 2.5 cm from the end of the colonoscope, but this can be varied during the procedure as necessary. The 135° angle-of-view chip on the end of the TER has been refined over several years and now provides a high-resolution image.

The first report of the initial prototype Retroscope appeared in 2007.[31] This bench test was designed to find simulated polyps placed behind folds in a colon model. A forward colonoscope found 12% of the simulated polyps that had been placed behind folds, and 81% of the hidden polyps were visualized with the TER device.

TER: CLINICAL STUDIES

The TER[32] was used clinically in 24 patients, and an additional 12% of polyps were found with the retrograde-viewing device but not seen with the standard forward-viewing colonoscope (**Fig. 4, Table 1**). During this study, 38 polyps were identified in 29 patients as the colonoscope and TER visualized the colon in both forward and retroview. Thirty of the polyps were seen with the colonoscope, 4 were visualized simultaneously by the colonoscope and the Retroscope, and an additional 4 were seen only with the Retroscope because they were located on the proximal aspect of folds. The sizes of the polyps found with the Retroscope varied from 0.2 to 0.7 cm.

A more recent prospective multicenter study in 249 patients at 8 locations[33] demonstrated an additional 13.2% increase in polyp detection, with an 11.0% increase in adenoma detection. Thirty-four polyps, including 15 additional adenomas, were located behind folds and were found only because they were detected in the retrograde view.

Of the total of 40 adenomas at least 6 mm in diameter, 32 were detected with the colonoscope and 8 more with the TER (25% additional yield). Of the 12 adenomas measuring at least 1 cm, 3 were first detected with the TER (33% additional yield). The mean size of adenomas detected with the TER was 5.2 mm compared with 4.4 mm for those detected with the colonoscope. The withdrawal phase of the examinations averaged 10.9 minutes, eliminating the time required for polyp removal.

These findings strikingly demonstrate that polyps may be located in areas difficult to detect by forward-viewing colonoscopy (Video 2). Colonoscopy is the best imaging

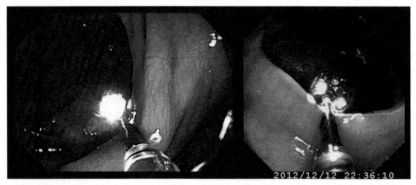

Fig. 4. A monitor view during a procedure with the image generated by the colonoscope on the left of the screen and that from the TER on the right where it shows the faceplate of the colonoscope and the area behind it. The bright light from the TER source illuminates well the usually dark area distal to the colonoscope tip.

Study	Preclinical Study[32]	Feasibililty[31]	Efficacy[33]	Learning Curve[38]	TERRACE[39]	TERRACE-2[40]
Patients	N/A	24	249	298	395	N/A
Investigators	10	2	14	17	21	—
Centers	1	1	8	9	9	—
Design	Models	One pass	One pass	One pass	Tandem	Subset analysis
ADR with TER (%)	12.0 c-scope 81.0 TER	11.8 for all polyps	11.0	25.0 after 15 procedures	23.0 after correcting for second pass effect	40.7 in patients more than avg risk

Table 1
Published studies on the TER

Abbreviations: ADR, adenoma detection rate; avg, average; c-scope, colonoscope; TERRACE, Third-Eye Retroscope Randomized Clinical Evaluation.

device currently available for the large bowel but may be an imperfect tool against colon cancer because neoplasms can be missed. Because modern guidelines[34–37] for colorectal cancer screening and surveillance depend on baseline colonoscopy findings, the need to identify all neoplasia in the colon has assumed even greater importance.

Another study focused on the impact of endoscopists' experience with the TER on adenoma detection rates.[38] In a multicenter study, the investigators found that the TER increased polyp detection and that the learning time for its use is relatively short.

Endoscopists with no previous experience with the TER participated in a prospective study at 9 sites to determine whether experience with the TER increases both polyp detection rates and procedure efficiency.

All polyps found during colonoscopic insertion were removed. The TER was inserted through the accessory channel of the colonoscope once the tip of the instrument reached the cecum. When a polyp was seen, the endoscopist indicated whether it could have been seen with a colonoscope using a routine withdrawal technique or if it could only have been detected with the TER. All polyps seen with the colonoscope or the TER were subsequently found with the colonoscope and removed.

In these 298 patients, 182 polyps including 100 adenomas were detected with the colonoscope and an additional 27 polyps including 16 adenomas were detected with the TER, for 14.8% and 16.0% increases, respectively. The results from 20 patients who were enrolled with each endoscopist were divided into quartiles, that is, the first 5 procedures constituted the first quartile, the second 5 procedures constituted the second quartile, and so forth. The learning curve was evaluated by comparing results among quartiles.

For all polyps, the additional detection rate for the TER was 17.8% in the first quartile and 17.0% in the fourth quartile. For adenomas, the additional detection rate by using the TER increased from 15.4% in the first quartile to 25% in the fourth quartile. The mean estimated size of all polyps detected with the TER was 6.5 mm, compared with 5.5 mm for those detected with the colonoscope alone. The TER detected 19% additional adenomas with a size of 10 mm or larger. These results suggest that there is a trend toward improvement of adenoma detection with increasing experience and that they require varying amounts of experience to develop optimal technique.

An international multisite (4 in Europe and 5 in the United States) study, called the Third-Eye Retroscope Randomized Clinical Evaluation (TERRACE),[39] involved a tandem-design trial that provided an immediate comparison of TER colonoscopy with standard colonoscopy. In this study, the retrograde-viewing device detected 23.2% additional adenomas, even after correction for the second-pass effect that invariably occurs in tandem studies. This effect has been shown to repeatedly occur; when a second look at the same area is accomplished, there are more polyps discovered that were not seen during the original view. This study corroborated previous studies with the TER and with virtual colonography showing that large polyps in addition to a significant number of smaller polyps are missed by standard colonoscopy.

The TERRACE investigators have recently published the results of post hoc subset analyses of their data looking at several variables that might have impacted their results.[40] The independent variables of gender, age, bowel prep quality, and withdrawal time did not significantly affect the relative risk of missing adenomas with standard colonoscopy versus TER colonoscopy. However, one set of variables, indications for procedures, showed highly significant differences when the TER was compared with standard colonoscopy; when the indication for colonoscopy was surveillance or for a diagnostic workup, the TER found additional adenoma and polyp detection rates of 35.7% and 55.4%, respectively. Pooling the results for those two groups of patients, who can be considered to have a more-than-average risk for colorectal cancer, TER colonoscopy showed 40.7% additional adenoma detection. In contrast, in average-risk people undergoing screening colonoscopy, TER colonoscopy detected only 4.4% additional adenomas.

During this highly controlled investigation, it became evident once again that standard colonoscopy can even miss large adenomas (>1 cm) at a rate of 11.8%, whereas the TER colonoscopy did not miss any large adenomas that could then be found during a second look with the forward colonoscope. The miss rate for large adenomas with standard colonoscopy in this series is almost identical to that found in 2 previously described studies that used other methods to look behind folds of the colon: Pickhardt and colleagues' 2004 CTC[28] study that demonstrated an 11.8% miss rate for large adenomas using standard colonoscopy and Hewett and Rex's 2011 report[16] that a second look with a retroflexed colonoscope following a previous straight view of the ascending colon found that 12% of large adenomas had been missed on the first examination.

The technique for retrograde viewing with the TER includes the following:

- Meticulously cleanse the fluid pools in the colon during intubation because the TER decreases the suction capacity of the standard colonoscope when it is positioned within the instrument/accessory channel of the colonoscope.
- When the cecum has been intubated with the colonoscope, the instrument is withdrawn several centimeters to allow the safe insertion of the TER.
- A locking mechanism permits stabilization of the tip of the TER once it has exited the instrument channel and has automatically flexed 180%. The TER does not have any controls for tip deflection but can be rotated to permit cleansing of the lens with the water jet from the mother colonoscope.
- The TER and the colonoscope are withdrawn together using standard colonoscopic techniques. In every study, all polyps initially found with the TER were subsequently located and removed with the standard colonoscope, even when the TER discovered a polyp hidden deep in a recess behind a fold.
- During withdrawal, the examiner has to pay strict attention to the side-by-side images on the monitor showing forward and retrograde views of the colon. Shifting the eyes between the 2 immediately adjacent images requires some acclimation but is not difficult.

- When negotiating the sigmoid colon, the TER is positioned closer to the faceplate of the colonoscope because of the multiple folds that would obscure vision of the TER if it remained in the extended mode several centimeters beyond the tip of the colonoscope.

SUMMARY

Retroview during colonoscopy reveals polyps hidden from the forward-viewing colonoscopic instruments. Being able to see fully the proximal side of interhaustral folds reveals more polyps than when the same area is examined in forward mode with the standard colonoscope. The increase in yield for retrograde colon examination for both polyps and adenomas is more than 10% and may be as high as 25%. The high numbers of missed lesions have implications for the recent reports stating that colonoscopy may not be as protective against right colon cancer. This decreased protection may be caused by the forward-viewing colonoscopy failing to detect polyps that are on the proximal side of folds, which is a problem that could be corrected when using a retroview to examine the colon.

SUPPLEMENTARY DATA

Supplementary data related to this article can be found at http://dx.doi.org/10.1016/j.gtc.2013.05.013.

REFERENCES

1. Saad A, Rex DK. Routine rectal retroflexion during colonoscopy has a low yield for neoplasia. World J Gastroenterol 2008;14:6503–5.
2. Cutler AF, Pop A. Fifteen years later: colonoscopic retroflexion revisited. Am J Gastroenterol 1999;94:1537–8.
3. Varadarajulu S, Ramsey WH. Utility of retroflexion in lower gastrointestinal endoscopy. J Clin Gastroenterol 2001;32:235–7.
4. García-Cano J, Jimeno-Ayllón C, Martínez-Fernández R, et al. Importance of retroflexion in the rectum during colonoscopy. Rev Esp Enferm Dig 2010;102:553–4.
5. Poon KK, Mills S, Booth IW, et al. Inflammatory cloacogenic polyp: an unrecognized cause of hematochezia and tenesmus in childhood. J Pediatr 1997;130: 327–9.
6. Coumaros D, Tsesmeli N. Retroflexion-assisted EMR in the colon with immediate closure of a procedure-related perforation. Gastrointest Endosc 2010;72:1332–3.
7. Tribonias G, Konstantinidis K, Theodoropoulou A, et al. Rectal perforation caused by colonoscopic retroflexion. Gastrointest Endosc 2010;71:662.
8. Katsinelos P, Kountouras J, Chatzimavroudis G, et al. Endoscopic closure of a large iatrogenic rectal perforation using endoloop/clips technique. Acta Gastroenterol Belg 2009;72:357–9.
9. Bechtold ML, Hammad HT, Arif M, et al. Perforation upon retroflexion: an endoscopic complication and repair. Endoscopy 2009;41:E155–6.
10. Quallick MR, Brown WR. Rectal perforation during colonoscopic retroflexion: a large, prospective experience in an academic center. Gastrointest Endosc 2009;69:960–3.
11. Ahlawat SK, Charabaty A, Benjamin S. Rectal perforation caused by retroflexion maneuver during colonoscopy: closure with endoscopic clips. Gastrointest Endosc 2008;67:771–3.

12. Fu K, Ikematsu H, Sugito M, et al. Iatrogenic perforation of the colon following retroflexion maneuver. Endoscopy 2007;39:E175.

13. Nakao SK, Fassler S, Sucandy I, et al. Colorectal cancer following negative colonoscopy: is 5-year screening the correct interval to recommend? Surg Endosc 2013;27(3):768–73.

14. Singh H, Nugent Z, Mahmud SM, et al. Predictors of colorectal cancer after negative colonoscopy: a population-based study. Am J Gastroenterol 2010;105:663–73.

15. Bressler B, Paszat LF, Chen Z, et al. Rates of new or missed colorectal cancers after colonoscopy and their risk factors: a population-based analysis. Gastroenterology 2007;132:96–102.

16. Hewett DG, Rex DK. Miss rate of right-sided colon examination during colonoscopy defined by retroflexion: an observational study. Gastrointest Endosc 2011;74:246–52.

17. Kessler WR, Rex DK. Impact of bending section length on insertion and retroflexion properties of pediatric and adult colonoscopes. Am J Gastroenterol 2005;100:1290–5.

18. Harrison M, Singh N, Rex DK. Impact of proximal colon retroflexion on adenoma miss rates. Am J Gastroenterol 2004;99:519–22.

19. Hurlstone DP, Sanders DS, Thomson M, et al. "Salvage" endoscopic mucosal resection in the colon using a retroflexion gastroscope dissection technique: a prospective analysis. Endoscopy 2006;38:902–6.

20. Rex DK, Khashab M. Colonoscopic polypectomy in retroflexion. Gastrointest Endosc 2006;63:144–8.

21. Pishvaian AC, Al-Kawas FH. Retroflexion in the colon: a useful and safe technique in the evaluation and resection of sessile polyps during colonoscopy. Am J Gastroenterol 2006;101:1479–83.

22. Hixson LJ, Fennerty MB, Sampliner RE, et al. Prospective blinded trial of the colonoscopic miss-rate of large colorectal polyps. Gastrointest Endosc 1991;37:125–7.

23. Rex DK, Cutler CS, Lemmel GT, et al. Colonoscopic miss rates of adenomas determined by back-to-back colonoscopies. Gastroenterology 1997;112:24–8.

24. Heresbach D, Barrioz T, Ponchon T. Miss rate for colorectal neoplastic polyps: a prospective multicenter study of back-to-back video colonoscopies. Endoscopy 2008;40:284–90.

25. Ahn SB, Han DS, Bae JH, et al. The miss rate for colorectal adenoma determined by quality-adjusted, back-to-back colonoscopies. Gut Liver 2012;6:64–70.

26. Bensen S, Mott LA, Dain B, et al. The colonoscopic miss rate and true one-year recurrence of colorectal neoplastic polyps. Polyp Prevention Study Group. Am J Gastroenterol 1999;94:194–9.

27. Soetikno RM, Kaltenbach T, Rouse RV, et al. Prevalence of nonpolypoid (flat and depressed) colorectal neoplasms in asymptomatic and symptomatic adults. JAMA 2008;299:1027–35.

28. Pickhardt PJ, Nugent PA, Mysliwiec PA, et al. Location of adenomas missed by optical colonoscopy. Ann Intern Med 2004;141:352–9.

29. Pickhardt PJ, Taylor AJ, Gopal DV. Surface visualization at 3D endoluminal CT colonography: degree of coverage and implications for polyp detection. Gastroenterology 2006;130:1582–7.

30. East JE, Saunders BP, Burling D, et al. Surface visualization at CT colonography simulated colonoscopy: effect of varying field of view and retrograde view. Am J Gastroenterol 2007;102:2529–35.

31. Triadafilopoulos G, Li J. A pilot study to assess the safety and efficacy of the Third Eye retrograde auxiliary imaging system during colonoscopy. Endoscopy 2008; 40:478–82.
32. Triadafilopoulos G, Watts HD, Van Dam J. A novel retrograde-viewing auxiliary imaging device (Third Eye Retroscope) improves the detection of simulated polyps in anatomic models of the colon. Gastrointest Endosc 2007;65:139–44.
33. Waye JD, Heigh RI, Fleischer DE, et al. A retrograde-viewing device improves detection of adenomas in the colon: a prospective efficacy evaluation (with videos). Gastrointest Endosc 2010;71:551–6.
34. U.S. Preventive Services Task Force. Screening for colorectal cancer: U.S. Preventive Services Task Force recommendation statement. Ann Intern Med 2008; 149:627–37.
35. Rex DK, Johnson DA, Anderson JC, et al, American College of Gastroenterology. American College of Gastroenterology guidelines for colorectal cancer screening 2009. Am J Gastroenterol 2009;104:739–50.
36. Davila RE, Rajan E, Baron TH, et al, Standards of Practice Committee, American Society for Gastrointestinal Endoscopy. ASGE guideline: colorectal cancer screening and surveillance. Gastrointest Endosc 2006;63:546–57.
37. Levin B, Lieberman DA, McFarland B, et al, American Cancer Society Colorectal Cancer Advisory Group, US Multi-Society Task Force, American College of Radiology Colon Cancer Committee. Screening and surveillance for the early detection of colorectal cancer and adenomatous polyps, 2008: a joint guideline from the American Cancer Society, the US Multi-Society Task Force on Colorectal Cancer, and the American College of Radiology. Gastroenterology 2008;134: 1570–95.
38. DeMarco DC, Odstrcil E, Lara LF, et al. Impact of experience with a retrograde-viewing device on adenoma detection rates and withdrawal times during colonoscopy: the Third Eye Retroscope study group. Gastrointest Endosc 2010;71: 542–50.
39. Leufkens AM, DeMarco DC, Rastogi A, et al, Third Eye Retroscope Randomized Clinical Evaluation [TERRACE] Study Group. Effect of a retrograde-viewing device on adenoma detection rate during colonoscopy: the TERRACE study. Gastrointest Endosc 2011;73:480–9.
40. Siersema PD, Rastogi A, Leufkens AM, et al. Retrograde-viewing device improves adenoma detection rate in colonoscopies for surveillance and diagnostic workup. World J Gastroenterol 2012;18:3400.

Water-aided Colonoscopy

Felix W. Leung, MD[a,b,]*

KEYWORDS

- Colonoscopy • Water-aided method • Discomfort • Pain • Adenoma detection rate
- Water immersion • Water exchange

KEY POINTS

- Water immersion and water exchange are characterized by removal of the infused water predominantly during withdrawal and insertion, respectively.
- Randomized controlled trial data suggest that water exchange may be superior to water immersion in minimizing insertion pain and optimizing adenoma detection, particularly in the proximal colon.
- Although simple, the novel techniques of water exchange require practice to master all of the maneuvers.

INTRODUCTION

Water-aided methods for colonoscopy have received renewed attention in the literature in recent years. There are 2 major categories, namely water immersion and water exchange. Water immersion was described in the English-language literature in 1984 as an adjunct to air insufflation to aid insertion.[1] The method was characterized by suction removal of the infused water during the withdrawal phase of colonoscopy. Water exchange is a recent modification of water immersion, first reported in 2007.[2] Water exchange is advocated currently as the sole modality to use air exclusion to aid insertion and is characterized by suction removal of the infused water, predominantly during the insertion phase of colonoscopy. The water method studies that did not show an advantage for water compared with air used primarily water immersion rather than water exchange.[3,4] The current article is intended to clarify these nuances by providing a description of the two major water-aided methods. Reference is made to studies other than randomized controlled trials (RCTs) to provide a

The study is supported in part by Veterans Affairs Medical Research Funds at Veterans Affairs Greater Los Angeles Healthcare System and an American College of Gastroenterology Clinical Research Award (FWL).

[a] Division of Gastroenterology, Department of Medicine, Sepulveda Ambulatory Care Center, Veterans Affairs Greater Los Angeles Healthcare System, 111G, 16111 Plummer Street, North Hill, CA 91343, USA; [b] David Geffen School of Medicine at UCLA, 10833 Le Conte Avenue, Los Angeles, CA 90095, USA
* Corresponding author. Division of Gastroenterology, Department of Medicine, Sepulveda Ambulatory Care Center, Veterans Affairs Greater Los Angeles Healthcare System, 111G, 16111 Plummer Street, North Hills, CA 91343.
E-mail address: felix.leung@va.gov

Gastroenterol Clin N Am 42 (2013) 507–519
http://dx.doi.org/10.1016/j.gtc.2013.05.006
0889-8553/13/$ – see front matter Published by Elsevier Inc.

gastro.theclinics.com

historical perspective. A comparison of recent RCTs of water-aided methods and traditional air insufflations is presented to support the possibility that one approach (water exchange) may be superior to the other (water immersion) in minimizing pain and optimizing adenoma detection. The comparative data call for further head-to-head RCTs to assess air insufflations, water immersion, and water exchange.

HISTORICAL PERSPECTIVE

Pioneer colonoscopists used air insufflations to distend the colonic lumen in unsedated patients. Despite traditional maneuvers of loop reduction, patient position change, and abdominal compression to minimize pain, these early colonoscopic examinations were associated with unavoidable discomfort. Sedation was introduced to increase patient tolerance and soon became the standard of practice in the United States and elsewhere. Cleaning of the mucosal surface for inspection involved boluses of water injected by a syringe through the biopsy channel. In 1984, water immersion was described as an adjunct to conventional air insufflations to facilitate passage through the sigmoid colon affected by severe diverticulosis.[1] Water immersion was reported to speed up passage through the left colon.[5] Use of warm water to counter spasm was described as simple, inexpensive, and effective.[6] Water immersion is characterized by removal of the infused water predominantly during the withdrawal phase of the colonoscopy.

In 2002, a nursing shortage curtailed the ability to routinely offer conscious sedation for colonoscopy at the author's institution. After a search of the literature, unsedated colonoscopy was offered to restore local access.[7] When the pros and cons of sedation versus no sedation were presented, about 30% of veterans accepted the scheduled unsedated option, primarily because of lack of escorts.[7,8] Using the same method as was used in sedated patients, the success rate of cecal intubation was only about 80%,[7–10] but comparable with the best reports on unsedated colonoscopy of the time.[11]

The limiting factor during insertion was pain brought on by lengthening of the colon caused by the insufflated air needed to expand the lumen for visualization, preventing cecal intubation in ~20% of the unsedated patients.[7–10] To complete the failed cases without sedation, the first clinical research question was whether cecal intubation could be accomplished without the use of air insufflations. Of all the modalities for reducing colonoscopy discomfort,[12] water immersion as an adjunct to conventional air insufflations seemed to be the most promising.[13] Subsequent work focused on whether cecal intubation with water infusion in lieu of air insufflations (water exchange) could be accomplished.[2,10] The results of a series of observational studies[2,10,14] and RCTs[15–17] confirmed the feasibility of water exchange to aid insertion and accomplish cecal intubation.

METHODOLOGICAL DETAILS OF WATER-AIDED METHODS

Water immersion used as an adjunct to conventional air insufflations does not require the acquisition of new skills or the use of new maneuvers. It entails distention of the colon by water that is removed predominantly during withdrawal,[1,5,6] but the method has varied in the literature. The water is infused by syringe or water pump through the biopsy channel. One RCT reported less colonic spasm by the use of warm-to-touch water[6]; however, a recent RCT showed no difference between warm water (35°–38°C) and cool water (20°–23°C) with regard to sedation requirement, pain or satisfaction scores, or cecal intubation times.[18] Other descriptions permitted insufflation of puffs of air as needed[4] or when water immersion was deemed a failure based on intention to treat.[3] Some studies using water immersion also described complete exclusion of air.[19–21]

Water exchange was modified from water immersion specifically to develop the least painful method[10,16] for use in scheduled, unsedated patients in the United States.[7–10] Water exchange involved complete exclusion of air (no air insufflations and suction of all residual air in the colonic lumen). Infusion of an unrestricted volume of water coupled with removal of residual feces to clear the view is used to identify the lumen during insertion. It requires acquisition of a new set of skills, and practice is necessary to master the maneuvers.[22,23] Unique to the approach is the following maneuver to distinguish water exchange from water immersion: the infused water is removed predominantly during insertion.[10,17,22,23] A detailed description of the pearls and pitfalls of water exchange is provided in **Box 1**.

RCTS COMPARING CONVENTIONAL AIR INSUFFLATIONS WITH WATER IMMERSION OR WATER EXCHANGE: IMPACT ON PAIN

The data from RCTs comparing traditional air insufflations with water immersion or water exchange from 2008 to 2011 were summarized in a recent systematic qualitative review.[24] In the current article, the data from 3 additional RCTs published in 2012[25–27] are added. The mean (standard deviation [SD]) or median (interquartile range [IQR]) pain score in the air insufflations and water-aided method groups are shown in **Table 1**. The reductions in mean or median pain scores of the water-aided method groups are presented as percentages of the air insufflation groups (see **Table 1**). The overall reduction of pain scores was qualitatively greater with water exchange compared with water immersion in patients not given full sedation (see **Table 1**).

Water immersion is difficult to perform if the colon is not prepared well.[21] Suctioning dirty water and replacing it with clean water during insertion is time consuming.[3] Water exchange evolved from water immersion to manage residual feces in the colonic lumen, which requires time but is also effective in providing salvage cleansing in patients prepared with non–split-dose[16] and split-dose[28] bowel regimens. The prolonged insertion time of the water exchange method in scheduled, unsedated patients[9] was deemed a major limitation to its widespread application[29]; in addition, the time needed to learn the necessary maneuvers makes it impractical when only 30 minutes or less are allotted for each colonoscopy in a typical clinical practice. However, the feasibility of water exchange in situations other than scheduled, unsedated patients is suggested by mean insertion times ranging from 5 to 13 minutes in these alternative settings, as summarized in a recent systematic qualitative review.[24] Overall, the data in **Table 1** show that, compared with traditional air insufflations, pain during colonoscopy is reduced by both water immersion and exchange. The reduction in pain scores was qualitatively smaller with water immersion compared with water exchange.[24,30] In settings in which full sedation is practiced, the pain reduction provided by water-aided methods is likely to be of less importance than in settings in which unsedated, on-demand sedation, or minimally sedated colonoscopy, is practiced.

RCTS COMPARING CONVENTIONAL AIR INSUFFLATIONS WITH WATER IMMERSION OR WATER EXCHANGE: IMPACT ON ADENOMA DETECTION

A recent systematic qualitative review assessed the impact of water-aided methods on adenoma detection rate (ADR).[24] **Tables 2** and **3** summarize the ADR in the air insufflations and water-aided method groups. With water immersion, the effect on ADR is inconsistent. With water exchange, there is a trend toward higher ADR. Compared

Box 1
Pearls and pitfalls (italicized) of water exchange method

1. The air and water pump on the colonoscope and the accessory water pump used to deliver water for water exchange are checked to confirm proper function.

2. The air pump is turned off to avoid inadvertent air insufflations, which can elongate the colon.

3. On insertion of the colonoscope through the anus, the location of the lumen is noted. All residual air is removed. Point the suction port at the tip of the colonoscope (located at the 5 o'clock position) into the air pocket. Apply suction to collapse the lumen (the steps are repeated in the rectal sigmoid junction, splenic flexure, hepatic flexure and cecum, and redundant segments to decrease angulations and minimize loop formation).

4. The tip of the colonoscope is directed to abut the slitlike opening ahead or where the folds converge (**Fig. 1**A). Water is infused to confirm that the lumen opens (see **Fig. 1**B). *The farther the tip is to the target the less effective the infused water will be in opening the lumen ahead.*

5. If there is no obvious opening ahead, move the tip of the colonoscope systemically in a 360° fashion while simultaneously infusing and suctioning water to clear the residual fecal debris.

6. Only a sufficient amount of water is infused to confirm that the lumen ahead opens to allow passage of the colonoscope. Water infusion is stopped if the lumen does not open. The tip of the colonoscope is pulled back from the mucosa, redirected, and the process is repeated.

7. Suction of the mucosa is avoided by adjusting the level of wall suction, and by initiating water infusion just before pressing the suction button. The suction port is pointed toward the center of the lumen, away from the mucosa on the right side, which translates into seeing more mucosa on the left side and upper portion of the monitor screen (see **Fig. 1**C).

8. Be patient if bowel preparation is suboptimal. Remove the suspended residual feces and infuse clean water for visualization of the lumen. If the colonoscope is equipped with a single working channel, the maneuvers are done in rapid sequence. If the colonoscope is equipped with 1 working and 1 accessory channel, the maneuvers can be done simultaneously. The process seems to take time during insertion. The paradox is that it is easier to clean the mucosa in a collapsed water-filled colon during insertion with water exchange than in a distended air-filled colon during withdrawal with the water jet followed by suction.

9. *It is important not to forget to remove the infused water by suction when the insertion is going smoothly. Failure to do so results in a water-distended colon. The distention caused by water increases discomfort for the patient and predisposes to loop formation. If the appearance of the lumen ahead is round rather than slitlike and narrowed, there is likely to be too much water in the colon., which is the signal to perform more suction than infusion.*

10. Recognition of the underwater appearance of diverticular openings is critical to avoid mistaking it for a true lumen and inappropriate infusion of excess water into the diverticulum.

11. Cecal intubation is suggested by finding characteristic red suction marks (**Fig. 2**A) after attempts to further advance the colonoscope fails, or intubation of the terminal ileum (see **Fig. 2**B), or observing the ileocecal valve facing the tip of the colonoscope (see **Fig. 2**C), and confirmed by observing the appendix opening under water (**Fig. 3**). Remove as much of the infused water in the cecum as possible before insufflating air to initiate the withdrawal phase.

12. Other integral components of the water exchange method include colonoscope-shortening maneuver, abdominal compression, and change of patient position. These maneuvers may be needed less often than when air insufflation is used but they are needed for the same reason (eg, lumen ahead cannot be seen, paradoxic movement occurs) to assist advancement.

Adapted from Refs.[22,23,48–50]

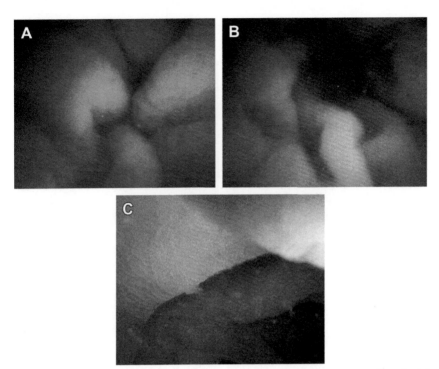

Fig. 1. (*A*) Slitlike appearance of the colonic lumen. (*B*) Water is infuse to confirm that the lumen opens. (*C*) Suction port positioned in the center of the colonic lumen (more mucosa is seen on the left side and upper portion of the monitor screen).

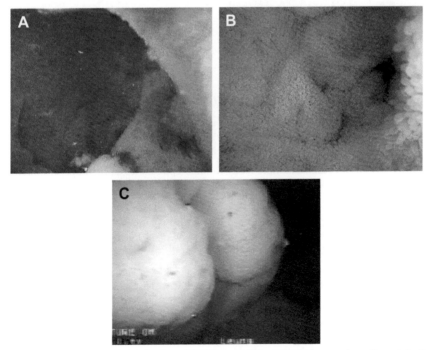

Fig. 2. Indication of cecal intubation. (*A*) Characteristic red suction marks adjacent to the appendix opening. (*B*) Water-filled terminal ileum. (*C*) Ileocecal valve facing the tip of the colonoscope.

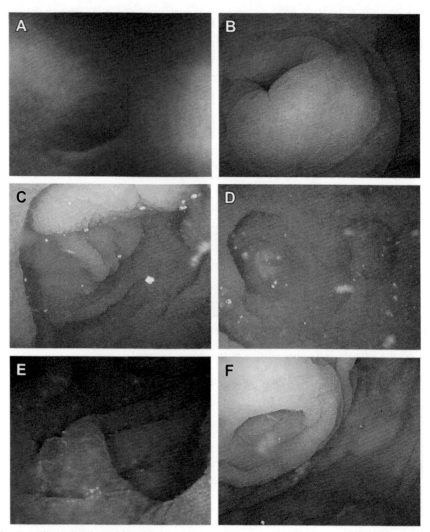

Fig. 3. Indication of cecal intubation. (A–L) Variable appearance of the appendix opening under water in different patients.

with air insufflations, no increase in ADR was shown for water immersion, but an increase was observed with water exchange, especially for diminutive adenomas in the proximal colon.[24,31]

IMPLICATIONS OF INCREASE IN ADR BY WATER EXCHANGE

Recent studies have raised concerns that colonoscopy may not be as effective in protecting against right-sided colon cancer as against left-sided colon cancer. An independent predictor of risk of interval colorectal cancer after screening colonoscopy is ADR but not cecal intubation rate.[32] These reports suggest that maneuvers that enhance detection of proximal lesions with malignant potential are needed to improve the quality and outcome of screening colonoscopy.

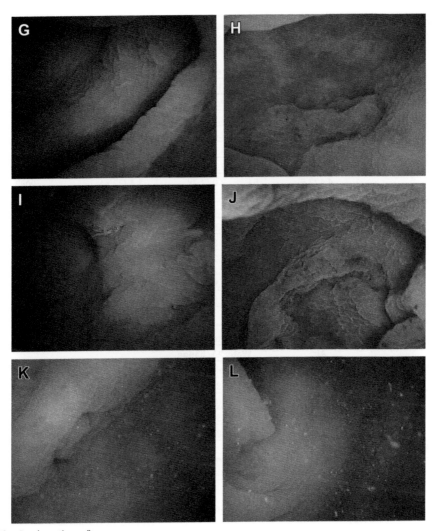

Fig. 3. (*continued*)

Water exchange was used in some but not in all of the RCTs of water-aided methods identified to date. A unique opportunity to determine whether water exchange has an impact on ADR is made possible by comparing the outcome of these studies summarized in a recent review.[24] Infusion and suction removal of water either in rapid sequence (single working channel) or simultaneously (dual working channels) during insertion creates turbulence in the vicinity of the tip of the colonoscope. The turbulence facilitates suspension of the residual feces adherent to the mucosal surface into the luminal water for suction removal. Water exchange in the collapsed colon during insertion is a more efficient maneuver to provide salvage cleansing of the mucosa compared with washing of the dirty mucosal surface with jets of water covering a small surface area in an air-filled lumen during withdrawal. The usefulness of the water exchange method rests with permitting visualization of the lumen for advancement of the colonoscope while maintaining minimal distention, and limiting discomfort even in the absence of sedation. The salvage cleansing effect of the water exchange method is

Table 1
RCT comparing air insufflations versus water immersion or water exchange: outcome related to reduction in pain score during colonoscopy

(A) Water Immersion: Removal of Infused Water Occurred Predominantly During Withdrawal

References	N	Air Pain Score	N	Water Immersion Pain Score	Pain Score Reduction	P
41,a,b	170	4.6 (1.8–9.2)[c]	170	2.9 (1.0–5.8)[c]	−1.7[d] (37%)	.001[e]
42,a,d	39	2.6 (2.2)	41	2.4 (2.2)[f]	−0.2 (7.7%)	.894
43,g,d	114	5.3 (2.7)	112	4.1 (2.7)	−1.2 (23%)	.001[h]
44,g,d	89	3.4 (2.8)	90	2.5 (2.5)	−0.9 (26%)	.021[h]
45,g,d	51	4.4 (2.6)	51	3.0 (2.2)[i]	−1.4 (32%)	.004[h]
			51	3.3 (2.4)[j]	−1.1 (25%)	.028[h]
4,k,b	114	3.9 (1.4–5.4)[c]	116	2.8 (1.2–4.4)[c]	−1.1[d] (28%)	.001[e]
46,g	31	5.5 (NR)	31	3.6 (NR)	−1.9 (35%)	<.05[h]
3,k	58	4.2 (2.3)	58	2.8 (1.9)	−1.3 (31%)	.01[l]
25,a	53	1.0 (2.0)	55	1.2 (2.5)[m]	+0.2 (−2%)	.920
			51	1.2 (2.5)[n]	+0.2 (−2%)	
			48	0.9 (1.9)[o]	−0.1 (1%)	
26,g	97	0 (0.24)	85	0 (0.22)	0 (0%)	NS
Average					19%	—

(B) Water Exchange: Removal of Infused Water Occurred Predominantly During Insertion

References	N	Air Pain Score	N	Water Exchange Pain Score	Pain Score Reduction	P
15,g,d	28	4.1 (3.4)	28	1.3 (1.8)	−2.8 (68%)	.0002[h]
16,a,b	40	6 (NR)	42	3 (NR)	−3 (50%)	.002[h]
17,k,d	50	4.9 (2.0)	50	2.3 (1.7)	−2.6 (53%)	.0012[h]
27,p	12	1.8 (0.8)	11	1.8 (1.0)	0 (0%)	NS
Average					43%	—

Abbreviations: NS, not significant; NR, not reported.
 [a] Unsedated.
 [b] Median score (interquartile range).
 [c] Converted from 0 to 100 scale to 0 to 10 scale for comparability of pain measures.
 [d] Mean score (SD).
 [e] Rank sum.
 [f] Converted from 0 to 5 scale (visual analogue scale) to 0 to 10 scale for comparability of pain measures.
 [g] Minimal sedation for premedication.
 [h] t-Test.
 [i] Limited-volume water infusion in the rectosigmoid colon only.
 [j] Large-volume water infusion throughout the colon during insertion.
 [k] On-demand sedation.
 [l] Mann-Whitney U.
 [m] 100 mL, room temperature.
 [n] 300 mL, room temperature.
 [o] 300 mL, warm.
 [p] Full sedation.

Table 2
Effect of water immersion or water exchange on overall ADR

	Overall ADR				Good to Excellent Bowel Prep (%)	
	Air	Water				
References	n/N (%)	n/N (%)	Difference (%)[a]	P[b]	Air	Water
Water Immersion						
43	44/114 (38.5)	47/112 (41.9)	3.4	NS	80	80
44	31/89 (34.8)	32/90 (35.6.)	0.8	NS	NR	
45	13/51 (25.5)	15/51 (29.4)	3.9	NS	69	63
4	46/114 (40.4)	29/116 (25.0)	−15.4	.013	95	94
46	10/31 (32.3)	9/31 (29.0)	−3.3	NS	NR	
3	15/58 (25.9)	19/58 (32.8)	6.9	NS	NR	
26	22/85 (25.9)	33/97 (34)	8.1	.334	74.2	78
Combined	181/542 (33.4)	184/555 (33.2)	—	NS	—	
Water Exchange						
16	9/40 (23)	15/42 (36)	13.2	NS	NR	
17	18/50 (36)	20/50 (40)	4.0	NS	NR	
47	88/191 (46)	101/177 (57)	10.9	.037	93	93
27	2/12 (17)	6/11 (55)	38	.057	NR	
Combined	117/293 (39.9)	142/280 (50.7)	—	.017	—	

Abbreviations: n, number of patients with adenoma; N, total number of patients in group.
[a] The difference between the water immersion and the water exchange group was significant (P<.05, rank sum test).
[b] Fisher exact test.

serendipitous, applicable to sedated patients as well (even though the maneuvers of water exchange were not initially intended for use with sedation) and is a plausible contributing factor to an enhanced examination. In addition, by performing water administration and suctioning during insertion, the endoscopist spends less time on

Table 3
Effect of water exchange on ADR in the proximal colon

	Air	Water		
References	n/N (ADR)	n/N (ADR)	Difference (%)	P[a]
Effect on Overall ADR in the Proximal Colon				
16	3/40 (7.5%)	7/42 (16.7%)	9.2	NS
17	12/50 (24.0%)	20/50 (40.0%)	16.0	NS
47	67/191 (35.1%)	81/177 (45.8%)	10.7	.043
Combined	82/281 (29.2%)	108/269 (40.1%)	—	.007
Effect on <10 mm ADR in the Proximal Colon				
16	3/40 (7.5%)	7/42 (16.7%)	9.2	NS
17	10/50 (20.0%)	19/50 (38.0%)	18.0	NS
47	59/191 (30.9%)	74/177 (41.8%)	10.9	.031
Combined	72/281 (25.6%)	100/269 (37.2%)	—	.004

The proximal colon refers to the segments proximal to the splenic flexure.
[a] Fisher exact test.

mucosal cleaning during withdrawal and potentially more time on inspection, which may contribute to the increased ADR in the proximal colon reported with water exchange (see **Table 3**). Additional studies in multiple settings and by different operators are required to confirm these observations.

Two recent meta-analyses[33,34] combined all the water-aided methods as water infusion colonoscopy and concluded that pain was reduced significantly compared with air insufflations, but adenoma detection was not enhanced. However, given the differences between water immersion and water exchange, future systematic reviews and meta-analyses should distinguish between the two modalities with regard to the outcome of adenoma detection.

RECENT DEVELOPMENTS

Several observational studies provide new insights into water-aided methods. With regard to the mechanism of pain reduction, magnetic endoscope imaging shows that significantly fewer loops are documented in the water exchange group compared with the air insufflations group.[35] A combination of indigo carmine with water exchange[36] and a combination of cap-assisted colonoscopy with water exchange[37] have both shown promise in significantly enhancing adenoma detection. Direct coaching is a feasible method for transfer of expertise of water exchange to experienced colonoscopists.[38]

SUMMARY

Both water immersion and water exchange attenuate patient discomfort during colonoscopy. Water immersion is easier to adopt because no additional skills are necessary when used as an adjunct to air insufflation. The pain reduction seems to be qualitatively larger with water exchange than with water immersion. The pain-alleviating effect of water-aided methods is likely to be less important in settings in which full sedation is routine than in settings in which unsedated, on-demand, or minimal-sedation colonoscopy is widely accepted. Water immersion does not seem to increase adenoma detection. In contrast, the observation that water exchange may increase ADR, especially in the proximal colon, is noteworthy and requires additional study for confirmation.[24,31,39] The increased yield is primarily for small and diminutive adenomas; however, a recent study revealed that polyps with features of high-grade dysplasia, adenocarcinoma, or advanced neoplasia were significantly smaller in the right versus left colon.[40] The hypothesis that the water exchange method may provide a strategy to improve prevention of right-sided colorectal cancer by improving detection of right-sided small, advanced polyps in screening colonoscopy is intriguing. A comparison of air insufflations, water immersion, and water exchange in a well-designed and adequately powered RCT of average-risk screening patients undergoing colonoscopy deserves to be considered. Such an RCT would help answer unresolved questions and determine the future role of water-aided colonoscopy.

REFERENCES

1. Falchuk ZM, Griffin PH. A technique to facilitate colonoscopy in areas of severe diverticular disease [letter]. N Engl J Med 1984;310:598.
2. Leung JW, Mann S, Leung FW. Option for screening colonoscopy without sedation – a pilot study in United States veterans. Aliment Pharmacol Ther 2007;26: 627–31.

3. Pohl J, Messer I, Behrens A, et al. Water infusion for cecal intubation increases patient tolerance, but does not improve intubation of unsedated colonoscopies. Clin Gastroenterol Hepatol 2011;9:1039–43.
4. Radaelli F, Paggi S, Amato A, et al. Warm water infusion versus air insufflation for unsedated colonoscopy: a randomized, controlled trial. Gastrointest Endosc 2010;72:701–9.
5. Baumann UA. Water intubation of the sigmoid colon: water instillation speeds up left-sided colonoscopy. Endoscopy 1999;31:314–7.
6. Church JM. Warm water irrigation for dealing with spasm during colonoscopy: simple, inexpensive, and effective. Gastrointest Endosc 2002;56:672–4.
7. Leung FW. Unsedated colonoscopy introduced as a routine option to ensure access is acceptable to a subgroup of US veterans. Dig Dis Sci 2008;53:2719–22.
8. Leung FW. Promoting informed choice of unsedated colonoscopy - patient-centered care for a subgroup of U.S. veterans. Dig Dis Sci 2008;53:2955–9.
9. Leung FW, Aharonian HS, Guth PH, et al. Involvement of trainees in routine unsedated colonoscopy - review of pilot experience. Gastrointest Endosc 2008;67:718–22.
10. Leung FW, Aharonian HS, Leung JW, et al. Impact of a novel water method on scheduled unsedated colonoscopy in U.S. veterans. Gastrointest Endosc 2009;69:546–50.
11. Thiis-Evensen E, Hoff GS, Sauar J, et al. Patient tolerance of colonoscopy without sedation during screening examination for colorectal polyps. Gastrointest Endosc 2000;52(2):606–10.
12. Leung FW. Methods of reducing discomfort during colonoscopy. Dig Dis Sci 2008;53:1462–7.
13. Leung FW. Water-related method for performance of colonoscopy. Dig Dis Sci 2008;53:2847–50.
14. Leung JW, Siao-Salera R, Toomsen L, et al. A pilot feasibility study of the method of water infusion without air insufflation in sedated colonoscopy. Dig Dis Sci 2009;54:1997–2001.
15. Leung JW, Mann SK, Siao-Salera R, et al. A randomized, controlled comparison of warm water infusion in lieu of air insufflation versus air insufflation for aiding colonoscopy insertion in sedated patients undergoing colorectal cancer screening and surveillance. Gastrointest Endosc 2009;70:505–10.
16. Leung FW, Harker JO, Jackson G, et al. A proof-of-principle, prospective, randomized controlled trial (RCT) demonstrating improved outcomes in scheduled unsedated colonoscopy by the water method. Gastrointest Endosc 2010;72:693–700.
17. Leung JW, Mann SK, Siao-Salera R, et al. A proof-of-concept RCT to confirm the beneficial effects of the water method on US veterans undergoing colonoscopy with the option of on demand sedation. Gastrointest Endosc 2011;73:103–10.
18. Lee BY, Katon R, Herzig D, et al. Warm water infusion during sedated colonoscopy does not decrease amount of sedation medication used. Gastrointest Endosc 2012;76:1182–7.
19. Vemulapalli KC, Rex DK. Water immersion simplifies cecal intubation in patients with redundant colons and previous incomplete colonoscopies. Gastrointest Endosc 2012;76:812–7.
20. Mizukami T, Yokoyama A, Imaeda H, et al. Collapse-submergence method: simple colonoscopic technique combining water infusion with complete air removal from the rectosigmoid colon. Dig Endosc 2007;19:43–8.

21. Friedland S. The water immersion technique for colonoscopy insertion. Gastroenterol Hepatol 2010;6:555–6.

22. Leung FW, Leung JW, Mann SK, et al. The water method significantly enhances patient-centered outcomes in sedated and unsedated colonoscopy. Endoscopy 2011;43:816–21.

23. Leung FW. Water exchange may be superior to water immersion for colonoscopy [editorial]. Clin Gastroenterol Hepatol 2011;9:1012–4.

24. Leung FW, Amato A, Ell C, et al. Water-aided colonoscopy: a systematic review. Gastrointest Endosc 2012;76:657–66.

25. Ryu KH, Huh KC, Kang YW, et al. An effective instillation method for water-assisted colonoscopy as performed by in-training endoscopists in terms of volume and temperature. Dig Dis Sci 2012;57:142–7.

26. Falt P, Liberda M, Smajstrla V, et al. Combination of water immersion and carbon dioxide insufflation for minimal sedation colonoscopy: a prospective, randomized, single-center trial. Eur J Gastroenterol Hepatol 2012;24:971–7.

27. Portocarrero DJ, Che K, Olafsson S, et al. A pilot study to assess feasibility of the water method to aid colonoscope insertion in community settings in the United States. J Interv Gastroenterol 2012;2:20–2.

28. Fischer LS, Lumsden A, Leung FW. Water exchange method for colonoscopy: learning curve of an experienced colonoscopist in a U.S. community practice setting. J Interv Gastroenterol 2012;2(3):136–40.

29. Wasan SK, Schroy PC. Water-assisted unsedated colonoscopy: does the end justify the means? Gastrointest Endosc 2009;69:551–3.

30. Leung FW, Harker JO, Leung JW, et al. Removal of infused water predominantly during insertion (water exchange) is consistently associated with a greater reduction of pain score – review of randomized controlled trials (RCTs) of water method colonoscopy. J Interv Gastroenterol 2011;1:114–20.

31. Leung FW, Harker JO, Leung JW, et al. Removal of infused water predominantly during insertion (water exchange) is consistently associated with an increase in adenoma detection rate – review of data in randomized controlled trials (RCTs) of water-related methods. J Interv Gastroenterol 2011;1(3):121–6.

32. Kaminski MF, Regula J, Kraszewska E, et al. Quality indicators for colonoscopy and the risk of interval cancer. N Engl J Med 2010;362:1795–803.

33. Jun WU, Bing HU. Comparative effectiveness of water infusion versus air insufflation in colonoscopy: a meta-analysis. Colorectal Dis 2013;15(4):404–9. http://dx.doi.org/10.1111/j.1463-1318.2012.03194.x.

34. Rabenstein T, Radaelli F, Zolk O. Warm water infusion colonoscopy: a review and meta-analysis. Endoscopy 2012;44:940–8.

35. Leung JW, Thai A, Yen A, et al. Magnetic endoscope imaging (ScopeGuide) elucidates the mechanism of action of the pain-alleviating impact of water exchange colonoscopy - attenuation of loop formation. J Interv Gastroenterol 2013;2:150–4.

36. Leung JW, Mann SK, Siao-Salera R, et al. Indigo carmine added to the water exchange method enhances adenoma detection - a RCT. J Interv Gastroenterol 2013;2:114–9.

37. Yen AW, Leung JW, Leung FW. A new method for screening and surveillance colonoscopy: combined water-exchange and cap-assisted colonoscopy. J Interv Gastroenterol 2013;2:122–7.

38. Leung FW, Cheung R, Fan RS, et al. The water exchange method for colonoscopy - effect of coaching. J Interv Gastroenterol 2013;2:130–3.

39. Leung FW, Leung JW, Siao-Salera RM, et al. The water method significantly enhances detection of diminutive lesions (adenoma and hyperplastic polyp combined) in the proximal colon in screening colonoscopy - data derived from two RCT in US veterans. J Interv Gastroenterol 2011;1:48–52.

40. Gupta S, Balasubramanian BA, Fu T, et al. Polyps with advanced neoplasia are smaller in the right than in the left colon: implications for colorectal cancer screening. Clin Gastroenterol Hepatol 2012;10:1395–401.

41. Brocchi E, Pezzilli R, Tomassetti P, et al. Warm water or oil-assisted colonoscopy: toward simpler examinations? Am J Gastroenterol 2008;103:581–7.

42. Park SC, Keum B, Kim ES, et al. Usefulness of warm water and oil assistance in colonoscopy by trainees. Dig Dis Sci 2010;55:2940–4.

43. Leung CW, Kaltenbach T, Soetikno R, et al. Colonoscopy insertion technique using water immersion versus standard technique: a randomized trial showing promise for minimal-sedation colonoscopy. Endoscopy 2010;42:557–62.

44. Hsieh YH, Lin HJ, Tseng KC. Limited water infusion decreases pain during minimally sedated colonoscopy. World J Gastroenterol 2011;17:2236–40.

45. Hsieh YH, Tseng KC, Hsieh JJ, et al. Feasibility of colonoscopy with water infusion in minimally sedated patients in an Asian community setting. J Interv Gastroenterol 2011;1:185–90.

46. Ransibrahmanakul K, Leung JW, Mann SK, et al. Comparative effectiveness of water vs. air methods in minimal sedation colonoscopy performed by supervised trainees in the US – a RCT. Am J Clin Med 2010;7:113–8.

47. Ramirez FC, Leung FW. The water method for aiding colonoscope insertion: the learning curve of an experienced colonoscopist. J Interv Gastroenterol 2011;1:97–101.

48. Leung FW. Is there a place for sedationless colonoscopy? J Interv Gastroenterol 2011;1:19–22.

49. Leung FW. Prevalence and predictors of interval colorectal cancers – what hypotheses should colonoscopists consider in planning studies to modify the undesirable outcome. Ann Gastroenterol 2012;25:178–80.

50. Leung FW. Magnetic endoscope imaging colonoscope – a new modality for hypothesis-testing in unsedated colonoscopy. Gastrointest Endosc 2012;75:1037–9.

Chromocolonoscopy

Deepika Devuni, MBBS[a], Haleh Vaziri, MD[a],
Joseph C. Anderson, MD[a,b,c],*

KEYWORDS

- Chromocolonoscopy • Flat adenomas • Adenoma detection rate
- Kudo classification • Inflammatory bowel disease • Aberrant crypt foci

KEY POINTS

- Dye staining has been shown to be useful in detecting and differentiating polyps.
- The increased yield is primarily for small polyps with less clinical significance.
- Chromoendoscopy increases procedure time.
- It may not be recommended for routine screening and surveillance.
- The increased yield of dysplasia in inflammatory bowel disease makes it a useful adjunct for surveillance in this population.

INTRODUCTION

Colonoscopy is the preferred method for colon cancer screening as recommended by the American College of Gastroenterology.[1] However, the use of conventional colonoscopy is associated with a lower colorectal cancer (CRC) protection for proximal versus distal tumors.[1–5] The phenomena known as interval cancers are associated with low adenoma detection rates (ADRs), and may be related to nonvisualized flat or nonpolypoid lesions.[6] Multiple adjunctive techniques and technologies have been studied to improve ADRs. These include narrow band imaging, high definition, magnified endoscopy, and chromoendoscopy. In this article, we review chromoendoscopy and its role as an adjunct to colonoscopy. We also discuss the role of chromoendoscopy for the detection of dysplasia in inflammatory bowel diseases (IBDs).

Chromoendoscopy is the application of dye on the colonic surface that allows for a more detailed analysis of mucosal abnormalities. In 1977, Tada and colleagues[7] used a dye-spraying method with indigo carmine (IC) and methylene blue in the lower

The contents of this work do not represent the views of the Department of Veterans Affairs or the United States Government.
Conflict of Interest: Guarantors of the article: Joseph C. Anderson.
[a] University of Connecticut School of Medicine, 263 Farmington Avenue, Farmington, CT 06030, USA; [b] White River Junction VAMC, 215 Main Street, White River Junction, VT 05001, USA; [c] The Geisel School of Medicine at Dartmouth Medical, Hanover, NH, USA
* Corresponding author. University of Connecticut Health Center, Farmington, CT.
E-mail address: joseph.anderson@dartmouth.edu

gastrointestinal tract. They demonstrated that the dye-spraying method was useful to detect small mucosal changes. Colonoscopy with dye spraying or chromoendoscopy has since become a standard diagnostic tool for gastroenterologists.

TECHNIQUE OF CHROMOENDOSCOPY

Chromocolonoscopy involves examining colonic mucosa after it is sprayed with dye. Dye staining may also be achieved by a capsule[8] that is ingested immediately after a polyethylene glycol (PEG) lavage. However, the more widely used method involves a dye-spray catheter. Many spray catheters are commercially available for single use or multiple uses. For most procedures, the spray catheter is introduced through the working channel in the colonoscope, the dye is sprayed onto the mucosal surface of the colon in a continuous spray, and then any extra pooled dye is aspirated. Most techniques involve segmental dye spraying,[9–11] in which the colon is stained in small sections, typically 10 cm at a time.

Other techniques for dye spraying have been described. In contrast to the traditional high-volume technique, Pohl and colleagues[12] used a low-volume spraying technique. During continuous extubation of the colonoscope, 0.4% IC was applied by an assistant to achieve diffuse coverage of the mucosa. The volume of dye used with this method was smaller and the average time required for the procedure was less than reported in other studies. Other dye-application techniques are discussed in subsequent sections.

An important requirement for chromoendoscopy is good bowel preparation. Although the luminal surface is usually cleaned with water or a mucolytic agent, such as N-acetylcysteine (NAC), large amounts of stool prohibit adequate staining and mucosal visualization.

Chromoendoscopy can be performed using pan-colonic or localized techniques. Pan-colonic chromoendoscopy is usually performed to increase detection of adenomas or dysplasia in IBD.[9,12–15] Targeted dye spraying is used to delineate a lesion's margins[16] or to differentiate neoplastic from non-neoplastic lesions.

There are 3 different kinds of stains: absorptive, contrast, and reactive. The most commonly used stains are methylene blue and IC.

Absorptive Stains

Absorptive stains are taken up by specific epithelial cells and allow for better characterization of the mucosa. Methylene blue, Lugol iodine, Toluidine blue, and Cresyl violet are the most commonly used absorptive stains. The application of absorptive and contrast dyes can be very different and this is illustrated in **Fig. 1**. In **Fig. 2**, a polyp is shown before and after the application of IC.

Following are brief descriptions of commonly used stains:

Methylene blue

This stain is actively absorbed by mucosa of small intestine and colonic epithelium. Methylene blue is poorly absorbed by damaged mucosa or by nonabsorptive surfaces like squamous epithelium, areas of active inflammation, and intraepithelial neoplasia. The level of absorption correlates with the amount of cytoplasm and goblet cells present.[17] Methylene blue chromoendoscopy requires the application of a mucolytic, such as NAC, because mucus prevents active absorption of the dye. Thus, a suggested algorithm for the application of methylene blue includes[18,19] the following:

- The patient's colon is prepped with a PEG solution
- The targeted mucosa is washed with water

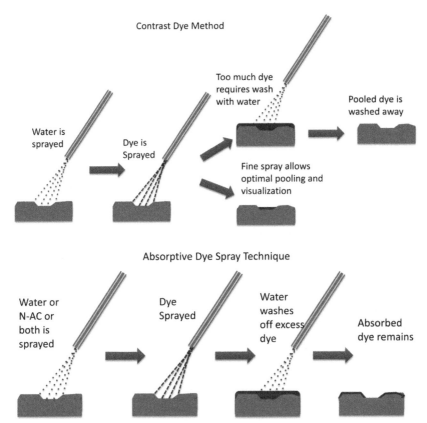

Contrast Dye Method

Too much dye
requires wash
with water

Pooled dye is
washed away

Water is
sprayed

Dye is
Sprayed

Fine spray allows
optimal pooling and
visualization

Absorptive Dye Spray Technique

Water or
N-AC or
both is
sprayed

Dye
Sprayed

Water
washes
off excess
dye

Absorbed
dye remains

Fig. 1. As compared with absorptive stains, pooling with contrast stains cannot be easily managed with water. Although the water will wash away excess stain in the former, it will wash away all of the latter dye.

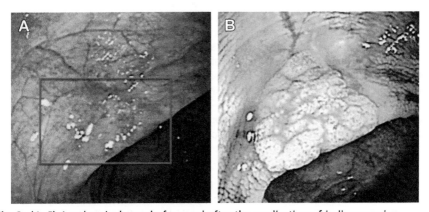

Fig. 2. (*A, B*) A polyps is shown before and after the application of indigo carmine.

- A mucolytic, such as NAC (10%–20%), is applied
- The mucosa is again washed with water
- The dye is sprayed at a concentration of less than 1%
- Excess dye is washed with water after 2 minutes of dye staining

Patients should be advised that the staining can last up to 24 hours and that they may have discolored stools. In addition, because it is an absorptive dye, they may experience discolored urine. Repici and colleagues[20] conducted an open-label trial of safety and efficacy of a methylene blue capsule in healthy volunteers. They administered 200 mg and 400 mg delayed release tablets of methylene blue in 22 healthy volunteers who had completed a PEG lavage. It was hypothesized that the tablets are better absorbed from colonic mucosa, as it is free from debris and fecal material. Peak levels of the active ingredient were seen in 16 hours. No serious adverse reactions were reported. The most common adverse event was elevated liver enzymes that returned to baseline in 15 days.

Methylene blue has some other attendant risks associated with its use as an absorptive stain. In vitro studies have demonstrated that white light and methylene blue can cause single-strand DNA breaks. Davies and colleagues[21] demonstrated that methylene blue and not IC caused DNA damage. More discussion regarding risks of methylene blue can be found in the IBD section.

Cresyl violet

Cresyl violet is as less commonly used dye that can be used in combination with IC to better delineate colonic lesions. Kudo and colleagues[22] used this agent with magnification colonoscopy to delineate pit patterns, which are discussed later in this article. Cresyl violet 0.2% is applied to the mucosa, which is previously stained with IC. This preferentially stains the pit margins and provides clear definition of each pit pattern.

Contrast Stains

Because contrast stains are not be absorbed by the mucosa, these stains pool in the mucosal grooves and crevices. This allows for better definition of colonic mucosa and neoplasms.

IC

IC is the most commonly used contrast dye for colonic staining. This stain is applied typically in concentrations that vary from 0.008% to 0.4%. Although it is usually applied with a spray catheter, Leung and colleagues[23] used a water method with IC to uniformly stain the mucosa and to prevent exclusion of patients with poor preparation. One disadvantage of contrast stains, such as IC, may be in the management of the dye pooling. In contrast to the absorptive stains, the contrast stains cannot be managed with water spray, which will wash away the stain. Thus, the dye needs to be sprayed carefully. **Fig. 1** demonstrates the difference between applying a contrast and an absorptive stain.

IC in particular is also an unstable compound and has a short half-life. Therefore it is best to prepare the dye just before application. However, one benefit is the good safety profile of this commonly used food dye. The suggested staining method for IC includes[14] the following:

- The patient's colon is prepped with a PEG solution
- Water is sprayed to clean the mucosa
- Indigo carmine is sprayed using a spray catheter in a 0.2%–0.4% concentration

- Given the mercurial pooling nature of this contrast stain, it may be prudent to find a catheter that atomizes well
- Another option is to use a stopcock with 2 syringes: one for dye to prime the catheter and one 60 mL with air to spray the dye

CHROMOENDOSCOPY FOR POLYP MORPHOLOGY

Multiple studies have examined the utility of chromoendoscopy in detection of adenomas during screening and surveillance colonoscopy. Selected trials are shown in **Table 1**. Many of these have been single-arm chromoendoscopy studies.[16,24–27] These trials demonstrated an increase in flat and small adenomas, many of which were often proximal.[26]

A review on chromocolonoscopy and adenoma detection requires a brief review of polyp morphology. Polyps can be classified as protruding or nonprotruding. One classification is the Japanese Research Society Classification (JRSC), which defines flat lesions as those with a height that is less than one-half the measured diameter.[28–30] The Paris classification classifies polyps into protruding and nonprotruding based on whether the lesion protrudes into the lumen a distance of at least 2.5 mm or the approximate width of a standard snare catheter or jaws of a closed biopsy forceps.[31,32] A representation of the Paris Classification is shown in **Table 2**. Although many polyps may be flat, there is a distinct clinical significance among those that are elevated, flat, or depressed. The less commonly seen IIc or depressed lesions have the highest likelihood of advanced pathology, such as high-grade dysplasia.[33]

Flat colorectal adenomas were first described by Muto and colleagues in 1985.[34] Mitooka and colleagues[8] demonstrated 37 minute flat lesions in 32 of 1152 patients who had a colonoscopy after swallowing an IC capsule. Rembacken and colleagues[25] examined 1000 patients for flat or depressed lesions. Any mucosal abnormality was sprayed with 0.2% IC: 36% (117) were flat and 0.6% (2) appeared depressed; 54% of the advanced neoplasms were flat or depressed.[25] Although such studies highlight the significance of depressed lesions, it should be noted that most adenomas are IIa or flat elevated and do not contain advanced pathology.[35]

CHROMOENDOSCOPY FOR POLYP DETECTION

Several randomized controlled studies examining pancolonic chromocolonoscopy were performed in high-risk patients who were symptomatic or had a family or personal history of colorectal neoplasia.[9,10,15,36,37] Brooker and colleagues[9] observed no increase in overall adenoma detection in one of the earliest randomized trials. However, the chromocolonoscopy group had more diminutive adenomas proximal to sigmoid colon, more patients with 3 or more adenomas, and more non-neoplastic lesions detected. The extubation time with chromocolonoscopy was also statistically significantly longer as compared with the control group.

Lapalus and colleagues[36] randomized 292 patients with a personal history of colorectal adenomas and/or family history of colorectal cancer. Patients received a conventional colonoscopy followed by randomization to repeat conventional colonoscopy or dye spraying with structural enhancement. There was no difference in the number of patients with at least one adenoma detected or in the number of detected adenomas. However, this study also observed an increase in detection of proximal adenomas and increased examination duration in the dye group.

In a trial by Hurlstone and colleagues,[15] the investigators controlled for extubation time and observed a statistically significant increase of detected adenomas in the chromocolonoscopy group. There were more diminutive adenomas smaller than

Table 1
Chromocolonoscopy studies examining polyp detection

Study	N	Design	Dye Used	Type of Chromo-colonoscopy	Extubation Time	Procedure Time	Results	Conclusions
Jaramillo et al,[27] 1995 Sweden	232 High Risk	Single arm w/HR colonoscopy and chromoendoscopy	0.5% IC	Targeted	Not reported	Not reported	Flat lesions seen in almost 25% of patients	Targeted chromocolonoscopy helps to identify the flat lesions
Rembacken et al,[25] 2000 UK	1000 High Risk	Single arm w/ conventional and magnifying chromocolonoscopy	0.2% IC	Targeted	Not reported	Not reported	More than half of the advanced neoplasia lesions were flat or depressed	Targeted chromocolonoscopy helps to identify the flat lesions
Brooker et al,[9] 2002 UK	259 High Risk	RCT: colonoscopy vs chromocolonoscopy	0.1% IC	Pancolonic	Chromocolonoscopy duration was longer	Not reported	Chromocolonoscopy detects more small proximal adenomas, patients with >2 adenomas, non-neoplastic lesions	Chromocolonoscopy increases detection of small proximal adenomas and patients with many adenomas but longer procedure time
Tsuda et al,[26] 2002 Sweden	371 High Risk	Single-arm chromocolonoscopy	0.1% IC	Targeted	Not reported	Not reported	Flat lesions were 6.8% of all lesions located mostly in right colon	Chromoendoscopy may detect lesions w/ central depression
Lee et al,[24] 2003 Korea	74 High Risk	Single-arm conventional colonoscopy followed by chromoendoscopy	0.2% IC	Left colon to 30 cm	Not reported	Not reported	Smaller and flat adenomas seen after IC spraying	Chromoendoscopy may detect flat or depressed adenomas in normal-appearing colon
Hurlstone et al,[15] 2004 UK	260 High Risk	RCT: pancolonic chromocolonoscopy vs targeted chromocolonoscopy	0.5% IC	Pan colonic	No difference	Not reported	Pan-colonic chromocolonoscopy detected more small/ flat/proximal/multiple adenomas hyperplastic polyps and advanced lesions	Chromocolonoscopy detects more small proximal adenomas but also lesions w/advanced pathology

Lecomte et al,[10] 2005 France	36 HNPCC patients	Single arm HR colonoscopy followed by chromoendoscopy	0.4% IC	Proximal colon	Not reported	Not reported	Chromoendoscopy increased detection of flat adenomas as well as proximal adenomas and HPs	Chromocolonoscopy may increase detection of adenomas and flat lesions in HNPCC
Lapalus et al,[36] 2006 France	300 High Risk	RCT: tandem conventional HR colonoscopy followed by conventional HR colonoscopy vs chromocolonoscopy w/structure enhancement	IC	Pancolonic	Not reported	Chromocolonoscopy longer	Chromocolonoscopy detected more diminutive and proximal (but not total) adenomas and hyperplastic polyps but increased examination duration	Chromoendoscopy w/structural enhancement not recommended in high-risk patients
Le Rhun et al,[37] 2006 France	203 High Risk	RCT: HR chromocolonoscopy vs conventional colonoscopy	0.4% IC	Pancolonic	Chromocolonoscopy was longer	Not reported	Chromocolonoscopy detected more polyps and flat (but not total) adenomas per patient but with increased time required	HRC requires more time with small increase in adenoma detection than colonoscopy
Trecca et al,[16] 2006 Italy	305 High Risk	Single-arm conventional chromocolonoscopy	0.2% IC	Targeted	Not reported	Not reported	Chromocolonoscopy detected flat lesions missed by conventional colonoscopy	Targeted chromoendoscopy in presence of suspicion may detect flat lesions
Raitu et al,[40] 2007 Romania	55 High Risk	HR conventional sigmoidoscopy followed chromo-sigmoidoscopy	0.27% IC	Left colon	Not reported	Not reported	Chromoendoscopy improved detection of diminutive but not larger adenomas	Routine IC application in flexible sigmoidoscopy could become a good option for screening.
Stoffel et al,[11] 2008 USA	50 High Risk	Randomized controlled tandem: conventional followed by intense inspection or chromoendoscopy	0.2% IC	Pancolonic	Not reported	2nd exam: Chromocolonoscopy was longer than intense inspection	Chromoendoscopy detected additional adenomas in more subjects than intensive inspection; these were smaller and proximal	Chromocolonoscopy improves detection of adenomas missed by conventional colonoscopy but increased number of normal biopsies

(continued on next page)

Table 1
(continued)

Study	N	Design	Dye Used	Type of Chromo-colonoscopy	Extubation Time	Procedure Time	Results	Conclusions
Park et al,[41] 2008 Korea	316	Randomized conventional colonoscopy with "2 passes" vs chromocolonoscopy	0.2% IC	Ascending colon	No difference	Not reported	Chromocolonoscopy identified higher number of additional polyps and more patients with at least one adenoma.	Chromocolonoscopy detects more polyps in AC and cecum.
Huneburg et al,[42] 2009 Germany	114 HNPCC	Two arms: Conventional colonoscopy followed by chromocolonoscopy and NBI followed by chromocolonoscopy	0.08% IC	Pancolonic	No difference	Chromocolonoscopy longer than colonoscopy or NBI	Compared with white light, chromocolonoscopy more flat adenomas. Compared with NBI, chromocolonoscopy detected more hyperplastic lesions, adenomas and flat adenomas.	Chromocolonoscopy improves detection rate of adenomas but with longer times
Kahi et al,[14] 2010 USA	660	Randomized high-definition colonoscopy w/ chromocolonoscopy vs high-definition colonoscopy w/white light colonoscopy	0.2% IC	Pancolonic	Not reported	Chromocolonoscopy longer	Chromocolonoscopy detected more flat adenomas per patient, small adenomas, and non-neoplastic lesions but total procedure time was longer.	High-definition chromocolonoscopy marginally increased flat and small adenoma detection but with longer time.
Hashimoto et al,[39] 2010 Japan	130	Randomized tandem; HR colonoscopy followed vs HR sigmoidoscopy w/chromo vs HR sigmoidoscopy	0.2% IC	Distal colon	Chromoendoscopy duration longer	Not reported	Chromoendoscopy increased withdrawal time with no significant difference in ADR	Chromoendoscopy did not detect more polyps in distal colon and increased withdrawal time

Pohl et al,[12] 2011 Germany	1008	Randomized HR colonoscopy vs HR chromoendoscopy	0.4% IC	Pancolonic	Chromocolonoscopy duration longer	Chromocolonoscopy duration longer	Chromocolonoscopy increased the overall ADR, detection rate of flat adenomas, and serrated adenomas and increased procedure time	Chromocolonoscopy superior to conventional in detection of lesions
Leung et al,[23] 2011 USA	150	Nonrandomized w/3 arms: colonoscopy w/air vs w/water vs w/ chromocolonoscopy and water	0.008% IC	Pan colonic: water w/dye	Not reported	IC/water: duration was longer than w/water which was longer than colon w/air	ADR was higher for IC/water method followed by water method then air method	Chromocolonoscopy with water method yields high ADR but longer procedure times

Abbreviations: ADR, adenoma detection rate; HNPCC, hereditary nonpolyposis colorectal cancer; HR, high resolution; IC, indigo carmine; NBI, narrow band imaging; RCT, randomized controlled trial; w/, with.

Table 2
Paris classification of polyp morphology

Type	Description	Representation
Ip	Pedunculated	
Is	Sessile	
Isp	Subpedunculated	
IIa	Flat elevated	
IIb	Flat nonelevated	
IIc	Flat depressed	

4 mm, diminutive and flat polyps in right colon, and an increased number of patients with multiple adenomas. They recommended use of chromocolonoscopy for index colonoscopies to risk stratify patients. Le Rhun and colleagues[37] observed in their randomized trial that chromocolonoscopy detected more polyps but it required longer procedure time. Stoffel and colleagues[11] conducted their study with high-risk patients who had at least one previous colon polyp and/or colorectal cancer. A major critique of chromoendoscopy trials is that the increased adenoma detection rates may result from an increased observation time. In the Stoffel and colleagues trial,[11] patients were randomized to chromoendoscopy versus conventional endoscopy with intense inspection to counter the time effect of dye spraying. The study concluded that chromoendoscopy detected additional adenomas in more subjects than intensive inspection (44% vs 17%) and identified significantly more missed adenomas per subject (0.7 vs 0.2, $P<.01$). The adenomas detected with chromoendoscopy were significantly smaller and more often right-sided. Chromoendoscopy took longer than conventional with intense inspection. One important observation was the increased number of normal biopsies in the patients who had chromocolonoscopy.

Based on the previously mentioned studies, Kahi and colleagues[14] randomized 660 average-risk screening patients to chromocolonoscopy with high-definition white light or high-definition white light only. They observed that chromocolonoscopy detected marginally more small and flat adenomas than white light alone. In addition, they observed a difference between study sites, implying that the benefit of chromoendoscopy may vary between endoscopists. Although this study controlled for mucosal examination time, the overall procedure time was greater in the chromocolonoscopy arm.

Using a novel dye-spraying technique as described previously, Pohl and colleagues[12] enrolled 1008 patients in the largest randomized controlled trial of pancolonic chromocolonoscopy. The proportion of patients with at least one adenoma was significantly higher in the chromocolonoscopy group. The pancolonic chromocolonoscopy group had an increased overall ADR with an increased detection of flat and serrated adenomas. Because serrated lesions may be implicated in interval cancers,[38] this benefit of chromocolonoscopy may be important clinically. There was a trend toward an increased rate for detection of advanced adenomas. Unlike the Kahi and colleagues' trial,[14] this group recommended chromocolonoscopy for average-risk individuals.

Other studies have examined the impact of chromocolonoscopy in targeted segments of the colon. Although some examine the distal colon,[24,39,40] others have examined the proximal colon.[41] These studies confirm the findings of pancolonic chromoendoscopy studies with regard to the small size of detected lesions and increased procedure time for the chromoendoscopy group.

CHROMOENDOSCOPY AND HEREDITARY NONPOLYPOSIS COLORECTAL CANCER

There are 2 published studies evaluating the use of chromoendoscopy in patients with hereditary nonpolyposis colorectal cancer (HNPCC). Lecomte and colleagues[10] enrolled 36 consecutive patients with HNPCC. Patients had a complete high-resolution colonoscopy and, after a second intubation of cecum, the second step was chromoendoscopy of proximal colon on withdrawal. Chromoendoscopy increased detection of flat adenomas compared with conventional. It also detected more adenomatous lesions in the proximal colon than regular colonoscopy.

Huneburg and colleagues[42] studied a total of 109 patients with HNPCC. Forty-seven patients had standard colonoscopy followed by chromocolonoscopy, and 62 patients had narrow band imaging (NBI) followed by chromocolonoscopy. In comparison with white light and NBI, chromocolonoscopy detected statistically significantly more lesions per patient. In particular, these were hyperplastic polyps and flat adenomas.

SUMMARY OF CHROMOCOLONOSCOPY AND POLYP DETECTION RATE

In the randomized trials that observed an increased detection rate, most of the polyps were hyperplastic or small proximal adenomas. Aside from one trial,[15] it has not been shown to increase detection of advanced adenomas. One study suggests that although chromocolonoscopy may benefit some endoscopists, this technique may not be useful in routine screening or surveillance colonoscopies.[14] There were a few trials that found that more patients with multiple adenomas were identified during chromocolonoscopy.[9,15] This aspect may have an impact on changing surveillance intervals in some patients from 5 to 3 years.

Routine use of chromoendoscopy has been shown to prolong procedure times. Newer staining methods, such as capsule ingestion or mixing the dye with water, may mitigate this issue, but will not reduce the time taken to sample the detected lesions.[8,23] As one study observed, the number of biopsies, especially normal tissue, were higher in the chromocolonoscopy group.[11] Thus, the attendant potential risks and increased procedural time associated with chromocolonoscopy may override the small benefit accrued from detecting small proximal adenomas.

DIFFERENTIATION OF POLYPS

Chromoendoscopy has been used to aid in the differentiation of hyperplastic from adenomatous polyps, as demonstrated in a small study of 36 patients (**Table 3**).[43] In that trial, an observation was made regarding the characteristics of the surface of

Table 3
Use of chromoendoscopy in differentiating adenomatous or neoplastic polyps from non-neoplastic polyps

Study	Kudo Used	N	Design	Dye Used	Findings	Conclusions
Kudo et al,[22] 1996 Japan	Yes	2050 lesions	Tandem: SM followed by chromocolonoscopy/ magnifying colonoscopy	0.2% IC 0.4% CV	Agreement SM and chromocolonoscopy/ magnifying 81.5%	Chromocolonoscopy/ magnifying colonoscopy predicts histology
Axelrad et al,[43] 1996 US	No	36 patients w/polyps <1 cm	Single arm w/HR chromocolonoscopy	0.2% IC	Distinct pit patterns for HPs: "orderly arranged "dots" APs: "grooves"/"sulci." Sensitivity/specificity distinguishing AP from NAP were 93% and 95% respectively	Chromocolonoscopy can predict histology, obviating removal.
Togashi et al,[47] 1999 Japan	Modified A–F	923 polyps	Single arm w/zoom chromocolonoscopy	0.2% IC 0.05% CV	Neoplastic changes (%): A (I) (10%); B (II) (15.9%); C (III$_L$) (93.7%); D (III$_L$) (100%); E (IV) (94.8%); F (V) (87.5%)	Chromocolonoscopy/ magnifying colonoscopy can aid in distinguishing NP from NNP
Kiesslich et al,[56] 2001 Germany	Yes	100	Single-arm HR chromocolonoscopy	0.4% IC	Chromocolonoscopy distinguishes AP (Types II–V) from NAP (Types I–II) with sensitivity of 92% and specificity 93%	Chromocolonoscopy helps to elucidate pit patterns and distinguish NP from NNP
Tung et al,[48] 2001 Taiwan	Yes	141 patients 175 polyps	Single arm w/zoom chromocolonoscopy	0.2% IC	Neoplasia (%) in I (0); II (12.2); III$_L$ (69.7); III$_S$ (80); IV (84.4); V (100)	Pit pattern can predict histology
Kato et al,[51] 2001 Japan	Modified	3438 lesions	Single-arm magnifying chromocolonoscopy	0.2% IC	Accuracy of chromocolonoscopy/ magnifying colonoscopy: NNP 75% (117/157), AP 94% (3006/ 3186), and invasive carcinomas 85% (81/95).	Magnifying chromocolonoscopy can aid in predicting lesions that can be removed endoscopically vs surgically

Study	Magnification	Patients/Polyps	Study design	IC	Results	Conclusion
Eisen et al,[55] 2002 US	No	299 patients 520 polyps	Single arm with HR chromocolonoscopy	0.2%–0.8% IC	Use of chromocolonoscopy to predict AP: Sens (82%); Spec (82%) and NPV (88%)	HR/IC aids endoscopist in differentiating AP from NAP
Konishi et al,[52] 2003 Japan	Yes	660 patients	Randomized magnifying chromocolonoscopy vs nonmagnifying chromocolonoscopy	0.2% IC	Accuracy chromocolonoscopy w/magnification to distinguish NP from NNP lesions (92%, 372/405) higher than for nonmagnifying chromocolonoscopy (68%, 278/407).	Chromocolonoscopy w/ magnifying colonoscopy superior to nonmagnifying
Su et al,[46] 2004 Taiwan	Yes	270 polyps	Single-arm magnifying chromocolonoscopy	0.2% IC	I/II vs III–V diagnostic accuracy 91.9% to distinguish NP from NNP	Flat lesions with II or I have little risk
Fu et al,[54] 2004 Japan	Yes	206 polyps ≤1 cm	Colonoscopy vs chromocolonoscopy vs magnifying chromocolonoscopy	0.2% IC	Overall diagnostic accuracies; C (84%), chromocolonoscopy (89.3%), chromocolonoscopy/ magnifying (95.6%)	Magnifying chromocolonoscopy most reliable to distinguish NP from NNP
Sonwalker et al,[57] 2006 UK	Yes	476 patients 709 polyps	Single-arm chromocolonoscopy with no magnification	0.2% IC	423/467 (91%) APs and 153/187 (82%) NAPs correctly identified	Magnification not always needed
Apel et al,[59] 2006 Germany	Yes	158 patients 273 polyps <5 mm	Tandem comparison: HR colonoscopy followed by chromocolonoscopy	0.4% IC	Predicting HP's HR colon vs IC: Sens (93 vs 94%); Spec (60 vs 64%) and overall accuracy (81 vs 83%)	Chromocolonoscopy adds little to HR
Tischendorf et al,[53] 2007 Germany	Yes	150 patients 200 polyps	Tandem: Magnifying conventional colonoscopy followed by: magnifying chromocolonoscopy vs NBI	0.3% IC	NBI and chromocolonoscopy/ magnifying performed equal with pit patterns but NBI better for capillary pattern	NBI aids in distinguishing NP from NNP through use of vascular pattern

(continued on next page)

Table 3
(continued)

Study	Kudo Used	N	Design	Dye Used	Findings	Conclusions
East et al,[60] 2007 UK	Yes	33 polyps <6 mm	High definition chromocolonoscopy vs NBI	0.1% MB	Pit patterns for MB and NBI differed in 12 and 20 of 33 polyps	Kudo classification may not be valid in NBI
Chiu et al,[50] 2007 Taiwan	Yes	133 patients 180 polyps	Conventional colonoscopy vs chromocolonoscopy (high and low magnifying) and NBI (h/l magnifying)	0.2% IC	Diagnostic accuracy of NBI and chromocolonoscopy (both high magnifying) superior to NBI/IC (low magnifying) or conventional	High and low magnifying NBI useful in distinguishing NP from NNP
Yamada et al,[49] 2009 Japan	Yes	208 patients	Magnifying chromocolonoscopy with SM examining impact of fixing on accuracy	0.2% IC	Adenomas with III$_L$ pattern correctly identified when fixed with SM	Magnifying chromocolonoscopy is accurate and perceived accuracy is limited by lack of fixation
Togashi et al,[58] 2009 Japan	Yes	107 polyps	CP in CC vs OBI (CP) vs pit pattern in chromocolonoscopy	0.2% IC	Overall accuracy for differentiating NP from NNP: CC CP (70%); OBI CP (87%) and chromocolonoscopy PP (86%)	OBI similar to chromocolonoscopy and both superior to CC in differentiating NP from NNP
Hasegawa et al,[62] 2011 Japan	Yes	145 serrated lesions	Magnifying chromoendoscopy	0.075% CV	TSAs more likely to have III$_L$ than SSA or HP but not statistically significant	Potential to differentiate serrated lesions with magnifying chromoendoscopy
Yano et al,[88] 2011 Japan	Yes	86 serrated lesions	Used HR chromocolonoscopy to classify 3 crypt types (hyperplastic, adenomatous, and mixed) by clinical, pathologic and molecular features	0.2% IC	Lesions w/HP pattern were in proximal colon and had CIMP (+) and lesions w/AP pattern were in the distal colon and KRAS(+)	Clinical, path/molecular features of SNs correlate with mucosal crypt patterns w/chromocolonoscopy

Study	Chromo	N	Technique	Design/Methods	Dye	Results	Conclusion
Kimura et al,[45] 2012 Japan	Yes	261 lesion	Magnifying chromoendoscopy		IC	Novel Type II open-shape pit pattern (Type II-O) was predictive of SSAs w/BRAF mutation and CIMP	Type II-O pit pattern predicts SSA (histo and molecular mutations)
Kuiper et al,[61] 2012 Netherlands	Yes	64 patients 154 lesions		Single-arm, colonoscopy followed by NBI examination, assessment of vascular pattern intensity, chromocolonoscopy and confocal endomicroscopy	0.2% IC	Accuracy of confocal microscopy less than NBI or chromocolonoscopy	Chromocolonoscopy accuracy as good or better than newer technology

Abbreviations: AP, adenomatous polyp; CC, conventional colonoscopy; CIMP, CpG island methylator phenotype; CP, capillary pattern; CV, crystal violet; HR, high resolution; HP, hyperplastic polyp; IC, indigo carmine; MB, methylene blue; NAP, non adenomatous polyp; NNP, non-neoplastic polyp; NP, neoplastic polyp; NPV, negative predictive polyp; OBI, optimal band imaging; PP, pit pattern; SSA, sessile serrated adenoma; Sens, sensitivity; Spec, specificity; SM, stereomicroscopy; TSA, traditional serrated adenoma; w/, with.

hyperplastic polyps and adenomas. Hyperplastic lesions had orderly arranged dots, whereas adenomas had "grooves" or "sulci." The morphologic appearance of the polyp surface or "pit pattern" has been characterized by Kudo and colleagues.[22] The Kudo classification divides polyps into 5 categories. These are shown in **Fig. 3**.

Each of the patterns may aid in predicting polyp pathology. The round Type I pattern is typically seen in normal mucosa. The stellate Type II pits are predictive of hyperplastic lesions and often appear round but are larger than surrounding the Type I found in normal mucosa. Types III to V are observed in adenomatous lesions. Although Type III$_L$ or grooved sulci and Type IV or cerebriform are relatively easy to characterize, the smaller Type III$_S$ and Type V may be more difficult to discern. A study using more than 200 photographs of polyps demonstrated good interobserver and intraobserver consistency in the assessment of pit patterns by experienced endoscopists.[44]

Type	Description	Representation
I	Normal (round)	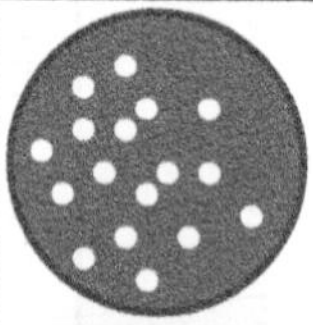
II	Asteroid/ stellar/ papillary	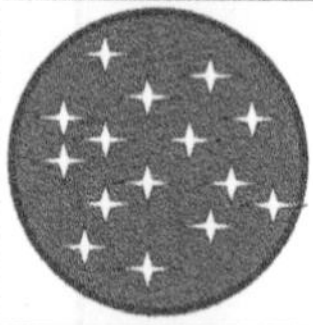
III-L	Tubular (smaller than type I)	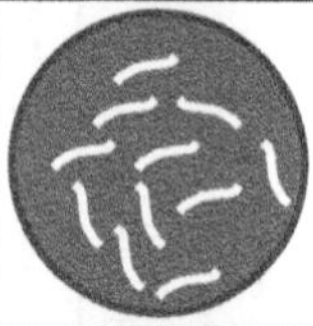
III-S	Round pit (smaller than type I)	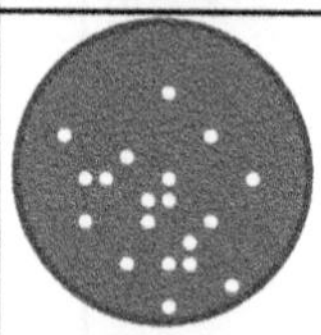
IV	Gyrus-like	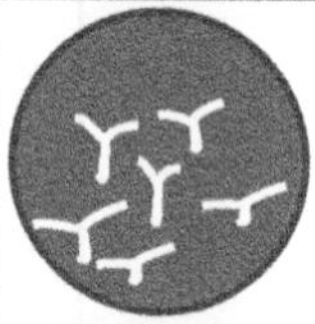
V	Irregular arrangements	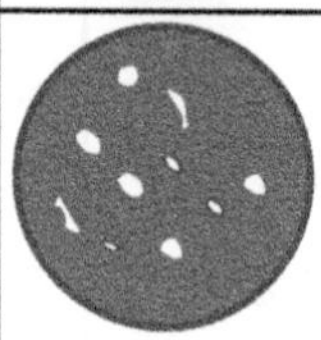

Fig. 3. Kudo classification for pit pattern.

Recently a Type II-O pattern has been shown to be associated with sessile serrated adenoma histology.[45]

An important aspect of chromocolonoscopy is the use of this technique to identify polyp pit patterns for the purpose of distinguishing neoplastic from non-neoplastic lesions. One obvious benefit is the potential reduction in the removal of insignificant lesions.[43] Using chromoendoscopy and the Kudo classification, multiple studies have observed that although Type I and Type II have low rates of neoplasia, Types III to V have much higher rates of dysplasia.[46–48] One investigator has also demonstrated that the perceived accuracy may be lower than the actual rate because of inadequate fixing of the pathology specimen.[49] Thus, identifying pit patterns with chromocolonoscopy may aid in determining the importance of detected polyps.

Much of the literature examining chromocolonoscopy and pit patterns has examined the efficacy of new technologies in conjunction or comparison with chromoendoscopy. Many studies have used or advocated the adjunctive use of zoom, magnifying, or high-definition colonoscopy.[46,48,50–54] Other investigators have found that the colonoscopes with conventional magnification have been adequate in predicting neoplasia.[43,55–59] New technology, such as NBI[60] and confocal endomicroscopy (CE), add other features, such as a superior examination of vascular patterns.[53] Many studies have shown that the accuracy of chromocolonoscopy compares favorably to NBI[50] or CE.[61]

In summary, chromocolonoscopy is a useful tool to examine pit patterns and predict neoplasia. However, the attendant issues of increased procedure time and cumbersomeness associated with chromocolonoscopy make newer technology more attractive. Other investigations regarding chromocolonoscopy may involve newer lesions, such as sessile serrated adenomas.[45,62]

CHROMOENDOSCOPY IN PATIENTS WITH IBD

Although the risk is lower than previously thought, colorectal cancer is one the most feared complications of long-standing IBD, especially if the disease is extensive.[63] The detection of early neoplastic lesions can be challenging, as these lesions grow in an infiltrating pattern. The current surveillance strategy of multiple random colonic biopsies throughout the colon in the management of patients with ulcerative colitis and Crohn colitis has been the subject of controversy because of the high cost and sampling error. Although it has been recommended to obtain 33 biopsies to have a 90% probability for detection of dysplasia,[64] studies have shown that most clinicians do not take the recommended number of biopsies.[65,66] On the other hand, on average, 1 dysplasia is detected for every 1266 random biopsies taken during nontargeted biopsies.[67] These data clearly demonstrate the need for a better surveillance program in this group of patients.

New advances in endoscopic imaging techniques may potentially help to increase dysplasia detection rates and lowering the cost and workload of the standard random biopsy approach. Chromoendoscopy can increase the rate of dysplasia detection when compared with conventional colonoscopy and random biopsies (**Table 4**). The SURFACE guidelines[68] give a helpful summary of how to optimize chromoendoscopy in patients with IBD. According to this guideline, this technique should be avoided in patients with active disease, or inadequate bowel preparation. A pancolonic examination rather than local staining is recommended. In addition, a spasmolytic should be used if necessary. The analysis of the detected lesions should be done according to the pit pattern classification[22] and targeted biopsies should be obtained from these lesions. Suggested targets include mucosa with Types III to V pit patterns,[69,70] fold

Table 4
Use of chromoendoscopy in irritable bowel disease

Study	Years with Colitis	No. of Patients	Dysplasia (No. of Patients)	Design	Dye	Type of Chromo-colonoscopy	Results
Kiesslich et al,[70] 2003 Germany	>8	165 (UC)	19	Randomized, 1:1	0.1% MB	PC	CE detected more patients w/dysplasia (32 vs 10) (P = .003)
Matsumoto et al,[89] 2003 Japan	>5	57 (UC)	12	Prospective cohort, WLE followed by CE	0.2% IC	PC	CE has higher sensitivity for dysplasia than WLE (85.7% vs 38.1%)
Rutter et al,[90] 2004 UK	>8	100 (UC)	7	Prospective cohort, WLE followed by CE	0.1% IC	PC	CE detected more biopsies w/dysplasia (9 vs 0) and more patients with dysplasia (7 vs 0) (P = .02) than WLE
Hurlstone et al,[71] 2004 UK	>8	324 (UC)	38	Prospective cohort	0.5% IC	Selective CE	CE detected more biopsies with dysplasia than WLE (42 vs 11) (P<.001)
Hurlstone et al,[91] 2005 UK	>8	700 (UC)	81	Prospective cohort	0.5% IC	Targeted	CE detected more patients with dysplasia than WLE (69 vs 24) (P<.0001[a])
Kiesslich et al,[92] 2007 Germany	>8	153 (UC)	15	Randomized 1:1	0.1% MB	PC	CE detected more patients with dysplasia than WLE (19 vs 4) (P = .005)
Marion et al,[93] 2008 USA	>8	102 (79 UC, 23 CD)	19	Prospective cohort, WLE followed by CE	0.1% MB	PC	CE detected more patients with dysplasia than WLE (17 vs 3) (P<.001)
Gunther et al,[94] 2011 Germany	>8	100 (95 UC, 5 CD)	2	Randomized 1:1:1[b]	0.1% IC	PC	CE group had more biopsies w/dysplasia than random WLE (2 vs 0)
Hlavaty et al,[69] 2011 Slovakia	>8 (PC) >15 (L-sided)	45 (29 UC, 16 CD)	7	Prospective cohort 2:1	0.4% IC	PC	CE group had more biopsies w/dysplasia than random WLE (12 vs 0) and more patients with dysplasia (7 vs 0 patients) (P = .002)

Abbreviations: CD, Crohn disease; CE, chromoendoscopy; IC, indigo carmine; MB, methylene blue; PC, pancolonic; UC, ulcerative colitis; WLE, white light endoscopy.
[a] 20/69 lesions in the chromocolonoscopy group were diagnosed during nontargeted biopsies.
[b] In this study, 150 patients were divided to 3 groups: (1) 50 in conventional colonoscopy, (2) 50 in chromoendoscopy, and (3) 50 in confocal endomicroscopy groups. For the purpose of this article, only the data from groups 1 and 2 are included in the table.

convergence, air-induced deformation, interruption of innominate grooves, or focal discrete color changes.[71]

Chromoendoscopy has some limitations, including the need for a longer examination, the risk of DNA damage to the colonocytes when using methylene blue,[21] and the difficulties in differentiating inflammation from neoplasia. One way to overcome the latter limitation is to avoid using this technique in patients with active inflammation. Regarding the risk of DNA damage by methylene blue, a prospective pilot study by Kiesslich and colleagues,[72] has shown that this risk is minimal and without a real biologic significance, but further larger studies are needed to confirm this result.

Chromoendoscopy has been adopted as the method of choice for screening patients with colitis according to the European Crohn's and Colitis Organization 2008[73] and British Society of Gastroenterology 2010.[74] Although the American College of Gastroenterology 2010 and American Gastroenterological Association 2010 guidelines recommend 4 quadrant biopsies at 10-cm intervals for a total of at least 33 biopsies, there is a trend toward the targeted biopsy strategy using chromoendoscopy in patients with long-standing colitis.

IDENTIFICATION OF ABERRANT CRYPT FOCI

Aberrant crypt foci (ACFs) are diminutive growths in the colon that can best be identified using chromoendoscopy. They were initially identified in postmortem examinations.[75,76] These lesions may be 2 crypts in size and are identified by their lumens that are larger than normal crypts that surround the ACF. Some investigators have proposed the use of ACFs as potential precursors or biomarkers. An initial use of ACFs was for biomarkers in chemopreventive trials[77] but enthusiasm for this use has waned after one trial demonstrated the highly labile nature of these lesions.[78,79]

Their frequency may also correlate with advanced colorectal neoplasia in patients.[19,80,81] Hurlstone and colleagues[82] observed an increase of ACFs in patients with flat adenomas. Risk factors for ACF include age, smoking, and family history of CRC.[81,83–85] Given the possibility that ACFs may represent surrogate biomarkers for advanced and flat colorectal neoplasia, it is reasonable to postulate that ACFs may provide clues regarding future colorectal neoplasia.[77] One recent trial observed that an increased frequency of ACFs detected in the distal 20 cm of the colorectum was independently associated with risk for metachronous advanced neoplasia on follow-up colonoscopy. Along with a previous history of advanced neoplasia, the frequency of ACF helped to predict the risk for future advanced neoplasia. Specifically, those subjects who had more than 6 ACFs were more likely to have an advanced lesion found on follow-up examination. This relationship appeared to be stronger in patients with a previous history of advanced adenomas. Thus, distal ACFs may serve as potential biomarkers for future advanced colorectal neoplasia.

Identifying ACFs can be accomplished by the following steps:

- Identifying ACFs requires dye staining with either methylene blue or IC. Given the subtle features in identifying these lesions, the absorptive stain is the preferred dye.
- ACFs are identified by 2 or more crypts that are darkly stained and have lumen diameters that are 1.5 to 2.0 times those of surrounding crypt lumens.
- On tangential view, ACFs should be raised above the mucosal surface.
- The following criteria should be used to confirm the identification of ACFs: round, dilated, slit, or star-shaped lumen, or thick crypt walls having compressed lumens.

- To ensure that ACFs were not double counted or missed, endoscopists use established inspection techniques, such as dividing the colon into quadrants or withdrawing the scope in a clockwise manner.

In summary, ACFs may be identified using chromoendoscopy and may serve as biomarkers or models for carcinogenesis.[86] With regard to clinical use, they may be limited due to their labile nature, difficulty to biopsy, and the onerous nature of staining.[87]

SUMMARY

Dye staining has been shown to be useful in detecting and differentiating polyps; however, the increased yield is primarily for small polyps with less clinical significance. In addition, chromoendoscopy increases procedure time. Therefore, it may not be recommended for routine screening and surveillance. The increased yield of dysplasia in IBD makes it a useful adjunct for surveillance in this population.

REFERENCES

1. Rex DK, Johnson DA, Anderson JC, et al. American College of Gastroenterology guidelines for colorectal cancer screening 2009 [corrected]. Am J Gastroenterol 2009;104:739–50.
2. Bressler B, Paszat LF, Chen Z, et al. Rates of new or missed colorectal cancers after colonoscopy and their risk factors: a population-based analysis. Gastroenterology 2007;132:96–102.
3. Brenner H, Hoffmeister M, Arndt V, et al. Protection from right- and left-sided colorectal neoplasms after colonoscopy: population-based study. J Natl Cancer Inst 2010;102:89–95.
4. Baxter NN, Warren JL, Barrett MJ, et al. Association between colonoscopy and colorectal cancer mortality in a US cohort according to site of cancer and colonoscopist specialty. J Clin Oncol 2012;30:2664–9.
5. Baxter NN, Goldwasser MA, Paszat LF, et al. Association of colonoscopy and death from colorectal cancer. Ann Intern Med 2009;150:1–8.
6. Kaminski MF, Regula J, Kraszewska E, et al. Quality indicators for colonoscopy and the risk of interval cancer. N Engl J Med 2010;362:1795–803.
7. Tada M, Katoh S, Kohli Y, et al. On the dye spraying method in colonofiberscopy. Endoscopy 1977;8:70–4.
8. Mitooka H, Fujimori T, Maeda S, et al. Minute flat depressed neoplastic lesions of the colon detected by contrast chromoscopy using an indigo carmine capsule. Gastrointest Endosc 1995;41:453–9.
9. Brooker JC, Saunders BP, Shah SG, et al. Total colonic dye-spray increases the detection of diminutive adenomas during routine colonoscopy: a randomized controlled trial. Gastrointest Endosc 2002;56:333–8.
10. Lecomte T, Cellier C, Meatchi T, et al. Chromoendoscopic colonoscopy for detecting preneoplastic lesions in hereditary nonpolyposis colorectal cancer syndrome. Clin Gastroenterol Hepatol 2005;3:897–902.
11. Stoffel EM, Turgeon DK, Stockwell DH, et al. Chromoendoscopy detects more adenomas than colonoscopy using intensive inspection without dye spraying. Cancer Prev Res (Phila) 2008;1:507–13.
12. Pohl J, Schneider A, Vogell H, et al. Pancolonic chromoendoscopy with indigo carmine versus standard colonoscopy for detection of neoplastic lesions: a randomised two-centre trial. Gut 2011;60:485–90.

13. Pohl J, May A, Rabenstein T, et al. Computed virtual chromoendoscopy: a new tool for enhancing tissue surface structures. Endoscopy 2007;39:80–3.
14. Kahi CJ, Anderson JC, Waxman I, et al. High-definition chromocolonoscopy vs. high-definition white light colonoscopy for average-risk colorectal cancer screening. Am J Gastroenterol 2010;105:1301–7.
15. Hurlstone DP, Cross SS, Slater R, et al. Detecting diminutive colorectal lesions at colonoscopy: a randomised controlled trial of pan-colonic versus targeted chromoscopy. Gut 2004;53:376–80.
16. Trecca A, Gaj F, Di Lorenzo GP, et al. Improved detection of colorectal neoplasms with selective use of chromoendoscopy in 2005 consecutive patients. Tech Coloproctol 2006;10:339–44.
17. Trivedi PJ, Braden B. Indications, stains and techniques in chromoendoscopy. QJM 2013;106(2):117–31.
18. Anderson JC, Swede H, Rustagi T, et al. Aberrant crypt foci as predictors of colorectal neoplasia on repeat colonoscopy. Cancer Causes Control 2012;23: 355–61.
19. Anderson JC, Pleau DC, Rajan TV, et al. Increased frequency of serrated aberrant crypt foci among smokers. Am J Gastroenterol 2010;105(7):1648–54.
20. Repici A, Di Stefano AF, Radicioni MM, et al. Methylene blue MMX tablets for chromoendoscopy. Safety tolerability and bioavailability in healthy volunteers. Contemp Clin Trials 2012;33:260–7.
21. Davies J, Burke D, Olliver JR, et al. Methylene blue but not indigo carmine causes DNA damage to colonocytes in vitro and in vivo at concentrations used in clinical chromoendoscopy. Gut 2007;56:155–6.
22. Kudo S, Tamura S, Nakajima T, et al. Diagnosis of colorectal tumorous lesions by magnifying endoscopy. Gastrointest Endosc 1996;44:8–14.
23. Leung JW, Ransibrahmanakul K, Toomsen L, et al. The water method combined with chromoendoscopy enhances adenoma detection. J Interv Gastroenterol 2011;1:53–8.
24. Lee JH, Kim JW, Cho YK, et al. Detection of colorectal adenomas by routine chromoendoscopy with indigocarmine. Am J Gastroenterol 2003;98:1284–8.
25. Rembacken BJ, Fujii T, Cairns A, et al. Flat and depressed colonic neoplasms: a prospective study of 1000 colonoscopies in the UK. Lancet 2000;355:1211–4.
26. Tsuda S, Veress B, Toth E, et al. Flat and depressed colorectal tumours in a southern Swedish population: a prospective chromoendoscopic and histopathological study. Gut 2002;51:550–5.
27. Jaramillo E, Watanabe M, Slezak P, et al. Flat neoplastic lesions of the colon and rectum detected by high-resolution video endoscopy and chromoscopy. Gastrointest Endosc 1995;42:114–22.
28. Kudo S, Kashida H, Tamura T. Early colorectal cancer: flat or depressed type. J Gastroenterol Hepatol 2000;15(Suppl):D66–70.
29. Kudo S, Lambert R, Allen JI, et al. Nonpolypoid neoplastic lesions of the colorectal mucosa. Gastrointest Endosc 2008;68:S3–47.
30. Kudo S, Tamura S, Hirota S, et al. The problem of de novo colorectal carcinoma. Eur J Cancer 1995;31A:1118–20.
31. The Paris endoscopic classification of superficial neoplastic lesions: esophagus, stomach, and colon: November 30 to December 1, 2002. Gastrointest Endosc 2003;58:S3–43.
32. Endoscopic Classification Review Group. Update on the Paris classification of superficial neoplastic lesions in the digestive tract. Endoscopy 2005;37: 570–8.

33. Bianco MA, Cipolletta L, Rotondano G, et al. Prevalence of nonpolypoid colorectal neoplasia: an Italian multicenter observational study. Endoscopy 2010; 42:279–85.

34. Muto T, Kamiya J, Sawada T, et al. Small "flat adenoma" of the large bowel with special reference to its clinicopathologic features. Dis Colon Rectum 1985;28: 847–51.

35. Rex DK, Helbig CC. High yields of small and flat adenomas with high-definition colonoscopes using either white light or narrow band imaging. Gastroenterology 2007;133:42–7.

36. Lapalus MG, Helbert T, Napoleon B, et al. Does chromoendoscopy with structure enhancement improve the colonoscopic adenoma detection rate? Endoscopy 2006;38:444–8.

37. Le Rhun M, Coron E, Parlier D, et al. High resolution colonoscopy with chromoscopy versus standard colonoscopy for the detection of colonic neoplasia: a randomized study. Clin Gastroenterol Hepatol 2006;4:349–54.

38. Arain MA, Sawhney M, Sheikh S, et al. CIMP status of interval colon cancers: another piece to the puzzle. Am J Gastroenterol 2010;105:1189–95.

39. Hashimoto K, Higaki S, Nishiahi M, et al. Does chromoendoscopy improve the colonoscopic adenoma detection rate? Hepatogastroenterology 2010;57: 1399–404.

40. Ratiu N, Gelbmann C, Rath HR, et al. Chromoendoscopy with indigo carmine in flexible sigmoidoscopy screening: does it improve the detection of adenomas in the distal colon and rectum? J Gastrointestin Liver Dis 2007;16:153–6.

41. Park SY, Lee SK, Kim BC, et al. Efficacy of chromoendoscopy with indigocarmine for the detection of ascending colon and cecum lesions. Scand J Gastroenterol 2008;43:878–85.

42. Huneburg R, Lammert F, Rabe C, et al. Chromocolonoscopy detects more adenomas than white light colonoscopy or narrow band imaging colonoscopy in hereditary nonpolyposis colorectal cancer screening. Endoscopy 2009;41: 316–22.

43. Axelrad AM, Fleischer DE, Geller AJ, et al. High-resolution chromoendoscopy for the diagnosis of diminutive colon polyps: implications for colon cancer screening. Gastroenterology 1996;110:1253–8.

44. Huang Q, Fukami N, Kashida H, et al. Interobserver and intra-observer consistency in the endoscopic assessment of colonic pit patterns. Gastrointest Endosc 2004;60:520–6.

45. Kimura T, Yamamoto E, Yamano HO, et al. A novel pit pattern identifies the precursor of colorectal cancer derived from sessile serrated adenoma. Am J Gastroenterol 2012;107:460–9.

46. Su MY, Ho YP, Chen PC, et al. Magnifying endoscopy with indigo carmine contrast for differential diagnosis of neoplastic and nonneoplastic colonic polyps. Dig Dis Sci 2004;49:1123–7.

47. Togashi K, Konishi F, Ishizuka T, et al. Efficacy of magnifying endoscopy in the differential diagnosis of neoplastic and non-neoplastic polyps of the large bowel. Dis Colon Rectum 1999;42:1602–8.

48. Tung SY, Wu CS, Su MY. Magnifying colonoscopy in differentiating neoplastic from nonneoplastic colorectal lesions. Am J Gastroenterol 2001; 96:2628–32.

49. Yamada T, Tamura S, Onishi S, et al. A comparison of magnifying chromoendoscopy versus histopathology of forceps biopsy specimen in the diagnosis of minute flat adenoma of the colon. Dig Dis Sci 2009;54:2002–8.

50. Chiu HM, Chang CY, Chen CC, et al. A prospective comparative study of narrow-band imaging, chromoendoscopy, and conventional colonoscopy in the diagnosis of colorectal neoplasia. Gut 2007;56:373–9.
51. Kato S, Fujii T, Koba I, et al. Assessment of colorectal lesions using magnifying colonoscopy and mucosal dye spraying: can significant lesions be distinguished? Endoscopy 2001;33:306–10.
52. Konishi K, Kaneko K, Kurahashi T, et al. A comparison of magnifying and nonmagnifying colonoscopy for diagnosis of colorectal polyps: a prospective study. Gastrointest Endosc 2003;57:48–53.
53. Tischendorf JJ, Wasmuth HE, Koch A, et al. Value of magnifying chromoendoscopy and narrow band imaging (NBI) in classifying colorectal polyps: a prospective controlled study. Endoscopy 2007;39:1092–6.
54. Fu KI, Sano Y, Kato S, et al. Chromoendoscopy using indigo carmine dye spraying with magnifying observation is the most reliable method for differential diagnosis between non-neoplastic and neoplastic colorectal lesions: a prospective study. Endoscopy 2004;36:1089–93.
55. Eisen GM, Kim CY, Fleischer DE, et al. High-resolution chromoendoscopy for classifying colonic polyps: a multicenter study. Gastrointest Endosc 2002;55:687–94.
56. Kiesslich R, von Bergh M, Hahn M, et al. Chromoendoscopy with indigo carmine improves the detection of adenomatous and nonadenomatous lesions in the colon. Endoscopy 2001;33:1001–6.
57. Sonwalkar S, Rotimi O, Rembacken BJ. Characterization of colonic polyps at conventional (nonmagnifying) colonoscopy after spraying with 0.2 % indigo carmine dye. Endoscopy 2006;38:1218–23.
58. Togashi K, Osawa H, Koinuma K, et al. A comparison of conventional endoscopy, chromoendoscopy, and the optimal-band imaging system for the differentiation of neoplastic and non-neoplastic colonic polyps. Gastrointest Endosc 2009;69:734–41.
59. Apel D, Jakobs R, Schilling D, et al. Accuracy of high-resolution chromoendoscopy in prediction of histologic findings in diminutive lesions of the rectosigmoid. Gastrointest Endosc 2006;63:824–8.
60. East JE, Suzuki N, Saunders BP. Comparison of magnified pit pattern interpretation with narrow band imaging versus chromoendoscopy for diminutive colonic polyps: a pilot study. Gastrointest Endosc 2007;66:310–6.
61. Kuiper T, van den Broek FJ, van Eeden S, et al. Feasibility and Accuracy of Confocal Endomicroscopy in Comparison With Narrow-Band Imaging and Chromoendoscopy for the Differentiation of Colorectal Lesions. Am J Gastroenterol 2012;107:543–50.
62. Hasegawa S, Mitsuyama K, Kawano H, et al. Endoscopic discrimination of sessile serrated adenomas from other serrated lesions. Oncol Lett 2011;2:785–9.
63. Ullman TA, Itzkowitz SH. Intestinal inflammation and cancer. Gastroenterology 2011;140:1807–16.
64. Rubin CE, Haggitt RC, Burmer GC, et al. DNA aneuploidy in colonic biopsies predicts future development of dysplasia in ulcerative colitis. Gastroenterology 1992;103:1611–20.
65. Eaden JA, Ward BA, Mayberry JF. How gastroenterologists screen for colonic cancer in ulcerative colitis: an analysis of performance. Gastrointest Endosc 2000;51:123–8.
66. Bernstein CN, Weinstein WM, Levine DS, et al. Physicians' perceptions of dysplasia and approaches to surveillance colonoscopy in ulcerative colitis. Am J Gastroenterol 1995;90:2106–14.

67. Rutter MD. Surveillance programmes for neoplasia in colitis. J Gastroenterol 2011;46(Suppl 1):1–5.
68. Kiesslich R, Neurath MF. Chromoendoscopy: an evolving standard in surveillance for ulcerative colitis. Inflamm Bowel Dis 2004;10:695–6.
69. Hlavaty T, Huorka M, Koller T, et al. Colorectal cancer screening in patients with ulcerative and Crohn's colitis with use of colonoscopy, chromoendoscopy and confocal endomicroscopy. Eur J Gastroenterol Hepatol 2011; 23(8):680–9.
70. Kiesslich R, Fritsch J, Holtmann M, et al. Methylene blue-aided chromoendoscopy for the detection of intraepithelial neoplasia and colon cancer in ulcerative colitis. Gastroenterology 2003;124(4):880–8.
71. Hurlstone DP, McAlindon ME, Sanders DS, et al. Further validation of high-magnification chromoscopic-colonoscopy for the detection of intraepithelial neoplasia and colon cancer in ulcerative colitis. Gastroenterology 2004; 126(1):376–8.
72. Kiesslich R, Burg J, Kaina B, et al. Safety and efficacy of methylene blue-aided chromoendoscopy in ulcerative colitis: a prospective pilot study upon previous chromoendoscopies. Gastrointest Endosc 2004;59:97.
73. Travis S, Van Assche G, Dignass A, et al. On the second ECCO Consensus on Crohn's disease. J Crohns Colitis 2010;4:1–6.
74. Cairns SR, Scholefield JH, Steele RJ, et al. Guidelines for colorectal cancer screening and surveillance in moderate and high risk groups (update from 2002). Gut 2010;59:666–89.
75. Pretlow TP, Barrow BJ, Ashton WS, et al. Aberrant crypts: putative preneoplastic foci in human colonic mucosa. Cancer Res 1991;51:1564–7.
76. Roncucci L, Stamp D, Medline A, et al. Identification and quantification of aberrant crypt foci and microadenomas in the human colon. Hum Pathol 1991;22:287–94.
77. Cho NL, Redston M, Zauber AG, et al. Aberrant crypt foci in the adenoma prevention with celecoxib trial. Cancer Prev Res (Phila) 2008;1:21–31.
78. Schoen RE, Mutch M, Rall C, et al. The natural history of aberrant crypt foci. Gastrointest Endosc 2008;67:1097–102.
79. Pinsky PF, Fleshman J, Mutch M, et al. One year recurrence of aberrant crypt foci. Cancer Prev Res (Phila) 2010;3:839–43.
80. Moxon D, Raza M, Kenney R, et al. Relationship of aging and tobacco use with the development of aberrant crypt foci in a predominantly African-American population. Clin Gastroenterol Hepatol 2005;3:271–8.
81. Mutch MG, Schoen RE, Fleshman JW, et al. A multicenter study of prevalence and risk factors for aberrant crypt foci. Clin Gastroenterol Hepatol 2009;7:568–74.
82. Hurlstone DP, Karajeh M, Sanders DS, et al. Rectal aberrant crypt foci identified using high-magnification-chromoscopic colonoscopy: biomarkers for flat and depressed neoplasia. Am J Gastroenterol 2005;100:1283–9.
83. Anderson JC, Latreille M, Messina C, et al. Smokers as a high-risk group: data from a screening population. J Clin Gastroenterol 2009;43:747–52.
84. Stevens RG, Swede H, Heinen CD, et al. Aberrant crypt foci in patients with a positive family history of sporadic colorectal cancer. Cancer Lett 2007;248:262–8.
85. Swede H, Rohan TE, Yu H, et al. Number of aberrant crypt foci associated with adiposity and IGF1 bioavailability. Cancer Causes Control 2009;20:653–61.
86. Rosenberg DW, Yang S, Pleau DC, et al. Mutations in BRAF and KRAS differentially distinguish serrated versus non-serrated hyperplastic aberrant crypt foci in humans. Cancer Res 2007;67:3551–4.

87. Gupta AK, Pinsky P, Rall C, et al. Reliability and accuracy of the endoscopic appearance in the identification of aberrant crypt foci. Gastrointest Endosc 2009;70:322–30.

88. Yano Y, Konishi K, Yamochi T, et al. Clinicopathological and molecular features of colorectal serrated neoplasias with different mucosal crypt patterns. Am J Gastroenterol 2011;106:1351–8.

89. Matsumoto T, Nakamura S, Jo Y, et al. Chromoscopy might improve diagnostic accuracy in cancer surveillance for ulcerative colitis. Am J Gastroenterol 2003; 98(8):1827–33.

90. Rutter MD, Saunders BP, Schofield G, et al. Pancolonic indigo carmine dye spraying for the detection of dysplasia in ulcerative colitis. Gut 2004;53(2): 256–60.

91. Hurlstone DP, Sanders DS, Lobo AJ, et al. Indigo carmine-assisted high-magnification chromoscopic colonoscopy for the detection and characterisation of intraepithelial neoplasia in ulcerative colitis: a prospective evaluation. Endoscopy 2005;37(12):1186–92.

92. Kiesslich R, Goetz M, Lammersdorf K, et al. Chromoscopy-guided endomicroscopy increases the diagnostic yield of intraepithelial neoplasia in ulcerative colitis. Gastroenterology 2007;132(3):874–82.

93. Marion JF, Waye JD, Present DH, et al. Chromoendoscopy-targeted biopsies are superior to standard colonoscopic surveillance for detecting dysplasia in inflammatory bowel disease patients: a prospective endoscopic trial. Am J Gastroenterol 2008;103(9):2342–9.

94. Gunther U, Kusch D, Heller F, et al. Surveillance colonoscopy in patients with inflammatory bowel disease: comparison of random biopsy vs. targeted biopsy protocols. Int J Colorectal Dis 2011;26(5):667–72.

Ancillary Imaging Techniques and Adenoma Detection

Zilla H. Hussain, MD[a], Heiko Pohl, MD[a,b],*

KEYWORDS

- Colonoscopy • Screening • NBI • Electron chromoendoscopy
- Digital chromoendoscopy • Adenoma detection • FICE • iScan
- Autofluorescence imaging

KEY POINTS

- Advancements in image technology have allowed recognition of mucosal architecture in more detail and may improve adenoma detection.
- This review provides a technical overview on individual imaging technologies and their effect on detection of adenoma.
- High-definition white light endoscopy improves detection of small adenomas.
- None of the digital chromoendoscopy technologies improves adenoma detection.
- Autoimmunfluorescence imaging in conjunction with high-definition endoscopy may improve detection of small adenomas.

The effector of benefit for all colorectal cancer (CRC) screening modalities is colonoscopy with adequate detection and resection of neoplastic polyps. It is therefore neoplasia detection that determines screening efficacy. However, several studies have shown that many adenomas are missed during a colonoscopy, with an overall miss rate of approximately 20%, ranging from 6% for large ($\geq$10 mm) adenomas to 13% for small (6–9 mm) and 26% for diminutive ($\leq$5 mm) adenomas.[1–3] Missing neoplastic lesions likely represents the major contributor to the development of post-colonoscopy or so-called interval cancers in as many as 70% to 80% of patients.[4] Minimizing miss rate and improving neoplasia detection may therefore be regarded as the most important task to improve the effectiveness of CRC screening. This objective has been well recognized by gastrointestinal societies, and adenoma detection rate is considered a key quality indicator of colonoscopy.

Considerable advancements in endoscopic imaging technology may improve detection. In 1869, when Adolf Kussmaul performed the first documented upper

Disclosure: The authors have no conflicts of interest to disclose.
[a] Dartmouth-Hitchcock Medical Center, 1 Medical Center Drive, Lebanon, NH 03756, USA; [b] VA Medical Center, 215 North Main Street, White River Junction, VT 05009, USA
* Corresponding author. VA Medical Center, 215 North Main Street, White River Junction, VT 05009.
E-mail address: heiko.pohl@dartmouth.edu

Gastroenterol Clin N Am 42 (2013) 547–565
http://dx.doi.org/10.1016/j.gtc.2013.05.007
0889-8553/13/$ – see front matter Published by Elsevier Inc.

endoscopy on a sword swallower, he did not have adequate light to recognize intestinal epithelium.[5] Through integrated lenses and mirrors (Schindler-Wolf gastroscope 1932), fiber-optic bundles (Hirshowitz 1957), and camera chips with transmission of digital images, we have entered a new phase in endoscopic imaging. We have now at our disposal high-resolution endoscopes with various imaging filters, capable of postimage processing with the common goal of better recognizing intestinal disease.

In this article, the following advanced imaging technologies are discussed:

- High-definition (HD) colonoscopy
- Narrow-band imaging (NBI) (Olympus Medical Systems, Tokyo, Japan)
- Fujinon Intelligence Chromoendoscopy (FICE) (Fujinon Inc, Saitama, Japan)
- i-Scan (Pentax, Tokyo, Japan)
- Autofluorescence imaging (AFI) (Olympus Medical Systems, Tokyo, Japan)

The goal is to provide a technological update and to summarize whether and to what extent these imaging modalities improve detection of neoplastic polyps. Each section reviews the technology, summarizes studies on adenoma detection, and provides an outlook for next steps and potential areas for research.

HIGH-DEFINITION ENDOSCOPY

When camera chips replaced fiber-optic bundles, the operator was able to view video-transmitted images in real time on a monitor. Camera chips are charged coupled devices (CCD) comprising several thousands of photo cells known as picture elements (pixels). Pixel density has substantially increased in recent years. Whereas first-generation video endoscopes were equipped with 200,000-pixel CCDs, current endoscopes contain chips with 1.4 million pixels, allowing high image resolution.

Current Olympus endoscopes use 1 of 2 imaging systems.[6] In the LUCERA system (Olympus 200 series, used in Asia and the United Kingdom) light from a xenon arc lamp is filtered through a rotating broadband red-green-blue filter to produce sequential light bursts in each spectrum. The reflected red, blue, and green images are sequentially captured by a monochromatic CCD and transmitted to a video processor to create a single composite picture in full color (**Fig. 1**A).

In contrast, the EXERA system (Olympus 100 series, used in North and South America and in many European countries) uses full-spectrum white light (WL) from a xenon lamp. The light is reflected off the mucosa and passes through a color filter mounted over the CCD. The filter selectively assigns each wavelength to a particular pixel, hence creating an image on the CCD surface. The image is then processed and displayed (see **Fig. 1**B).

To enhance image acquisition and processing, high-resolution images can be shown on HD monitors. The standard broadcasting systems (PAL [phase alternating line] and NTSC [National Television Standard Committee]) generate approximately 48 to 576 scanning lines on a screen, whereas the new HD monitors generate up to 1080 scanning lines. These HD endoscopy systems (high-resolution endoscopy combined with HD screens) therefore allow examination of the mucosal architecture in the gastrointestinal tract.

Summary of Studies on High-Definition Colonoscopy and Adenoma Detection

Because HD colonoscopy shows mucosal surface in greater detail, it is plausible that it may improve neoplasia detection. Of 8 published studies (**Table 1**) 3 were randomized controlled trials (RCTs) and 2 did not shown a significant benefit[7,8]; however, both RCTs seem to have been underpowered. For instance a clinically meaningful

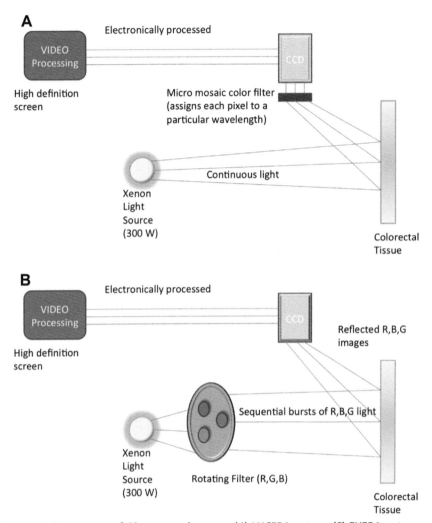

Fig. 1. Imaging systems of Olympus endoscopes: (*A*) LUCERA system. (*B*) EXERA system.

improvement in adenoma detection rate (ADR) from 50% to 58% with HD in the study by Tribonias and colleagues[8] was not statistically significant. A third randomized trial by Rastogi and colleagues[9] found an improved ADR from 39% to 46%, but again this was not significant (*P* = .17). This study found a significant increase of flat adenomas (9% vs 2%, *P* = .01) and right-sided adenomas (34% vs 19%, *P* = .01), but there was no benefit of HD for detection of advanced adenomas.

The remaining 5 studies had different designs. Two were prospective,[10,11] and 3 retrospective.[12–14] Only 1 study examined non-Olympus colonoscopes, and compared an HD Fujinon with a standard-definition (SD) Pentax colonoscope.[14] This study did not find a difference in adenoma detection. Despite a nonrandomized design, all studies attempted to compare groups that were similar to each other. For instance, one of the retrospective studies by Burke and colleagues[13] compared 852 patients who were assigned to different scopes by availability. In this study, HD colonoscopes did not improve adenoma detection. Another retrospective study by Buchner and

Table 1
Studies that compared adenoma detection with HD colonoscopy with standard-definition (SD) colonoscopy

Study	Method	Endoscopist (Center)	Patients	Population	ADR (%)			Mean Number of Adenomas per Patient		
					HD	SD	P	HD	SD	P
HD										
Pellise et al,[7] 2008	RCT	7 (1)	620	Average	26	25	.96	0.45	0.43	.87
Tribonias et al,[8] 2010	RCT	1 (1)	300	Average	58	50	.16	1.4	1.1	.10
Rastogi et al,[9,a] 2011	RCT	6 (2)	420	Average	46	39	.17	1.13	0.69	.02
East et al,[10] 2008	Prospective nonrandomized	1 (1)	130	Average	71	60	.20	1.6	1.2	n.s.
Adler et al,[11] 2012	Prospective nonrandomized	27 (23)	1656	Average	22	18	<.01	0.33	0.27	<.01
Buchner et al,[12] 2010	Retrospective	18 (1)	2430	Average	29	24	.02	0.51	0.44	.01
Burke et al,[13] 2010	Retrospective	Multiple (1)	852	Average	25	22	.36	0.4	0.3	.13
Erim et al,[14] 2011	Retrospective (HD Fujinon vs SD Pentax)	3 (1)	900	Average	19	18	.56	0.41	0.42	.82

Average: Average-risk patients, who presented for a colonoscopy for screening, surveillance, or because of symptoms.
Abbreviations: ADR, adenoma detection rate (patients with ≥1 adenoma/all patients); n.s., not significant.
[a] 3 arms: HD, NBI, and SD (see **Table 2**).

colleagues[12] analyzed more than 1400 patients who were assigned to rooms with or without HD scopes. In this study, HD colonoscopy increased overall ADR from 24% to 29% ($P = .02$), but it did not improve detection of advanced adenomas. Similar results were reported by Adler and colleagues,[11] in a large prospective study from Germany, which compared 1256 patients from 5 clinical practices equipped with HD colonoscopes with 1400 patients from 18 practices using older SD colonoscopes. HD increased ADR from 18% to 22% ($P<.01$), with a marginally significant increase in detection of adenomas with high-grade dysplasia from 0.6% to 1.2% ($P = .06$).

Although nonrandomized, the major strength of these studies is the large sample size and the participation of multiple endoscopists, which reflects how these new colonoscopes fare in clinical practice. A recent meta-analysis[15] systematically summarized 5 of the discussed studies. HD colonoscopy improved ADR in pooled analysis by 3.5% (95% confidence interval [CI] 0.9–6.1), largely related to an increased detection of diminutive adenomas. When also considering studies that were not included in the meta-analysis, the gain in ADR with HD would be even greater (crude increase of 4.4%).

The HD colonoscopes also come with an increased visual angle from 140° with prior Olympus scopes to 170° with HD scopes. Although it seems plausible that the increased angle may enhance adenoma detection, 3 studies that have examined wide-angle colonoscopy[16–18] did not find that it improved adenoma detection.

High-Definition Colonoscopy: Summary and Outlook

Studies on HD colonoscopy showed the following main results:

1. HD endoscopy improves adenoma detection.
2. The increased adenoma detection is related to an improved detection of small adenomas. It does not improve detection of large or advanced lesions.

It may be argued that the reported increase in ADR is marginal. However, the approximate 4% absolute increase translates to a relative increase of 16% (from 28% to 33%). When we consider an adenoma miss rate of 20%,[1–3] an increased adenoma detection by 16% with HD colonoscopy seems relevant.

Most endoscopy units have moved to HD systems and the next generation of HD endoscopy has been introduced. Although it is important to continue to assess whether they improve adenoma detection, studies should also examine whether higher-resolution colonoscopes might help to better recognize sessile serrated adenomas/polyps.

DIGITAL CHROMOENDOSCOPY

Light absorption and reflection are dependent on mucosal characteristics. Selecting certain wavelengths of reflected light or image processing may therefore contrast neoplastic from nonneoplastic tissue. Resultant images appear in a different color reminiscent of chromoendoscopy, therefore these electronically modified imaging modalities are also called electronic, virtual, or digital chromoendoscopy. Available systems differ in their technology, but result in a similar effect: enhancement of mucosal contrast. NBI filters light before image processing. In contrast, FICE and i-Scan manipulate light using postprocessing computer algorithms.

NBI

Conventional WL endoscopy uses the entire spectrum of visible light (400–700 nm) and allows viewing of mucosa in its natural color.[19] NBI (Olympus) uses a light filter to achieve an increased proportion of blue light (that allows its passage) and a decreased proportion of red light (that does not allow its passage) (**Fig. 2**). Therefore, it narrows standard WL to a bandwidth of blue light (390–445 nm) and green light (530–550 nm). This narrowed band spectrum corresponds to the main peaks on the absorption spectrum of hemoglobin; it is preferentially absorbed by hemoglobin and appears dark (not reflected), thus enhancing tissue microvasculature from its surrounding. In addition, the shorter wavelength of blue light has a more shallow tissue penetration than the longer wavelength of red light. Therefore, NBI enhances structures in the surface, especially those with hemoglobin content. Because adenomas have an increased vascular density and abnormal vascular pattern, NBI should help to improve detection of adenomatous polyps.

Studies on NBI and Adenoma Detection

At least 11 fully published randomized studies have examined whether NBI improves detection of adenoma or decreases the adenoma miss rate when compared with high definition white light (HDWL), either in average-risk screening and surveillance populations[9,17,20–26] or in higher-risk individuals (**Table 2**).[27,28] The fact that at least 5 meta-analyses have been published on the subject highlights the interest in understanding whether NBI increases adenoma detection. The most recent is a Cochrane meta-analysis,[29] which also includes 3 studies published only as an abstract. The overall results are clear: NBI does not improve adenoma detection and does not decrease the adenoma miss rate. In fact, none of the studies found a significant benefit of NBI compared with HDWL. One of the initial studies suggested that the use of NBI may assist in learning to better recognize adenomas with WL.[21] The investigators observed an increasing ADR with WL during the study period. However, this was not supported by later studies. For instance, Rex and Helbig[17] reported a very high ADR (66%) with

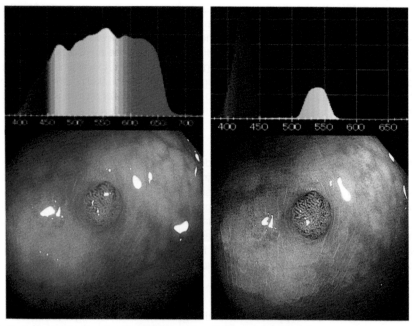

Fig. 2. Adenomatous polyp in HDWL imaging (*left*) and NBI (*right*).

Table 2
Studies that compared adenoma detection HD NBI colonoscopy with HDWL colonoscopy

Study	Method	Endoscopist (Center)	Patients	Population	ADR (%)			Mean Number of Adenomas per Patient		
					NBI	WL	P	NBI	WL	P
Rex & Helbig,[17] 2007	RCT	1 (1)	434	Average	65	67	.61	1.9	1.8	.68
Inoue et al,[22] 2008	RCT	6 (1)	243	Average	42	34	.20	0.84	0.54	<.05
Adler et al,[21] 2008	RCT	7 (1)	401	Average	23	17	.13	0.33	0.26	.12
Adler et al,[20] 2009	RCT	6 (5)	1256	Average	22	22	n.s.	0.32	0.34	n.s.
Paggi et al,[27] 2009	RCT	6 (1)	211	High risk[a]	57	58	.88	1.95	1.83	.69
Pisello et al,[23] 2009	RCT	– (1)	120	Average	n.a.	n.a.		0.85	0.82	
Sabbagh et al,[24] 2011	RCT	3 (2)	482	Average	n.a.	n.a.		0.19	0.20	n.s.
Rastogi et al,[9] 2011	RCT[b]	6 (2)	443	Average	46	46	n.s.	1.13	1.12	n.s.
East et al,[28] 2012	RCT	3 (1)	214	High risk[c]	73	66	.30	2	1.8	.42
Kaltenbach et al,[26] 2008	RCT-tandem (nonblinded)	6 (1)	276	Average	50	44	.29	1.1	0.87	n.s.
Ikematsu et al,[25] 2012	RCT-tandem (nonblinded)[d]	27 (6)	782	Average	42	42	.67	0.79	0.79	.98

Average: average-risk patients, who presented for a colonoscopy for screening, surveillance, or because of symptoms.

Abbreviations: ADR, adenoma detection rate (patients with ≥1 adenoma/all patients); n.a., not assessed; n.s., not significant.

[a] Positive fecal immune-chemistry testing.

[b] 3 arms: HD, NBI, and SD (see **Table 1**).

[c] Positive fecal occult blood test, personal history of CRC or advanced adenoma.

[d] Study included the examination of only the right colon (proximal to splenic flexure).

either technology in a study by a single endoscopist. Such ADR in an average screening population was unprecedented and was higher than historical controls by the same endoscopist. The investigators speculate that it is not NBI alone, but rather HD imaging (with or without NBI) that improves adenoma detection. The benefit seems to be in finding more small and diminutive adenomas, which is also supported by studies comparing HD with SD colonoscopy (as discussed earlier). NBI did seem to improve the detection of flat adenomas in 2 studies,[27,28] but showed a lower flat ADR in a third study.[20] No effect was seen in the detection of small adenomas or advanced adenomas, or with respect to location in the colon. Some studies have noted a longer withdrawal time with NBI, yet no difference in adenoma detection,[17,20,23] indicating that WL viewing was dominant over NBI (same number of adenomas in a shorter time).

Few studies have measured the miss rate using a tandem colonoscopy design. Of the 2 fully published studies, Kaltenbach and colleagues[26] did not find a difference, with a miss rate of 12% using NBI and 13% using WL. A larger study by Ikematsu and colleagues[25] reported a significantly lower miss rate (21 vs 28%), which was attributed to improved detection of small adenomas. However, this study limited its NBI examination to the right colon. A much smaller study of 22 patients with hereditary nonpolyposis colorectal cancer also detected a lower miss rate with NBI when compared with WL (0% vs 30%).[30] One meta-analysis[31] systematically reviewed studies regarding miss rates, included 2 studies published in abstract form. This analysis did not find that NBI significantly decreases the adenoma miss rate, with a summary odds ratio of 0.65 (95% CI 0.40–1.06).

NBI: Summary and Outlook

Studies on HD NBI colonoscopy showed the following main results:

1. HD NBI colonoscopy does not improve adenoma detection or decrease adenoma miss rate when compared with HDWL colonoscopy.
2. The new-generation endoscopes with combined NBI and HD capabilities seem to achieve a higher adenoma detection than previous standard-definition white light (SDWL) systems.

The latter fact is interesting for 2 reasons. First, it suggests that the overall adenoma miss rate of 20% that was assumed primarily based on tandem colonoscopy studies[1–3] may be too low. This suggestion also explains why some studies found a higher miss rate in the control group between 28% and 49%.[25,30,32] Second, HD NBI colonoscopes allow the detection of more small adenomas in average-risk patients, hence increasing the pool of adenoma-bearing patients who would require a surveillance colonoscopy by current guidelines.[33]

FICE

FICE applies so-called computerized spectral estimation to the conventional endoscopic image. It takes the original image and arithmetically processes it to a dedicated wavelength of light. There are 10 preprogrammed FICE filters or settings that can be switched on the keyboard, each of which has a different setting for estimated red, green, and blue wavelengths (**Fig. 3**).

The concept is based on the fact that minute details of superficial patterns and color differences depend on the characteristics of light diffusion and absorption. Image colors vary as different wavelengths are applied (eg, shorter wavelengths for surface structures and longer for underlying blood vessels).

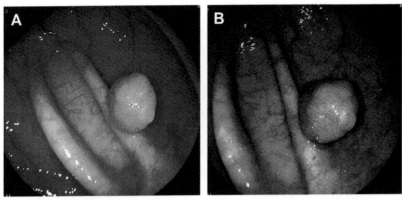

Fig. 3. Adenomatous polyp with HDWL (*A*) and FICE (*B*). (with special thanks to Alireza Aminalai, MD, F.E.B.G. Berlin, Germany.)

Studies on FICE and Adenoma Detection

Table 3 summarizes published randomized trials.[34–37] Only 1 study[35] showed an increased adenoma detection with FICE. This small study enrolled 128 patients and was conducted by a single endoscopist. The overall ADR was not significantly different (49% with FICE and 35% with WL), but FICE found significantly more diminutive adenomas (44% vs 22%). Despite randomization, the FICE groups included more men and had a higher proportion of nonscreening procedures, suggesting a possible higher adenoma risk for the FICE group. Two large multiendoscopist studies from Germany[37,38] did not show a benefit of using FICE over WL for adenoma detection. Pohl and Ell[38] enrolled 764 patients at 5 medical centers and found an almost identical ADR with FICE (36%) or WL (35%). The study by Aminalai and colleagues[37] reported similar results in a different setting. A total of 1318 patients were enrolled in 6 private gastroenterology practices. The ADR with FICE was not significantly different from WL (20.2% vs 16.5%), and both modalities detected a similar mean number of adenomas per patient (0.28). A large study by Chang and colleagues[36] followed a randomized tandem design. In addition to a similar ADR in both groups, these investigators did not find a lower miss rate (6.6% for FICE and 8.3% with WL). None of the studies showed any benefit for detection of advanced neoplasia.

FICE: Summary and Outlook

Studies on HD FICE colonoscopy showed the following main results:

1. FICE colonoscopy does not improve adenoma detection or decrease adenoma miss rate.

Although there have been only a few studies, 3 were of high quality (large, multiple centers/endoscopists) and the overall negative results are conclusive. All studies have used a similar FICE setting (mode 4 or D); however, some investigators argue that it may be worthwhile to investigate whether other settings may provide improved polyp recognition. Some of these studies have also examined the accuracy of real-time polyp prediction, with promising results, and similar to other digital chromoendoscopy modalities, this may be a niche for its application. Further study of adenoma detection using FICE does not seem warranted.

Table 3
Studies that compared adenoma detection with FICE with HDWL colonoscopy

Study	Method	Endoscopist (Center)	Patients, n	Population	ADR (%)			Mean Number of Adenomas per Patient		
					FICE	WL	P	FICE	WL	P
Pohl et al,[52] 2009	RCT	15 (5)	764	Average[a]	36	35	1.0	0.64	0.68	.92
Aminalai et al,[37] 2010	RCT	8 (6)	1318	Average	20	16	.09	0.28	0.28	.95
Chung et al,[53] 2010	RCT-tandem	5 (1)	359	Average	34	30	.74	0.64	0.55	.65
Cha et al,[35] 2010	RCT	1 (1)	128	Average	49	35	.12	0.68	0.69	.43

Abbreviation: ADR, adenoma detection rate (patients with ≥1 adenoma/all patients).
[a] Average: patients presenting for a colonoscopy for screening, surveillance, or because of symptoms.

Table 4
Studies that compared adenoma detection with i-Scan with HDWL colonoscopy

Study	Method	Endoscopist (Center)	Patients (n)	Population	ADR (%)			Mean Number of Adenomas per Patient		
					i-Scan	WL	P	i-Scan	WL	P
Hong et al,[39] 2012	RCT-tandem	3 (1)	389	Average	36[a] 33[b]	32	.74	0.63[a] 0.16[b]	0.54	n.s.
Hoffman et al,[40] 2010	RCT	6 (1)	200	Average	38[c]	13	<.01	0.8[c]	0.16	<.01

Abbreviations: ADR, adenoma detection rate (patients with ≥1 adenoma/all patients); n.s., not significant.
[a] Mode that combines surface enhancement 2+ and contrast enhancement 2+.
[b] Mode that combines mode[a] with tone enhancement.
[c] Mode of surface enhancement 4+.

i-SCAN

i-Scan combines high-resolution endoscopy with 3 adjustable modes of image enhancement[39]: (1) surface enhancement of a lesion through recognition of the edges, (2) contrast enhancement of depressed areas and of differences in structure through color representation, and (3) tone enhancement tailored to individual organs. These enhancement features are similar to NBI, which analyzes individual red, green, and blue components of a normal range and combines the color frequencies to show minute mucosal details with subtle color changes (**Fig. 4**).

Studies on i-Scan and Adenoma Detection

Only 2 studies have examined the effect of i-Scan on adenoma detection (**Table 4**). Both studies have applied a different image mode. The initial study by Hoffman and colleagues[40] used a surface enhancing setting, whereas the second study by Hong used a combination between surface and vascular enhancing modes.[39] The former compared HD-i-Scan with SDWL and found a significant improvement in ADR (38% vs 13%). i-Scan also detected significantly more adenomas per patient (0.80 vs 0.13) and a higher rate of flat adenomas. Such a large difference is unexpected and is likely partly caused by the low ADR in the control group. Although both groups had similar baseline characteristics, it is still possible that the adenoma prevalence in each group was different, otherwise a miss rate far beyond 50% in the control group would have to be assumed. An alternative explanation for such a difference may be related to the unblinded design of the study. In contrast, the second study did not find an improved adenoma detection with i-Scan. The tandem design allowed evaluation of the miss rate, which was not significantly different between both imaging modalities. Both studies were limited by a small sample size. A third retrospective study report a higher rate of mucosal lesions with HD-i-Scan compared with SDWL but failed to report on detection of neoplastic lesions.

i-Scan: Summary and Outlook

Studies on i-Scan colonoscopy showed the following main results:

1. Based on the limited available data, it is unclear whether i-Scan improves adenoma detection or decreases adenoma miss rates.

Although more studies should be performed, the lack of benefit with other contrast-enhancing modalities makes it less likely that postprocessing imaging modification with i-Scan would lead to improved adenoma detection.

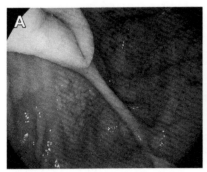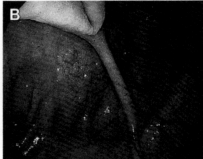

Fig. 4. Adenomatous polyp with HDWL (*A*) and i-Scan (*B*). (with special thanks to Klaus Mönkemüller, MD, Birmingham, AL, USA)

AUTOFLUORESCENCE IMAGING

The human colon contains naturally fluorescent molecules. Some light energy that enters the colonic mucosa is absorbed and excites electrons to a higher energy level. When returning to the ground state, light is emitted (fluorescence) dependent on tissue and its fluorescent characteristics. Neoplastic lesions are less autofluorescent because of a different distribution of collagen, increased mucosal thickness, and glandular density.[22]

Endoscopes that are capable of recognizing autofluorescence have a special CCD chip in addition to the WL chip (AFI). These chips can easily be switched by pushing a button on the scope handle. A real-time autofluorescent pseudocolored image is produced from images after blue light excitation (395–475 nm), combined with green reflectance (540–560 nm) alone (see trimodal imaging system) or in combination with red reflectance (600–620 nm) (8). Colorectal neoplastic lesions for instance are shown as purple. These lesions contrast with green-appearing normal colonic mucosa (**Fig. 5**).

Studies on AFI and Adenoma Detection

Five studies have examined whether AFI improves adenoma detection (**Table 5**). All studies used a tandem colonoscopy design. Outcomes were expressed as miss rates with AFI compared with WL. A large study by Kuiper and colleagues[41] compared AFI followed by HDWL with back to back HDWL. AFI detected 28% additional adenomas, similar to HDWL 29%. Similarly, van den Broeck and colleagues[42] did not find a significantly different miss rate (AFI 20%, HDWL 29%, $P = .351$). In contrast, a significantly greater adenoma detection with AFI was suggested by 2 other studies. The single-endoscopist study by Matsuda and colleagues[43] reported a lower miss rate with AFI compared with HDWL (29% vs 47%). A smaller study with 75 high-risk patients[44] reported a miss rate of 8% with AFI versus 32% with WL. Additional adenomas were more likely small and located in the proximal colon. A small nonrandomized study that only looked at the effect of AFI in the rectosigmoid colon found a lower miss rate, but the difference was exclusively attributed to examinations performed by less experienced endoscopists (ADR of 5.9%).[45] The small sample size in some of the studies is a major limitation. A meta-analysis may overcome such limitation, but this has not been performed.

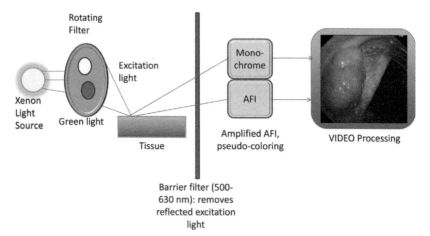

Fig. 5. AFI.

Table 5
Studies that compared adenoma detection and miss rate with AFI and WL colonoscopy

Study	Method	Endoscopist (Center)	Patients	Population	ADR with First Pass (%)			Adenoma Miss Rate		
					AFI	WL	P	AFI	WL	P
AFI										
Kuiper et al,[41] 2011	RCT-tandem (nonblinded), HDWL-AFI vs HDWL-HDWL	8 (6)	234	Average	36	39	n.s.	29	28	n.s.
van den Broek et al,[42] 2009	RCT-tandem (nonblinded), AFI-HDWL vs HDWL-AFI	3 (1)	100	Average	28[a]	38[a]	n.s.	24[a]	27[a]	.35
Matsuda et al,[43] 2008	RCT-tandem (nonblinded), AFI-HDWL vs HDWL-AFI	1 (1)	167	Average	–	–	–	29	47	.02
Ramsoekh et al,[44] 2010	RCT-tandem (blinded), AFI-SDWL vs SDWL-AFI	2 (1)	75	High risk[b]	–	–	–	8	32	<.01
Moriichi et al,[45] 2012	Nonrandomized tandem (blinded), HDWL-AFI[c]	8 (1)	88	Average	26	18	<.05	3	28	<.05

Abbreviations: ADR, adenoma detection rate (patients with ≥1 adenoma/all patients); n.s., not significant; SDWL, standard-definition white light.
[a] Includes sessile serrated adenomas/polyps.
[b] High-risk patients: Lynch syndrome or families with familial CRC.
[c] Study limited to examination of the rectosigmoid colon.

AFI: Summary and Outlook

Studies on HD AFI colonoscopy showed the following main results:

1. AFI in conjunction with HDWL seems to improve adenoma detection.
2. An increase in adenoma detection is related to an improved detection of small adenomas.

Because of limited data from (in part) small studies, no final conclusions can be drawn. The results suggest that it is worthwhile engaging in larger studies, performed by multiple endoscopists in average-risk patients, with special attention to flat right-sided polyps. Such studies should also address practicality. Considering that AFI is beneficial, how would the ideal examination be performed? A combination of AFI plus WL should probably be compared with WL only to reflect clinical practice.[41] AFI seems to require increased examination time because of frequent switching between imaging modalities to distinguish neoplasia from remaining stool material, which appears in the same color. Therefore, future studies should also address possible challenges for clinical practice. However, AFI remains experimental, because the colonoscopes with trimodal imaging are all prototypes based on the LUCERA system (Olympus 200 series) and are not commercially available.

SUMMARY

Although digital chromoendoscopy enhances mucosal contrast and allows examination of intestinal disease in greater detail, it does not improve adenoma detection or decrease adenoma miss rate. There is conclusive evidence that neither NBI nor FICE significantly improves adenoma detection. Data on i-Scan are still limited; however, the lack of benefit with NBI and FICE make it doubtful that a different contrast-enhancing technology would improve detection of adenomas. In contrast to imaging processing modalities, tissue autofluorescence may improve adenoma detection and decrease miss rates. Data on AFI are still limited, and the trimodal imaging endoscopes (including NBI ability) are available only as prototypes as part of the LUCERA system (Olympus 200 series). Given that AFI requires a longer examination time (because of frequent switching between AFI and WL), future studies should also consider application in clinical practice.

One possible explanation of the lack of benefit is that the new-generation endoscopes not only provide digital chromoendoscopy, but all come with integrated high-resolution imaging and HD monitors. Studies that only compared HD with SDWL colonoscopy showed an overall 4% improved adenoma detection, representing a relative increase of 16%. HD imaging alone seems to be accurate, and the addition of digital chromoendoscopy may not further improve recognition of neoplastic lesions.

Studies on advanced imaging share similar limitations. Clearly, retrospective studies are inherently flawed by selection bias. Even RCTs may lead to different study cohorts, especially if the number of subjects is small. Further, studies that are performed by 1 endoscopist, and to a lesser extent at 1 center, are also prone to bias, especially if blinding to various imaging modalities is difficult or impossible. The most rigorous design to study ADR or miss rate is a tandem design with a second endoscopist, who is blinded to the first pass. There are few such studies.

Many studies seem to be underpowered to show a clinically relevant difference as significant. Sample size calculations should be based on an expected improvement in adenoma detection. Tandem colonoscopy studies suggest an overall miss rate of

20%.[1-3] Studies designed to examine adenoma detection should therefore not expect a higher gain. Even if considering a 20% increased detection, a typical RCT would require at least 800 participants (approximately half for a tandem design). It would therefore be helpful if other outcome measures to assess quality of colon inspection were developed, for instance an objective assessment of the colonic surface.[46]

Some technical aspects may account for disappointing results. Electronic image alteration changes the color of the viewed mucosa, which may reduce brightness of the image, especially when surveying a larger area of the colonic lumen. Remaining intestinal fluid may also appear darker and impair the view to a greater extent than with light. Optimal use of digital chromoendoscopy may require an even more pristine colon cleansing than with WL.

The higher yield described in adenoma detection with HD imaging seems primarily related to the detection of lower-risk diminutive adenomas (adenomas with a less than 0.1% risk of prevalent cancer and a low risk of transition to cancer).[4,47,48] Although the pool of adenoma-bearing patients increases, the overall disease burden of CRC in the population does not. Put differently, we find more abnormalities that likely do not matter. From a different perspective, finding more adenomas is associated with a lower risk of interval cancers.[49] Therefore a high ADR, including those of small lesions, can be seen as a surrogate marker for high-quality colonoscopy, and is therefore recommended to be tracked as a main quality indicator.[50]

All studies focused on the detection of adenomatous polyps. More recently, sessile serrated adenomas/polyps have been implicated as neoplastic lesions following a different pathway to cancer.[51] These lesions are more subtle than adenomatous polyps, and digital chromoendoscopy may not enhance contrast between these lesions and surrounding mucosa, although there is some suggestion of increased recognition with NBI.[30] As more is learned about the clinical relevance of sessile serrated adenomas/polyps, future studies on improving detection of these lesions may be worthwhile.

Imaging modalities may perform differently depending on operator experience. Therefore, these technologies may be beneficial as a learning tool,[21] and may aid trainees and less experienced gastroenterologists to better discriminate neoplasia from normal tissue. However, once the maximum benefit of improved imaging is reached (similar to a ceiling effect), technique combined with a meticulous examination likely remain the most important components for adequate neoplasia detection.

Research Questions:
- Does AFI improve neoplasia detection and decrease neoplasia miss rate?
- Do digital chromoendoscopy imaging modalities (NBI, FICE, i-Scan, AFI) improve detection of sessile serrated adenomas/polyps?
- Can digital chromoendoscopy aid trainees to recognize neoplasia?
- Can digital chromoendoscopy decrease variation in neoplasia detection between endoscopists?

Rapidly evolving imaging technology has introduced a series of improvements in endoscopic imaging. HD colonoscopy systems allow minute examination of normal and abnormal intestinal mucosa. This development has improved detection of adenoma, predominantly of smaller lesions. However, the addition of digital chromoendoscopy to HD imaging has not been shown to improve detection of adenomas. Future studies should focus on the detection of sessile serrated adenomas/polyps and examine whether and how imaging technology may decrease variation in detection of neoplasia across endoscopists.

REFERENCES

1. van Rijn JC, Reitsma JB, Stoker J, et al. Polyp miss rate determined by tandem colonoscopy: a systematic review. Am J Gastroenterol 2006;101(2):343–50.
2. Pickhardt PJ, Choi JR, Hwang I, et al. Computed tomographic virtual colonoscopy to screen for colorectal neoplasia in asymptomatic adults. N Engl J Med 2003;349(23):2191–200.
3. Pickhardt PJ, Nugent PA, Mysliwiec PA, et al. Location of adenomas missed by optical colonoscopy. Ann Intern Med 2004;141(5):352–9.
4. Pohl H, Robertson DJ. Colorectal cancers detected after colonoscopy frequently result from missed lesions. Clin Gastroenterol Hepatol 2010;8(10): 858–64.
5. Modlin IM. A brief history of endoscopy. Milan (Italy): MultiMed; 2000.
6. Rey JF, Tanaka S, Lambert R, et al. Evaluation of the clinical outcomes associated with EXERA II and LUCERA endoscopes. Dig Endosc 2009;21(Suppl 1): S113–20.
7. Pellise M, Fernandez-Esparrach G, Cardenas A, et al. Impact of wide-angle, high-definition endoscopy in the diagnosis of colorectal neoplasia: a randomized controlled trial. Gastroenterology 2008;135(4):1062–8.
8. Tribonias G, Theodoropoulou A, Konstantinidis K, et al. Comparison of standard vs high-definition, wide-angle colonoscopy for polyp detection: a randomized controlled trial. Colorectal Dis 2010;12(10 Online):e260–6.
9. Rastogi A, Early DS, Gupta N, et al. Randomized, controlled trial of standard-definition white-light, high-definition white-light, and narrow-band imaging colonoscopy for the detection of colon polyps and prediction of polyp histology. Gastrointest Endosc 2011;74(3):593–602.
10. East JE, Stavrindis M, Thomas-Gibson S, et al. A comparative study of standard vs. high definition colonoscopy for adenoma and hyperplastic polyp detection with optimized withdrawal technique. Aliment Pharmacol Ther 2008;28(6):768–76.
11. Adler A, Aminalai A, Aschenbeck J, et al. Latest generation, wide-angle, high-definition colonoscopes increase adenoma detection rate. Clin Gastroenterol Hepatol 2012;10(2):155–9.
12. Buchner AM, Shahid MW, Heckman MG, et al. High-definition colonoscopy detects colorectal polyps at a higher rate than standard white-light colonoscopy. Clin Gastroenterol Hepatol 2010;8(4):364–70.
13. Burke CA, Choure AG, Sanaka MR, et al. A comparison of high-definition versus conventional colonoscopes for polyp detection. Dig Dis Sci 2010;55(6):1716–20.
14. Erim T, Rivas JM, Velis E, et al. Role of high definition colonoscopy in colorectal adenomatous polyp detection. World J Gastroenterol 2011;17(35):4001–6.
15. Subramanian V, Mannath J, Hawkey CJ, et al. High definition colonoscopy vs. standard video endoscopy for the detection of colonic polyps: a meta-analysis. Endoscopy 2011;43(6):499–505.
16. Fatima H, Rex DK, Rothstein R, et al. Cecal insertion and withdrawal times with wide-angle versus standard colonoscopes: a randomized controlled trial. Clin Gastroenterol Hepatol 2008;6(1):109–14.
17. Rex DK, Helbig CC. High yields of small and flat adenomas with high-definition colonoscopes using either white light or narrow band imaging. Gastroenterology 2007;133(1):42–7.
18. Deenadayalu VP, Chadalawada V, Rex DK. 170 degrees wide-angle colonoscope: effect on efficiency and miss rates. Am J Gastroenterol 2004;99(11): 2138–42.

19. Song LM, Adler DG, Conway JD, et al. Narrow band imaging and multiband imaging. Gastrointest Endosc 2008;67(4):581–9.
20. Adler A, Aschenbeck J, Yenerim T, et al. Narrow-band versus white-light high definition television endoscopic imaging for screening colonoscopy: a prospective randomized trial. Gastroenterology 2009;136(2):410–416.e1 [quiz: 715].
21. Adler A, Pohl H, Papanikolaou IS, et al. A prospective randomised study on narrow-band imaging versus conventional colonoscopy for adenoma detection: does narrow-band imaging induce a learning effect? Gut 2008;57(1):59–64.
22. Inoue T, Murano M, Murano N, et al. Comparative study of conventional colonoscopy and pan-colonic narrow-band imaging system in the detection of neoplastic colonic polyps: a randomized, controlled trial. J Gastroenterol 2008; 43(1):45–50.
23. Pisello F, Geraci G, Arnone E, et al. Endoscopic surveillance of colon-rectum in the narrow band imaging era. G Chir 2009;30(10):440–4 [in Italian].
24. Sabbagh LC, Reveiz L, Aponte D, et al. Narrow-band imaging does not improve detection of colorectal polyps when compared to conventional colonoscopy: a randomized controlled trial and meta-analysis of published studies. BMC Gastroenterol 2011;11:100.
25. Ikematsu H, Saito Y, Tanaka S, et al. The impact of narrow band imaging for colon polyp detection: a multicenter randomized controlled trial by tandem colonoscopy. J Gastroenterol 2012;47(10):1099–107.
26. Kaltenbach T, Friedland S, Soetikno R. A randomised tandem colonoscopy trial of narrow band imaging versus white light examination to compare neoplasia miss rates. Gut 2008;57(10):1406–12.
27. Paggi S, Radaelli F, Amato A, et al. The impact of narrow band imaging in screening colonoscopy: a randomized controlled trial. Clin Gastroenterol Hepatol 2009;7(10):1049–54.
28. East JE, Ignjatovic A, Suzuki N, et al. A randomized, controlled trial of narrow-band imaging vs high-definition white light for adenoma detection in patients at high risk of adenomas. Colorectal Dis 2012;14(11):e771–8.
29. Nagorni A, Bjelakovic G, Petrovic B. Narrow band imaging versus conventional white light colonoscopy for the detection of colorectal polyps. Cochrane Database Syst Rev 2012;(1):CD008361.
30. Boparai KS, van den Broek FJ, van Eeden S, et al. Increased polyp detection using narrow band imaging compared with high resolution endoscopy in patients with hyperplastic polyposis syndrome. Endoscopy 2011;43(8):676–82.
31. Pasha SF, Leighton JA, Das A, et al. Comparison of the yield and miss rate of narrow band imaging and white light endoscopy in patients undergoing screening or surveillance colonoscopy: a meta-analysis. Am J Gastroenterol 2012;107(3):363–70 [quiz: 371].
32. Gross SA, Buchner AM, Crook JE, et al. A comparison of high definition-image enhanced colonoscopy and standard white-light colonoscopy for colorectal polyp detection. Endoscopy 2011;43(12):1045–51.
33. Lieberman DA, Rex DK, Winawer SJ, et al. Guidelines for colonoscopy surveillance after screening and polypectomy: a consensus update by the US Multi-Society Task Force on colorectal cancer. Gastroenterology 2012;143(3): 844–57.
34. Pohl J, Lotterer E, Balzer C, et al. Computed virtual chromoendoscopy versus standard colonoscopy with targeted indigocarmine chromoscopy: a randomised multicentre trial. Gut 2009;58(1):73–8.

35. Cha JM, Lee JI, Joo KR, et al. A prospective randomized study on computed virtual chromoendoscopy versus conventional colonoscopy for the detection of small colorectal adenomas. Dig Dis Sci 2010;55(8):2357–64.

36. Chang CC, Hsieh CR, Lou HY, et al. Comparative study of conventional colonoscopy, magnifying chromoendoscopy, and magnifying narrow-band imaging systems in the differential diagnosis of small colonic polyps between trainee and experienced endoscopist. Int J Colorectal Dis 2009;24(12):1413–9.

37. Aminalai A, Rosch T, Aschenbeck J, et al. Live image processing does not increase adenoma detection rate during colonoscopy: a randomized comparison between FICE and conventional imaging (Berlin Colonoscopy Project 5, BECOP-5). Am J Gastroenterol 2010;105(11):2383–8.

38. Pohl J, Ell C. Impact of virtual chromoendoscopy at colonoscopy: the final requiem for conventional histopathology? Gastrointest Endosc 2009;69(3 Pt 2):723–5.

39. Hong SN, Choe WH, Lee JH, et al. Prospective, randomized, back-to-back trial evaluating the usefulness of i-SCAN in screening colonoscopy. Gastrointest Endosc 2012;75(5):1011–21.e2.

40. Hoffman A, Sar F, Goetz M, et al. High definition colonoscopy combined with i-Scan is superior in the detection of colorectal neoplasias compared with standard video colonoscopy: a prospective randomized controlled trial. Endoscopy 2010;42(10):827–33.

41. Kuiper T, van den Broek FJ, Naber AH, et al. Endoscopic trimodal imaging detects colonic neoplasia as well as standard video endoscopy. Gastroenterology 2011;140(7):1887–94.

42. van den Broek FJ, Fockens P, Van Eeden S, et al. Clinical evaluation of endoscopic trimodal imaging for the detection and differentiation of colonic polyps. Clin Gastroenterol Hepatol 2009;7(3):288–95.

43. Matsuda T, Saito Y, Fu KI, et al. Does autofluorescence imaging videoendoscopy system improve the colonoscopic polyp detection rate?–a pilot study. Am J Gastroenterol 2008;103(8):1926–32.

44. Ramsoekh D, Haringsma J, Poley JW, et al. A back-to-back comparison of white light video endoscopy with autofluorescence endoscopy for adenoma detection in high-risk subjects. Gut 2010;59(6):785–93.

45. Moriichi K, Fujiya M, Sato R, et al. Back-to-back comparison of autofluorescence imaging (AFI) versus high resolution white light colonoscopy for adenoma detection. BMC Gastroenterol 2012;12:75.

46. Varayil JE, Enders F, Tavanapong W, et al. Colonoscopy: what endoscopists inspect under optimal conditions. Gastroenterology 2011;140(5):S-718.

47. Butterly LF, Chase MP, Pohl H, et al. Prevalence of clinically important histology in small adenomas. Clin Gastroenterol Hepatol 2006;4(3):343–8.

48. Rex DK, Overhiser AJ, Chen SC, et al. Estimation of impact of American College of Radiology recommendations on CT colonography reporting for resection of high-risk adenoma findings. Am J Gastroenterol 2009;104(1):149–53.

49. Kaminski MF, Regula J, Kraszewska E, et al. Quality indicators for colonoscopy and the risk of interval cancer. N Engl J Med 2010;362(19):1795–803.

50. Rex DK, Petrini JL, Baron TH, et al. Quality indicators for colonoscopy. Am J Gastroenterol 2006;101(4):873–85.

51. Huang CS, Farraye FA, Yang S, et al. The clinical significance of serrated polyps. Am J Gastroenterol 2011;106(2):229–40 [quiz: 241].

52. Pohl J, Lotterer E, Balzer C, et al. Computed virtual chromoendoscopy versus standard colonoscopy with targeted indigocarmine chromoscopy: a randomised multicentre trial. Gut 2009;58(1):73–8.

53. Chung SJ, Kim D, Song JH, et al. Efficacy of computed virtual chromoendoscopy on colorectal cancer screening: a prospective, randomized,
back-to-back trial of Fuji Intelligent Color Enhancement versus conventional colonoscopy to compare adenoma miss rates. Gastrointest Endosc
2010;72(1):136–42.

Real-time Histology in Colonoscopy

Martin Goetz, MD, PhD

KEYWORDS

- Histology • Colonoscopy • Endoscopy • Endomicroscopy
- Virtual chromoendoscopy • Chromoendoscopy

KEY POINTS

- High-definition white light endoscopy reveals an increasing amount of mucosal details.
- Light filters (narrow-band imaging) or digital filters (i-scan, Fuji Intelligent Chromo Endoscopy) provide tools to support analysis of suspicious lesion by highlighting tissue and vessel patterns. Studies from expert centers suggest a good accuracy for differentiation of nonneoplastic from neoplastic lesions.
- Endocytoscopy is an adaption of light microscopy that reveals cellular epithelial details after topical dye application, which may allow not only analysis of the surface of the lesion but also prediction of depth of invasion.
- Endomicroscopy has been widely studied and permits a detailed analysis of the mucosal microarchitecture. Neoplastic lesions of the colorectum can be visualized with high accuracy.
- For all these techniques, thorough training and ongoing evaluation in clinical trials should be sought to further corroborate their value in gastrointestinal endoscopy.

INTRODUCTION

Twenty years ago, studies showed for the first time that histology could be predicted during endoscopy by magnification chromoendoscopy with a high degree of confidence based on pit pattern analysis.[1] Chromoendoscopy is covered elsewhere in this issue, but it has set the stage for the aim of the endoscopist "to establish an immediate endoscopic diagnosis that is virtually consistent with the histologic diagnosis."[2] Such analysis by magnifying chromoendoscopy is based on the morphology of crypts (**Fig. 1**), but not on cellular or microarchitectural imaging. It therefore comes close to virtual histology, but still relies on prediction rather than visualization of ultrastructural changes. The recent introduction of high-definition (HD) endoscopy with virtual chromoendoscopy has similarly revealed many fine details of colonic lesions during ongoing endoscopy that can be used for immediate decision making on

Innere Medizin I, Universitätsklinikum Tübingen, Otfried-Müller-Street 10, Tübingen 72076, Germany
E-mail address: martin.goetz@med.uni-tuebingen.de

Gastroenterol Clin N Am 42 (2013) 567–575
http://dx.doi.org/10.1016/j.gtc.2013.05.004
0889-8553/13/$ – see front matter © 2013 Elsevier Inc. All rights reserved.

gastro.theclinics.com

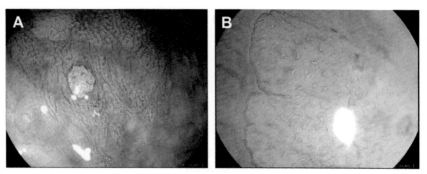

Fig. 1. Chromoendoscopy with methylene blue 0.1% in the colorectum unmasked a small lesion. (*A*) High-definition (HD) magnification endoscopy showed type II pit pattern and a clear margin. (*B*) The lesion was neither biopsied nor resected based on in vivo analysis.

therapeutic strategies. Autofluorescence imaging (AFI) follows a different path and tries to predict the nature of a lesion on a molecular or functional basis more than on morphologic grounds. Endocytoscopy (EC) is an adaption of white light microscopy that enables intravital contact microscopy at the mucosal surface with a high degree of accuracy. Endomicroscopy uses miniaturized laser scanning devices for fluorescent cellular imaging on, but also below, the mucosal surface and can even provide visualization of molecular changes to characterize colonic lesions. The intention of all these techniques is to provide an on-site analysis of histology that should translate into an immediate, tissue-based therapeutic decision.

HD ENDOSCOPY AND VIRTUAL CHROMOENDOSCOPY

HD white light endoscopy (WLE) became possible after introduction of technical improvements from digital broadcasting to endoscopy. In digital imaging, resolution is a function of pixel density, and is improved by incorporating high–pixel density charge-coupled device (CCD) chips. Although standard-definition endoscopes incorporated approximately 200,000 to 400,000 pixels on 576 lines, HD endoscopes provide more than 2×10^6 pixels on 1080 lines, which results in visualization of subtle mucosal details (**Fig. 2**).

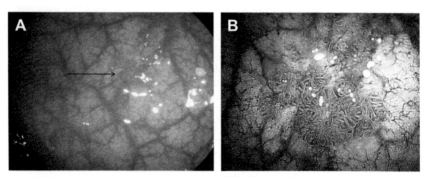

Fig. 2. A subtle irregularity of few millimeters on HD-WLE (*A, arrow*) was further analyzed by i-scan (*B*). the gyriform pattern of the lesion (corresponding with type IIIL pit pattern in chromoendoscopy) was clearly visible. Mucosal resection was performed, and histopathology confirmed the presence of a small low-grade adenoma.

Magnification or zoom endoscopy is obtained by a user-controlled movable lens in the endoscope tip and provides a continuously adaptable degree of magnification from 1.5-fold to 160-fold (see **Fig. 1**). This facility is different from electronic zooms, which enlarge the image without increasing pixel density at the trade-off of lower resolution despite software-based interpolation algorithms. HD endoscopes offer filter techniques (virtual chromoendoscopy) through the switch of a button on the endoscope, such as narrow-band imaging (NBI; Olympus, Japan), i-scan (Pentax, Japan), and Fuji Intelligent Chromo Endoscopy (FICE; Fujinon, Japan).[3]

NBI

Although WLE uses the complete spectrum of visible light, this spectrum is narrowed around the blue and green band by a rotating filter in NBI. Because blue light is absorbed by hemoglobin, the false colored NBI image pronounces the mucosal vessel structure (in contrast with real chromoendoscopy, which highlights pit patterns). Initial hopes that NBI enhances adenoma detection rates in screening colonoscopy have not been fulfilled.[4–6] Following these early trials, several classification systems have been developed for the use of NBI to predict histology (reviewed in Ref.[7]). These systems have recently been unified in the joint Japanese-European-American NBI International Colorectal Endoscopic (NICE) classification. This classification can be used with magnification or without, if close observation is accomplished with HD endoscopes. The NICE classification is based on color, vessel, and surface pattern. Type 1 shows the same or lighter color than the background, none or isolated lace vessels on the surface, and uniform surface pattern, and probably corresponds with a hyperplastic lesion. Type 2 is browner than the background (its color should arise from the vessels) and has thick brown vessels surrounding oval, tubular, or branched white structures (probable diagnosis is adenoma). Type 3 shows a (dark) brown color, areas with distorted or missing vessels, and areas of distorted or absent pattern, and indicates deep submucosal-invasive cancer.[7]

Early trials have reported impressive accuracy rates of NBI for characterization of polyps with[8] and without[9,10] magnification, when high-confidence diagnoses were considered. Those trials were performed by expert endoscopists. However, accuracy rates have decreased in some trials, when endoscopists with less experience with in vivo diagnosis were asked to predict histology in vivo: in a Dutch multicenter trial at 6 nonacademic centers, accuracy rates were 75%.[11] Thirteen US community gastroenterologists had 81% in vivo accuracy rates for diminutive adenomas.[12] Considerable variation between different gastroenterologists and different batches of lesions within the study period was observed. Lower accuracy rates for in vivo (vs ex vivo) characterization were noted, potentially pointing to the importance of technical issues during colonoscopy, such as good visualization of the lesion for thorough on-site analysis.

FICE and i-scan

FICE and i-scan and use software-based post–image acquisition algorithms to display the endoscopic image in false colors. Different modalities either enhance the tissue surface or the vessel structure through the push of a button (**Fig. 3**). Similar to NBI, virtual chromoendoscopy with digital filters has mainly contributed to better polyp characterization, whereas mucosal contrast enhancement in combination with HD imaging resulted in higher adenoma detection rates in some trials. In an expert center pilot study, i-scan with electronic filters, but without optical zoom, performed as well as chromoendoscopy for characterization of diminutive polyps of the rectum.[13] In a follow-up trial with patients screened by colonoscopy, i-scan showed an accuracy

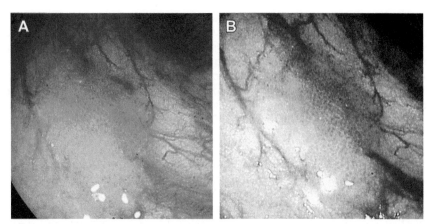

Fig. 3. In the ascending colon, a flat lesion with a sticky mucus cap was identified. HD-WLE was augmented by surface enhancement (*A*) and by virtual chromoendoscopy (*B*), revealing wide-open crypt lumina typical of serrated adenomas.[41] Histopathology confirmed the intravital diagnosis.

rate of 98% to differentiate nonneoplastic from neoplastic lesions.[14] Similar results were obtained for FICE: adenomas were correctly classified with 93% sensitivity and 61% specificity. This result was not significantly different from results obtained for chromoendoscopy in this study.[15]

AFI

The initial concept of AFI was to serve as a red-flag technology for detection of suspicious lesions. However, AFI relies on the characterization of lesions based on alterations in the contents of endogenous fluorophores such as hemoglobin, nicotinamide adenine dinucleotide (reduced form), and collagen. In AFI, sequential illumination of the mucosa with red and green light (for reflectance) and blue light (for excitation of fluorophores) results in a pseudocolored image in which neoplasia is depicted in purple against a green background of healthy mucosa. Many of the changes of tissue autofluorescence are not limited to neoplasia, but may also occur in inflammation, and thus may negatively affect specificity.[16] Therefore, the diagnostic accuracy of AFI has been unsatisfactory: Accuracy was only 55% and 65% for differentiating hyperplastic polyps from serrated adenomas or adenomas, respectively.[17] Therefore, AFI has recently been combined in an approach termed endoscopic trimodal imaging: HD-WLE and AFI are used for detection, and NBI for subsequent analysis of the suspicious areas,[18] but the use of AFI for characterization of lesions has not been subject of recent studies.

EC

EC is an adaption of light microscopy that provides ultrahigh magnification on contact with the mucosa of a fixed-focus, high-power lens projecting images to a CCD chip.[19] Probe-based[20] and integrated-type[21] EC systems (Olympus, Japan) have been evaluated that enable in vivo microscopic imaging in 450-fold to 1400-fold magnification after topical staining of the mucosa (eg, with methylene blue for delineation of nuclei, and crystal violet or toluidine blue for cytoplasmic staining). With this, the uppermost layers of the mucosa become visible. With probe-based EC, a short cap is often used to stabilize the probe on the mucosa.

Different classification systems have been published. In a first study using the probe-based system, Sasajima and colleagues[20] were able to predict histology on 113 patients with an overall accuracy of 93% and good agreement between EC and histopathology (kappa 0.91). In a study by Rotondano and colleagues,[22] EC corresponded completely with histopathology in differentiating nonneoplastic from neoplastic lesions. EC was even able to detect dysplasia in aberrant crypt foci within the colon.[23] In the last study, the mean time for EC was 44 ± 12 minutes.

Most recently, Kudo and colleagues[21] grouped 3 types of lesions based on the shape of the crypt lumina and the nuclear morphology. EC1 describes nonneoplastic lesions: EC1a has roundish lumina and fusiform basal nuclei, and corresponds with normal mucosa; and EC1b corresponds with serrated lumina (hyperplastic). EC2 shows slitlike smooth lumina with uniform nuclei (dysplasia). EC3a has irregular, rough lumina and an increased number of nuclei (high-grade dysplasia or superficial submucosal cancers), whereas EC3b is characterized by undefined crypt architecture and agglomeration of distorted nuclei as a sign of massive submucosal-invasive cancers. In vivo imaging with this simplified classification had 100% sensitivity and specificity to differentiate nonneoplastic from neoplastic tissue. Furthermore, non-resectable lesions (group EC3b) were predicted with a sensitivity and specificity of more than 90%. Therefore, in this study, EC was not only able to provide in vivo histology with high accuracy but also to predict depth of invasion and to guide endoscopic versus surgical therapy.

CONFOCAL LASER ENDOMICROSCOPY

Confocal laser endomicroscopy (CLE) is fundamentally different from EC through the use of laser light instead of visible light. This difference enables microscopic visualization not only on the tissue surface but also below the surface after the application of a fluorescent agent. Up to 1000-fold magnification is obtained, and subcellular details can be visualized. Two systems are currently available, both using excitation with blue laser light of 488 nm: one is endoscope-integrated (eCLE; Pentax, Japan), and the other is probe based (pCLE; MKT, France). The two systems differ with regard to resolution, imaging plane depth adaption, image acquisition rate, and field of view, as well as compatibility with different clinical indications (reviewed in Refs.[24–26]). In a similar way to EC, CLE provides optical sections parallel to the tissue surface.

The first publication, in 2004, established a classification system based on the tissue and vessel microarchitecture to differentiate between normal mucosa, regenerative (ie, hyperplastic or inflammatory), and neoplastic mucosa (**Fig. 4**).[27] With this classification, neoplasia could be predicted with 99% accuracy. This high level of accuracy has also been confirmed in ulcerative colitis,[28] and it has been confirmed that endoscopists are able to microscopically evaluate tissue in vivo. When fluorescein is injected for CLE, nuclei are not routinely discernible. Therefore, alternative staining protocols have been evaluated: Use of cresyl violet for simultaneous chromoendoscopy and CLE has yielded indirect (negative) nuclear visualization.[29] The combined use of systemic fluorescein and topical acriflavine even permitted differentiation of high-grade versus low-grade adenomas.[30] For pCLE, a classification system has recently been developed that will undergo further evaluation.[31]

A formal comparison between eCLE and pCLE has not been performed, but it may be anticipated from studies in the upper gastrointestinal (GI) tract that the accuracy rate may be higher for eCLE because of its higher resolution (higher specificity). In a

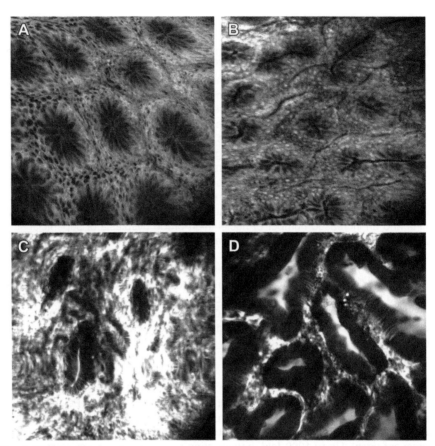

Fig. 4. With confocal endomicroscopy, normal crypts are round and coated with a regular layer of goblet cells containing dark mucin in an epithelial optical section that runs parallel to the tissue surface (*A*). In a hyperplastic lesion (*B*), the crypt opening is typically star shaped, and goblet cells are still present in large numbers. In inflammation (*C*), crypts are pushed apart by edema and cellular infiltration, and fewer crypts are visible per field of view (475 × 475 μm). Bright white fluorescein exudations within the lamina propria indicate enhanced vessel leakiness. Enhanced vascularity is present (intraluminal dark bands correspond with stacks of unstained erythrocytes). In neoplasia (*D*), crypt lumina are irregular, and the epithelial height may vary. All glandular epithelium is still contained by a clear-cut basal membrane; no infiltration into the lamina propria is visible. Goblet cells are scarce.

direct comparison of virtual chromoendoscopy (NBI, FICE) with pCLE for characterization of colorectal polyps, a higher sensitivity for pCLE was found with similar specificity.[32] Similar accuracy rates for NBI and pCLE, of 79% and 82%, respectively, have been reported recently.[33] Tumor infiltration below the mucosa cannot be directly visualized with CLE despite its ability to image below the tissue surface, because imaging plane depth is limited by laser light scattering (decreased signal/noise ratio) with blue laser light in deeper sections. However, the submucosa and muscle layer become visible after endoscopic resection. Nerves of the Meissner plexus were recently visualized with CLE,[34] which may facilitate the study of colonic motility disorders, an area that has only been incompletely amenable to diagnostic tools.

PERSPECTIVES

Most of the methods described earlier rely on gross morphologic alterations of the tissue. Driven by progress in molecular targeted therapies for GI cancer or inflammation, molecular imaging has been a major focus of research in GI endoscopy.[35,36] Apart from wide-field detection of colonic lesions,[37] molecular labeling has been used for characterization of lesions based on their molecular fingerprints.[38,39] Larger studies are awaited.

All of the approaches of optical biopsies listed earlier are designed to optimize polyp characterization, which is currently used for visual guidance of biopsies (few so-called smart biopsies instead of multiple untargeted biopsies). However, as endoscopists detect more and more lesions with the advent of the new endoscopes and modalities, and on-site characterization during ongoing endoscopy becomes more reliable, the optimal management of such lesions is intensely discussed. The American Society for Gastrointestinal Endoscopy Preservation and Incorporation of Valuable Endoscopic Innovations statement[40] proposed a resect-and-discard strategy for diminutive colorectal lesions if a 90% or higher agreement on recommendation of screening intervals can be correctly based on visual analysis of polyps rather than histopathologic analysis. Furthermore, diminutive lesions of the rectosigmoid can be left in place without biopsy or resection if a negative predictive value of more than 90% for adenoma can be achieved. This proposal is only applicable to lesions with optimal visualization and image documentation and high examiner confidence, and requires the endoscopists to be familiar and well trained in novel imaging approaches.

SUMMARY

Diagnostic endoscopy has progressed considerably in recent years with respect to characterization of lesions and on-site microscopic imaging. Starting from magnification chromoendoscopy, HD-WLE augmented by virtual chromoendoscopy techniques significantly eased detailed endoscopic imaging. EC has provided ultrahigh light magnification. Endomicroscopy has brought confocal laser scanning microscopy into the endoscopy suite and proved its value in multiple studies. Together these tools help to optimize screening and surveillance of patients and to individualize targeted treatment.

REFERENCES

1. Kudo S, Hirota S, Nakajima T, et al. Colorectal tumours and pit pattern. J Clin Pathol 1994;47:880–5.
2. Kudo S, Tamura S, Nakajima T, et al. Diagnosis of colorectal tumorous lesions by magnifying endoscopy. Gastrointest Endosc 1996;44:8–14.
3. Sauk J, Hoffman A, Anandasabapathy S, et al. High-definition and filter-aided colonoscopy. Gastroenterol Clin North Am 2010;39:859–81.
4. Rex DK, Helbig CC. High yields of small and flat adenomas with high-definition colonoscopes using either white light or narrow band imaging. Gastroenterology 2007;133:42–7.
5. Adler A, Aschenbeck J, Yenerim T, et al. Narrow-band versus white-light high definition television endoscopic imaging for screening colonoscopy: a prospective randomized trial. Gastroenterology 2009;136:410–6.e1 [quiz: 715].
6. Adler A, Pohl H, Papanikolaou IS, et al. A prospective randomised study on narrow-band imaging versus conventional colonoscopy for adenoma detection: does narrow-band imaging induce a learning effect? Gut 2008;57:59–64.

7. Oba S, Tanaka S, Sano Y, et al. Current status of narrow-band imaging magnifying colonoscopy for colorectal neoplasia in Japan. Digestion 2011;83:167–72.

8. Sano Y, Ikematsu H, Fu KI, et al. Meshed capillary vessels by use of narrow-band imaging for differential diagnosis of small colorectal polyps. Gastrointest Endosc 2009;69:278–83.

9. Rastogi A, Keighley J, Singh V, et al. High accuracy of narrow band imaging without magnification for the real-time characterization of polyp histology and its comparison with high-definition white light colonoscopy: a prospective study. Am J Gastroenterol 2009;104:2422–30.

10. Rex DK. Narrow-band imaging without optical magnification for histologic analysis of colorectal polyps. Gastroenterology 2009;136:1174–81.

11. Kuiper T, van den Broek FJ, Naber AH, et al. Endoscopic trimodal imaging detects colonic neoplasia as well as standard video endoscopy. Gastroenterology 2011; 140:1887–94.

12. Ladabaum U, Fioritto A, Mitani A, et al. Real-time optical biopsy of colon polyps with narrow band imaging in community practice does not yet meet key thresholds for clinical decisions. Gastroenterology 2013;144(1):81–91.

13. Hoffman A, Kagel C, Goetz M, et al. Recognition and characterization of small colonic neoplasia with high-definition colonoscopy using i-Scan is as precise as chromoendoscopy. Dig Liver Dis 2010;42:45–50.

14. Hoffman A, Sar F, Goetz M, et al. High definition colonoscopy combined with i-Scan is superior in the detection of colorectal neoplasias compared with standard video colonoscopy: a prospective randomized controlled trial. Endoscopy 2010;42: 827–33.

15. Pohl J, Lotterer E, Balzer C, et al. Computed virtual chromoendoscopy versus standard colonoscopy with targeted indigocarmine chromoscopy: a randomised multicentre trial. Gut 2009;58:73–8.

16. van den Broek FJ, van Soest EJ, Naber AH, et al. Combining autofluorescence imaging and narrow-band imaging for the differentiation of adenomas from non-neoplastic colonic polyps among experienced and non-experienced endoscopists. Am J Gastroenterol 2009;104:1498–507.

17. Boparai KS, van den Broek FJ, van Eeden S, et al. Hyperplastic polyposis syndrome: a pilot study for the differentiation of polyps by using high-resolution endoscopy, autofluorescence imaging, and narrow-band imaging. Gastrointest Endosc 2009;70:947–55.

18. van den Broek FJ, Fockens P, van Eeden S, et al. Endoscopic tri-modal imaging for surveillance in ulcerative colitis: randomised comparison of high-resolution endoscopy and autofluorescence imaging for neoplasia detection; and evaluation of narrow-band imaging for classification of lesions. Gut 2008;57:1083–9.

19. Neumann H, Fuchs FS, Vieth M, et al. Review article: in vivo imaging by endocytoscopy. Aliment Pharmacol Ther 2011;33:1183–93.

20. Sasajima K, Kudo SE, Inoue H, et al. Real-time in vivo virtual histology of colorectal lesions when using the endocytoscopy system. Gastrointest Endosc 2006;63:1010–7.

21. Kudo SE, Wakamura K, Ikehara N, et al. Diagnosis of colorectal lesions with a novel endocytoscopic classification - a pilot study. Endoscopy 2011;43:869–75.

22. Rotondano G, Bianco MA, Salerno R, et al. Endocytoscopic classification of pre-neoplastic lesions in the colorectum. Int J Colorectal Dis 2010;25:1111–6.

23. Cipolletta L, Bianco MA, Rotondano G, et al. Endocytoscopy can identify dysplasia in aberrant crypt foci of the colorectum: a prospective in vivo study. Endoscopy 2009;41:129–32.

24. Goetz M, Watson A, Kiesslich R. Confocal laser endomicroscopy in gastrointestinal diseases. J Biophotonics 2011;4:498–508.
25. Kiesslich R, Goetz M, Neurath MF. Confocal laser endomicroscopy for gastrointestinal diseases. Gastrointest Endosc Clin North Am 2008;18:451–66, viii.
26. De Palma GD, Wallace MB, Giovannini M. Confocal laser endomicroscopy. Gastroenterol Res Pract 2012;2012:216209.
27. Kiesslich R, Burg J, Vieth M, et al. Confocal laser endoscopy for diagnosing intraepithelial neoplasias and colorectal cancer in vivo. Gastroenterology 2004;127: 706–13.
28. Kiesslich R, Goetz M, Lammersdorf K, et al. Chromoscopy-guided endomicroscopy increases the diagnostic yield of intraepithelial neoplasia in ulcerative colitis. Gastroenterology 2007;132:874–82.
29. Goetz M, Toermer T, Vieth M, et al. Simultaneous confocal laser endomicroscopy and chromoendoscopy with topical cresyl violet. Gastrointest Endosc 2009;70: 959–68.
30. Sanduleanu S, Driessen A, Gomez-Garcia E, et al. In vivo diagnosis and classification of colorectal neoplasia by chromoendoscopy-guided confocal laser endomicroscopy. Clin Gastroenterol Hepatol 2010;8(4):371–8.
31. Kuiper T, van den Broek FJ, van Eeden S, et al. New classification for probe-based confocal laser endomicroscopy in the colon. Endoscopy 2011;43: 1076–81.
32. Buchner AM, Shahid MW, Heckman MG, et al. Comparison of probe-based confocal laser endomicroscopy with virtual chromoendoscopy for classification of colon polyps. Gastroenterology 2010;138:834–42.
33. Shahid MW, Buchner AM, Heckman MG, et al. Diagnostic accuracy of probe-based confocal laser endomicroscopy and narrow band imaging for small colorectal polyps: a feasibility study. Am J Gastroenterol 2012;107:231–9.
34. Sumiyama K, Kiesslich R, Ohya TR, et al. In vivo imaging of enteric neuronal networks in humans using confocal laser endomicroscopy. Gastroenterology 2012; 143:1152–3.
35. Mahmood U. Optical molecular imaging approaches in colorectal cancer. Gastroenterology 2010;138:419–22.
36. Goetz M, Wang TD. Molecular imaging in gastrointestinal endoscopy. Gastroenterology 2010;138:828–33.e1.
37. Liu Z, Miller SJ, Joshi BP, et al. In vivo targeting of colonic dysplasia on fluorescence endoscopy with near-infrared octapeptide. Gut 2013;62(3):395–403.
38. Hsiung PL, Hardy J, Friedland S, et al. Detection of colonic dysplasia in vivo using a targeted heptapeptide and confocal microendoscopy. Nat Med 2008;14:454–8.
39. Goetz M, Ziebart A, Foersch S, et al. In vivo molecular imaging of colorectal cancer with confocal endomicroscopy by targeting epidermal growth factor receptor. Gastroenterology 2010;138:435–46.
40. Rex DK, Kahi C, O'Brien M, et al. The American Society for Gastrointestinal Endoscopy PIVI (Preservation and Incorporation of Valuable Endoscopic Innovations) on real-time endoscopic assessment of the histology of diminutive colorectal polyps. Gastrointest Endosc 2011;73:419–22.
41. Kimura T, Yamamoto E, Yamano HO, et al. A novel pit pattern identifies the precursor of colorectal cancer derived from sessile serrated adenoma. Am J Gastroenterol 2012;107:460–9.

The Modern Bowel Preparation in Colonoscopy

Ala I. Sharara, MD*, Rachel R. Abou Mrad, MD

KEYWORDS

- Colonoscopy • Quality • Preparation • Cleaning

KEY POINTS

- Adequate bowel preparation is essential for optimal performance of colonoscopy.
- There are several effective formulations with a good safety profile and these may be used interchangeably in patients without significant comorbidities depending on the patient profile and physician preference.
- Polyethylene glycol-electrolyte solution is the preferred regimen in patients with cardiac, renal, or liver disease because of its limited effect on plasma volume and electrolyte homeostasis.
- Regardless of choice, split dosing is an important and established concept that should be implemented whenever possible in an effort to enhance tolerance and adherence, and improve mucosal visibility and overall quality of the examination.
- The burden of the preparation on patients including dietary modifications and disturbance of daily routine and sleep should be taken into consideration.
- Proper patient education regarding the different steps of the proposed preparation and the need for compliance and adherence are essential.

INTRODUCTION

Colonoscopy is the preferred procedure for investigating large-bowel and terminal ileal disease in adults and children. In addition, colonoscopy is the current gold standard for colorectal cancer screening because of its high diagnostic sensitivity and specificity and its unique capability to permit sampling and removal of polyps. For optimal performance and visualization of mucosal lesions and details, however, adequate bowel preparation is essential. This is of particular importance in the screening setting where the objective is identification and removal of all resectable polyps including flat lesions. Colonoscopy preparations are generally poorly tolerated,

Disclosure: The authors have no personal conflicts of interest to declare.
Division of Gastroenterology, Department of Internal Medicine, American University of Beirut Medical Center, Beirut, Lebanon
* Corresponding author. Division of Gastroenterology, American University of Beirut Medical Center, PO Box 11-0236/16-B, Beirut, Lebanon.
E-mail address: as08@aub.edu.lb

Gastroenterol Clin N Am 42 (2013) 577–598
http://dx.doi.org/10.1016/j.gtc.2013.05.010
0889-8553/13/$ – see front matter © 2013 Elsevier Inc. All rights reserved.

disliked and, consequently, serve as an impediment to colorectal cancer screening and surveillance. Mounting evidence suggests that the fear of bowel preparation is a key reason many avoid colonoscopy.[1] Patients who have undergone colonoscopy state that the bowel preparation was the worst part of the experience, and, as a result, are sometimes reluctant to undergo the procedure again or recommend it to others.[2] In addition, patients commonly experience adverse events of the bowel preparation, including bloating, nausea, vomiting, and abdominal pain, which may lead to interruption or incomplete adherence. This may result in suboptimal bowel cleansing leading to incomplete examination, poor visualization of the mucosa, and missed colon pathology.[3]

Adequate bowel preparation, defined by the ability to detect polyps 5 mm or larger,[4] is crucial for the effectiveness of colonoscopy as a screening tool. This definition may be useful as a benchmark for screening examinations but in essence indicates the ability to achieve proper and complete mucosal inspection. Despite the unquestionable need for adequate colon cleansing, suboptimal bowel preparation occurs with surprising frequency in as many as 25% to 40% of cases.[1,5] Inadequate bowel preparation is associated with canceled procedures, prolonged procedure time, incomplete examination, increased cost and possibly complications, physician frustration and patient anxiety, but most importantly, with missed pathology (**Table 1**). The latter may be associated with the potential for medicolegal liability when an interval cancer is diagnosed before a timely repeat proper examination.

Some studies have suggested that suboptimal colon preparation significantly decreases the ability to detect colon polyps but not necessarily colon cancer.[6,7] In a study by Harewood and colleagues,[7] small colonic polyps (<9 mm) were more frequently detected during colonoscopies performed in patients with adequate bowel preparation than in those with inadequate preparation (22% vs 19%, respectively; $P<.0001$). However, larger polyps (>9 mm) were detected at the same rate (7%) irrespective of the quality of the preparation. Other studies reported high miss rates of adenomas and advanced lesions, as high as 34% to 42% and 18% to 27% respectively, when preparation for screening colonoscopy was unsatisfactory.[8,9] A large European prospective observational multicenter study, involving 5832 patients, found that all polyps were more likely to be discovered in an adequately prepared colon than in an inadequately prepared colon.[6] Furthermore, other important outcomes of colonoscopy were also found to significantly improve with higher cleansing quality (**Box 1**). As mentioned earlier, suboptimal bowel preparation is associated not only with decreased adenoma detection rate but also with increased cost of colonoscopy by virtue of decreased interval to repeat examination.[10] Therefore, efforts to improve the quality of bowel preparation are critical. In this review, the different colonoscopy

Table 1			
Effects of bowel preparation on colonoscopy outcome measures			
Outcome	**Low-Quality Preparation**	**High-Quality Preparation**	**P Value**
Mean time to cecum (min)	16.1	11.9	<.001
Mean withdrawal time (min)	11.3	9.8	<.001
Polyps of any size (%)	23.9	29.4	.007
Polyps >10 mm detected (%)	4.3	6.4	.016

Data from Froehlich F, Wietlisbach V, Gonvers JJ, et al. Impact of colonic cleansing on quality and diagnostic yield of colonoscopy: the European Panel of Appropriateness of Gastrointestinal Endoscopy European multicenter study. Gastrointest Endosc 2005;61:378–84.

> **Box 1**
> **Implications of a poor colonic preparation**
>
> Prolonged procedure time
>
> Increased potential for missed pathology
>
> Incomplete colonoscopy
>
> Possible increased complications (eg, perforation of an inadequately prepared bowel)
>
> Increased cost (decreased interval to repeat examination)
>
> Potential for medicolegal liability (if timely repeat colonoscopy is not undertaken and an interval colon cancer is diagnosed within a short time period)

preparation regimens are compared, and the modern bowel preparations and ways to optimize such an important variable are discussed.

THE IDEAL BOWEL PREPARATION

The ideal bowel preparation should be simple to administer, palatable, well tolerated, and effective in adequately cleansing the colon without altering colonic mucosa or plasma fluid and electrolyte homeostasis. Moreover, it should be free of other significant adverse effects and have no important contraindications for use in special populations such as patients with heart, liver, or kidney disease, pregnant women, or children. Although bowel preparations are traditionally described in terms of the solution administered (eg, sodium sulfate, sodium phosphate [NaP], and so forth.), many additional elements are involved in the process (**Box 2**). These include various dietary modifications and time of intake of the solution leading to important adjustments in the patient's social and work schedule and affecting the immediate preprocedural quality of life, which often goes unregistered in clinical trials. When evaluating studies examining the efficacy of a certain preparation, these factors should be taken into consideration. Therefore, the ideal bowel preparation should be one that has the least impact on patients' lifestyle. A one-type-cleans-all formulation does not exist at this stage and even the best regimen invariably fails in some patients. Customizing the preparation is sometimes necessary in particular situations such as in patients with severe constipation, those receiving psychotropic or anticholinergic drugs, and, intuitively, in patients with a history of inadequate bowel preparation at previous colonoscopy.

> **Box 2**
> **Burden of bowel preparation on patients**
>
> At scheduling: comprehend detailed explanation of the preparation including dietary restrictions using information leaflets, cartoons, and videos
>
> Day −1: Trigger reminder of colonoscopy appointment and initiate dietary changes
>
> Day −1: Adjust work and social schedule
>
> Day −1: Expect to feel hungry and experience possible sleep disturbance
>
> Day 0*: Restrict long-distance commute before procedure
>
> Day 0: Ensure easy access to restrooms
>
> * Day 0, day of colonoscopy.

EVOLUTION OF THE BOWEL PREPARATION

Colonoscopy preparations have evolved significantly over time. Early preparations were patient unfriendly, time consuming, and associated with fluid and electrolyte disturbances. In 1980, polyethylene glycol-electrolyte (PEG-E) solutions were introduced by Davis and colleagues[11] and became the most commonly used purgatives for colonic cleansing. These are nonabsorbable isosmotic solutions and thus do not induce any substantial shifts in plasma fluid and electrolyte levels. Traditionally, 4 L PEG-E solutions were given 1 day before colonoscopy. Their main disadvantages were the large volume, poor palatability, and the need to adhere to dietary restrictions. This led to poor adherence prompting further modifications of the PEG-E solutions, such as fruit-flavoring and low-salt formulations, as well as the search for alternatives.[12–19] NaP solutions were introduced in the late 1980s as a low-volume substitute for PEG-E, and were shown to result in effective colon cleansing when compared with conventional preparations.[18,20–23] Subsequent reports of phosphate nephropathy led to development of other small volume non–phosphate-containing solutions based on sodium sulfate or sodium picosulfate with magnesium. Reduced volume PEG-E with ascorbic acid or adjuvant bisacodyl were similarly shown to be effective means of bowel cleansing with improved tolerance and adherence.

ASSESSMENT OF QUALITY OF BOWEL PREPARATION

In clinical practice, the quality of bowel preparation is naturally determined during colonoscopy. Studies have shown that patients' own perception of the quality of the preparation is often inaccurate.[24,25] Questions regarding the color and quality of the last fecal effluent may be helpful before examination. Patients who report poor adherence to the prescribed regimen and/or a turbid or brown last fecal effluent may be better rescheduled for another date using a different or modified preparation regimen.[26] This preexamination assessment is probably money saving by avoiding the possibility of an aborted examination and the potential financial obligations of a repeat colonoscopy.

Clinical trials assessing the efficacy of modern bowel preparations have relied on several validated bowel preparation scales including the modified Aronchick scale, the Ottawa scale, and the Boston Bowel Preparation Scale (BBPS). These scales vary in complexity from a relatively simple 5-point rating for the modified Aronchick scale (poor to excellent) based on residual stool and fluid consistency to the BBPS, which assesses each colonic segment separately including attention to residual mucosal staining, to the more complex Ottawa scale, which is a calculated numerical score (range 0–14 points) based on segmental presence or absence and quality of any residual fluid and the need for wash and suction. There are a limited number of studies evaluating the agreement or concordance between these scales[27] but they could be complementary. **Fig. 1** illustrates the potential for discrepancy between the aforementioned scales when significant residual mucosal staining in the absence of liquid or solid stools may not be specifically accounted for, or given enough weight, in 1 scale versus another. In addition, there is no standardization of whether a preparation should be scored during the insertion or the withdrawal phase of the examination. In clinical practice, however, the quality of preparation is often based on a global assessment by the performing endoscopist. Despite a relatively low likelihood of investigator bias,[28] studies have shown fair to good interobserver and intraobserver agreement regarding the quality of bowel preparations.[24,29] Thus, there seems to be a need for proper standardization of the quality of bowel preparation in future trials as well as in clinical practice.

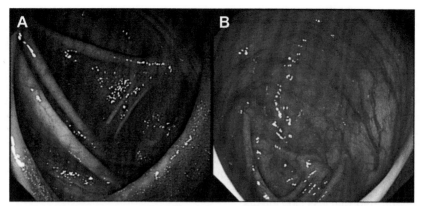

Fig. 1. Effect of split dosing on the quality of colonoscopy. Endoscopic images of the cecum after (A) day-before 4 L PEG-E and (B) split-dose 4 L PEG-E with 2 L consumed 2 to 3 hours before the examination.

DIETARY MODIFICATIONS IN BOWEL PREPARATION

As discussed earlier, diet is a central and integral part of bowel preparation with important effects on the quality of the preparation as well as the immediate preprocedural quality of life of patients. A clear liquid diet was traditionally recommended before colonoscopy and influenced both patient compliance and resulting cleanliness of the bowel preparation. A clear liquid diet is recommended by most manufacturers starting at or before lunch the day before colonoscopy. This was challenged in several randomized controlled trials that showed that the efficacy of the bowel preparation was unaltered by low-residue diet using PEG-E,[30,31] NaP,[32] and magnesium citrate plus bisacodyl[33] preparations. Although a low-residue diet is better tolerated than a liquid diet, the need to adhere to a low-residue diet remains an unwelcome burden for patients (see **Box 1**) and compliance is usually poor, particularly when recommended for 2 or 3 days before the scheduled colonoscopy.[34,35] In our experience, patients rank dietary modifications and restrictions as an important negative aspect of the procedure, second only to the volume and taste of the preparation. A randomized controlled trial by Aoun and colleagues[29] showed that an unrestricted diet and split-dose PEG-E was superior to 4 L PEG-E with a liquid diet. The validity of this strategy was confirmed in a recent trial showing good or excellent colon cleansing in 86 of 99 patients (87%) receiving a regular unrestricted diet for breakfast and lunch, a full liquid dinner and 4 L split-dose PEG-E.[36]

MODERN BOWEL PREPARATIONS
PEG-E

PEG-based solutions consist of a high-molecular-weight nonabsorbable polymer in a dilute electrolyte solution. PEG-E solutions are designed to be osmotically balanced, limiting the exchange of fluid and electrolytes across the colonic membrane. A variety of PEG-E preparations are currently available for bowel cleansing before colonoscopy. These differ with respect to volume, electrolyte content, molecular weight of the polymer, artificial flavorings, and the presence of artificial sweeteners. Sulfate-free PEG-E is less salty, more palatable, but comparable with PEG-E in terms of effective colonic cleansing and overall patient tolerance.[13] Traditionally, 4 L of PEG-E were used 1 day before colonoscopy. The recommended dosing of most PEG-E is 240 mL every 10 min until completion or a persistently clear rectal effluent. It is estimated, however, that 5% to 15% of patients are unable to consume the full dose of PEG-E because of palatability and/or adverse effects including bloating, nausea, and vomiting. The timing of PEG-E doses and its relationship to the time of colonoscopy has proved to be important both for tolerability of patients and the quality of the bowel preparation. PEG-E taken in divided or split doses (2 L the evening before and 2 L the morning of the procedure) was demonstrated in multiple randomized trials to be better tolerated and more effective than the standard 4-L dose given 1 day before, with good or excellent preparation achieved in 80% to 90% of patients.[24,29,37,38] The improved outcome with split dosing led to testing and development of split-dose low-volume PEG-E formulations containing ascorbic acid or supplemented with adjuvant bisacodyl. Randomized controlled trials showed that these lower volume formulations were equivalent to standard 4 L PEG-E, and even split-dose PEG-E, and were generally associated with less side effects.[29,34,37,39–47]

Two recent meta-analyses[48,49] have demonstrated that split-dose PEG-E results in much higher rates of adequate bowel preparation than the standard full-dose regimen, partly because of fewer discontinuations and lower incidence of nausea but perhaps, more importantly, because of the timing of the final dose in relation to the colonoscopy (discussed later). In their meta-analysis, Enestvedt and colleagues[49] showed that 4 L split-dose PEG-E is superior to other bowel preparation comparators for bowel cleansing (including split dose of either 2 L PEG-E + ascorbic acid, NaP, or Mira-LAX/Gatorade) and suggested that it be considered the standard against which new bowel preparations are compared.

Reduced-Volume PEG-E + Ascorbic Acid

PEG–E plus ascorbic acid and sodium sulfate is a low-volume PEG-based formulation. The megadose of ascorbic acid used is not completely absorbed, remaining in the colonic lumen, where it exerts an osmotic effect thereby reducing the necessary effective volume of colon cleansing solution to 2 L. Each liter of PEG-E + ascorbic acid contains 100 g macrogol 3350, 7.5 g sodium sulfate, 2.7 g sodium chloride, 1 g potassium chloride, 4.7 g ascorbic acid, 5.9 g sodium ascorbate, and lemon flavoring. Patients scheduled for a morning colonoscopy are instructed to take the 2 L preparation in the afternoon and evening the day before the colonoscopy. Those scheduled in the afternoon take 1 L the evening before and 1 L early in the morning on the day of colonoscopy. With every liter of PEG-E + ascorbic acid, patients should also take at least half a liter of a clear fluid to avoid dehydration. The efficacy of 2 L PEG-E + ascorbic acid was evaluated in several randomized controlled trials. Coporaal and colleagues[50] compared 2 L PEG-E + ascorbic acid with 4 L split-dose PEG-E and found that both preparations were equally effective. These results are in line with those from Ell and colleagues[43] who demonstrated successful bowel cleansing in 88.9% of patients receiving PEG-E + ascorbic acid versus 94.8% of patients prepared with PEG-E. Similarly, compared with NaP, PEG-E + ascorbic acid provided successful bowel cleansing in 72.5% of cases versus 63.9% with NaP.[51] PEG-E + ascorbic acid has also been investigated versus sodium picosulfate + magnesium citrate.[52] Again, both preparations produced similar success rates of 84.4% with PEG-E + ascorbic acid and 72.7% with sodium picosulfate + magnesium citrate.

NaP

NaP preparations are available in aqueous and tablet forms. Several randomized controlled trials have compared NaP and standard 4 L PEG-E suggesting they are equally effective with better tolerance and acceptability of NaP. A meta-analysis by

Tan and Tjandra[53] concluded that NaP was more effective in bowel cleansing than standard PEG-E or sodium picosulfate and comparable in terms of adverse events. A recent large prospective randomized trial by Lawrance and colleagues[54] comparing NaP, PEG-E, and sodium picosulfate preparations showed that NaP gave the worst results for morning procedures, whereas all 3 preparations were similarly effective for afternoon procedures. Most studies comparing NaP with PEG-E did so against standard 4 L PEG-E administered the day before colonoscopy. A randomized trial by Seo and colleagues[55] compared head-to-head NaP with split-dose PEG-E without strict dietary restrictions and showed no significant difference in efficacy between the 2 preparations. Split-dose PEG-E was, however, associated with significantly less nausea and vomiting. The dose of aqueous NaP is 45 mL taken in divided doses, 10 to 12 hours apart with 1 of the doses taken on the morning of the procedure. Proper hydration and consumption of clear fluids and water is recommended. A particular concern with the use of NaP is the potential risk of acute phosphate nephropathy (discussed later).

The tablet form of NaP was designed to improve taste and limit the volume of liquid required. The recommended dosage is 32 to 40 tablets taken as 20 tablets the evening before and 12 to 20 tablets the day of the procedure (3–5 hours earlier). The 20 tablets are taken as 4 tablets every 15 minutes with 240 mL of clear liquid. Each 2 g tablet contains 1500 mg of active ingredients (monobasic and dibasic NaP) and 460 mg of microcrystalline cellulose as a tablet binder. The latter is a nonabsorbable inert polymer and remains insoluble in the gastrointestinal tract. Initially, 2 large multicenter randomized controlled trials compared NaP tablets with conventional 4 L PEG-E regimens and found that they were equally effective in terms of colon cleansing.[56] The quality of the bowel preparation was excellent or good in 84.3% of patients in the NaP tablet group and in 76.7% in the PEG-E group. Patient compliance was greater in the tablet group, and there were significantly fewer gastrointestinal side effects in this group. However, the use of NaP tablets has some shortcomings in that the inactive microcrystalline cellulose ingredient produces a residue that obscures the mucosal surface and a large number of tablets need to be ingested over a short period of time. These drawbacks have been partly addressed by reducing the amount of microcrystalline cellulose per tablet[57] as well as the number of NaP tablets to be ingested from 32 to 28 to improve compliance and tolerability.[58]

Oral Sodium Sulfate

An oral sodium sulfate (OSS)-based solution was developed as a new low-volume alternative to NaP. This solution does not contain phosphate and is therefore unlikely to cause phosphate nephropathy. Only 2 randomized trials have been published to date[59,60] comparing OSS with 2 L PEG-E + ascorbic acid[59] or with standard 4 L PEG-E.[60] OSS was found to be superior to 4 L PEG-E, equally effective as 2 L PEG-E + ascorbic acid, and to have an acceptable safety profile. The preparation (consisting of 17.5 g sodium sulfate, 3.13 g potassium sulfate, and 1.6 g magnesium sulfate in each 1.8 L bottle) is used in split doses; each bottle is administered as 480 mL of diluted solution with an additional 1 L of water. A light breakfast only and/or clear fluids are recommended the day before the procedure.

Sodium Picosulfate/Magnesium Oxide/Citric Acid Preparations

Sodium picosulfate combined with magnesium citrate (P/MC) acts locally in the colon as both stimulant and osmotic laxative. Sodium picosulfate is a prodrug hydrolyzed by bacteria in the colon into its active metabolite, which acts as a stimulant laxative causing transfer of fluid and electrolytes to the bowel lumen. It is used commercially with magnesium oxide and citric acid to improve taste and cathartic effect. P/MC has better tolerability and acceptability than PEG-E or NaP.[61,62] Similar to all afore-mentioned regimens, using P/MC in a split-dose regimen was shown to be superior to the traditional dosing regimen for bowel preparation for colonoscopy.[63] More recently, a large randomized multicenter assessor-blinded study of day-before split-dose P/MC versus 2 L PEG-E + bisacodyl was published.[64] P/MC provided superior overall colon cleansing compared with day-before PEG-E + bisacodyl (84.2% vs 74.4%), as well as in each segment of the colon. The instructions are as follows: 2 sa-chets of P/MC are reconstituted in 150 mL of water each and taken as split doses, 1 day before colonoscopy, starting between 4 and 6 PM with the second dose taken after 6 hours, but no later than 9 hours before the procedure. On the day before the procedure, all patients were limited to a clear liquid diet. Despite its small volume and good acceptance and palatability, the burden of this particular preparation regimen on the individual daily schedule and sleep may be more substantial than other preparations given its relatively delayed onset of action, the time difference between doses (the second dose was taken after 10 PM), and the need for continued proper hydration with clear fluids throughout the preparation period. A true split-dosing regimen on consecutive days may be friendlier, with the second dose taken 4 hours before the examination,[63] but would be useful mostly in patients scheduled for late morning or afternoon colonoscopy. Oral P/MC is generally well tolerated. Adverse events are primarily gastrointestinal in nature and usually mild to moderate in intensity.

MiraLAX/Gatorade Combination

MiraLAX (PEG 3350) (Schering-Plough Healthcare Products, Inc, Kenilworth, NJ) is a laxative approved for the treatment of mild or occasional constipation. When used as a laxative, MiraLAX can cause excessive volume depletion and is not recommended in patients with kidney disease. Furthermore, it carries an even greater risk of volume depletion and potential electrolyte disturbances when taken as a bowel preparation at a dose 14 times (238 g) higher than the recommended laxative dose. MiraLAX does not contain a built-in electrolyte replacement solution, so the diarrhea it induces correlates with volume depletion and electrolyte imbalance. In an attempt to limit this problem, MiraLAX is often administered in combination with a hydrating sports drink (eg, Gatorade; PepsiCo, Purchase, NY) to boost electrolytes. Hjelkrem and col-leagues[65] found that split-dose MiraLAX in 2 L of Gatorade is not as effective as 4 L split-dose PEG-E in bowel cleansing. This finding was corroborated by another trial by Enestvedt and colleagues.[66] However, MiraLAX/Gatorade was better tolerated in both studies. A prospective randomized controlled study evaluating the efficacy, toler-ability, and safety of whole-dose and split-dose regimens of MiraLAX/Gatorade versus PEG-E found that split-dose MiraLAX/Gatorade and split-dose PEG-E were more effective than whole-dose PEG-E. MiraLAX/Gatorade was preferred over PEG-E by the study participants.[67] Bowel preparation with MiraLAX/Gatorade did not lead to any clinically significant electrolyte changes or clinically adverse event in any of the low-risk patients in this study. The combination of MiraLAX/Gatorade is not approved by the US Food and Drug Administration (FDA) for bowel cleaning before colonoscopy.

TIMING OF ADMINISTRATION OF THE BOWEL PREPARATION

The timing of bowel preparation in relation to endoscopy is an increasingly important consideration. Church[68] compared full-volume PEG-E taken on the morning of an af-ternoon colonoscopy with the same preparation taken the day before, showing that the quality of bowel preparation was significantly better with the shorter time interval.

The concept of split dosing was introduced in an attempt to refine bowel preparation by improving tolerance and adherence to 4 L PEG-E and to allow next-day examination of patients when required.[29,37] Dose splitting (2 L the evening before and 2 L the morning of the procedure) was found to be superior to the conventional 4 L day-before preparation, in terms of quality and tolerability of the preparation, and obviated the need for significant dietary restriction. Multiple randomized trials[16,29,37,63,68,69] and meta-analyses[48,49] have subsequently demonstrated that a split-dosing regimen, irrespective of the bowel preparation used, is more effective than its full-dose counterpart, partly because of less preparation discontinuations and lower incidence of nausea. Improved visualization of the right colonic mucosa was perhaps the biggest advantage of split-dose preparations. In patients who take the last purgative dose 8 to 12 hours before colonoscopy, new small bowel effluent accumulates in the right colon staining the mucosa and making visualization of mucosal details difficult (see **Fig. 1**).[69] One study showed that split-dose NaP resulted in better bowel cleansing and significantly lower fecal material in the right colon compared with the full dose taken the day before (4% vs 30%).[16] The bowel fluid was more translucent in the split-dosing group and more opaque in the day-before group. Parra-Blanco and colleagues[70] compared the cleansing quality of PEG-E and NaP with different schedules of administration. Patients receiving the preparation on the same day as the colonoscopy were significantly more likely to have good or excellent global cleansing scores than those receiving day-before preparations. Flat lesions, but not flat adenomas, were also more frequent in patients prepared on the same day. These data suggest that the timing of the second dose in relation to the procedure is more important than the time between the first and second doses. Studies have confirmed that consumption of PEG-E less than 5 hours before the procedure is associated with the highest scores for bowel cleansing.[71] Same-day bowel cleansing with all the solution consumed on the day of examination was recently shown to be superior to a split-dose PM/AM regimen[72] but is arguably impractical except for afternoon procedures or in controlled settings.

Two theoretic barriers to the preferential use of split-dose regimens have been raised. The first is the concern about risk of sedation or anesthesia in patients consuming fluids close to procedure time. However, studies have shown that minimal fluid ($\leq$20 mL) remains in the stomach 90 minutes after ingestion of 200 mL of water or full-fat milk[73,74] or in patients undergoing concomitant esophagogastroduodenoscopy as early as 90 minutes after a last dose of PEG-E.[29] The American Society of Anesthesia guidelines recommend that patients should fast for a minimum of 2 hours after consuming clear liquids before the administration of sedation.[75] The second point of contention is that patients are not willing to wake up earlier on the day of colonoscopy for the second purgative dose. A survey conducted in 2008 revealed that 83% of patients would be willing to wake up as early as 3 AM to take the second dose.[76] In a comparative study,[77] a significantly higher percentage of the split-dose group reported no or minimal difficulty completing the bowel preparation compared with the single-dose group (81% vs 55% respectively). In addition, significantly more patients in the split dose regimen were satisfied with the bowel preparation compared with the single-dose group (63% vs 46%, respectively). There was also no significant difference in the percentage of patients who stopped for a bowel movement on their way to colonoscopy. When asked which regimen was more convenient and less difficult to complete, 19% of patients in the PM/AM split-dosing group versus 44% in the single-dose group found that the regimen was hard to complete.

The data suggest that patients accept a split-dosing regimen better, are able to complete the preparation with no or minimal difficulty, and are willing to wake up early if convinced the timing of the second dose will enhance the outcome of their colonoscopy. An increase in patient compliance with the preparation, and hence improved mucosal visualization, may lead to enhanced polyp detection, greater patient satisfaction and uptake of colonoscopy, as well as potential cost savings.[78] Split dosing, where at least half of the preparation is given on the day of colonoscopy, is recommended in the American College of Gastroenterology guidelines for colorectal cancer screening.[79]

SAFETY OF BOWEL PREPARATIONS

In addition to high efficacy, safety is a paramount feature of the ideal bowel preparation. Generally, all bowel preparations are safe for use in healthy individuals without comorbid conditions. Care must be taken, however, when choosing a bowel preparation agent for patients with cardiac, liver, or renal diseases. PEG-E is safer than other osmotic laxatives including NaP, sodium sulfate, and sodium picosulfate, and is preferable in such patients. All current bowel preparations are associated with some mild adverse events such as nausea, bloating, headache, and vomiting. Occasionally, however, serious adverse events may develop. The administration of large-volume isosmotic, or low-volume hyperosmolar solutions as purgatives can lead to electrolyte disturbances by a variety of mechanisms, primarily through hypovolemia and increased antidiuretic hormone (ADH) levels. These are, for the most part, subclinical and rapidly reversible. Rare episodes of acute hyponatremic encephalopathy have been described with different regimens of bowel preparation including PEG-E, NaP, and off-label use of MiraLAX/Gatorade.[80–82] In a study by Cohen and colleagues,[83] 40 patients were followed from initial bowel preparation with PEG-E to 1 hour after colonoscopy and assessed for hyponatremia by measuring serum sodium and ADH levels. After bowel cleansing, and immediately before colonoscopy, 25% of patients had developed increased ADH levels. After colonoscopy, 7.5% experienced a decrease in serum sodium concentration to less than 130 mmol/L. Care must be taken when using NaP or sodium picosulfate/magnesium citrate bowel preparation in patients with a low seizure threshold, the elderly, or those with comorbidities. Seizures caused by electrolyte abnormalities associated with these bowel preparations have been described.[81,84]

Several reports have demonstrated more adverse events with the use of NaP-based bowel preparation regimens, particularly with respect to kidney injury.[85–88] Although usually asymptomatic, hyperphosphatemia is seen in as many as 40% of healthy patients completing NaP preparations, but this may be significant in patients with kidney disease.[89] The use of a single oral dose of NaP in 13 healthy volunteers receiving proper hydration resulted in significant increases in serum phosphorus at 120 min and a significant decrease in 12-h urinary calcium concentrations, an effect that was more pronounced in individuals of lower weight.[90] In addition, NaP has been shown to cause hypokalemia, increased blood urea nitrogen levels, decreased exercise capacity, increased plasma osmolality, and hypocalcemia, which can all be attributed to dehydration.[91] Although mild and transient in most patients, these electrolyte disturbances could be more pronounced in hospitalized patients, the elderly, in patients with hypoparathyroidism or chronic kidney disease, and in those with slow gastrointestinal transit or on vitamin D supplements.[92,93]

In a large retrospective cohort study involving 2352 patients without preexisting kidney disease, 4% of patients receiving a NaP preparation experienced renal impairment versus 3% for PEG-E.[94] However, in an accompanying editorial, the potential for selection bias whereby individual baseline patient characteristics may have influenced whether patients were prescribed NaP or PEG-E- in favor of NaP was raised.[95] Another retrospective cohort[96] identified 9799 patients who underwent colonoscopy and had serum creatinine values recorded within 365 days before and after the procedure. Acute kidney injury (defined as $\geq$50% increase from baseline serum creatinine) was identified in 114 patients (1.16%). Of those patients, 73% had received NaP and 27% had received PEG-E. Using a multiple logistic regression model, the use of oral NaP solutions was associated with increased risk for acute kidney injury (odds ratio 2.35; 95% confidence interval 1.51 to 3.66; $P<.001$).

Table 2 shows the patterns of acute kidney injury associated with oral NaP preparations.[97] Acute renal failure associated with NaP-based bowel preparations is a serious condition known as acute phosphate nephropathy (APN).[88] APN is characterized by the precipitation of calcium phosphate crystals in the renal tubules and may lead to chronic irreversible kidney injury. Patients with preexisting renal insufficiency or taking medications that affect kidney function such as diuretics, angiotensin-converting enzyme inhibitors, angiotensin receptor blockers, are most susceptible to complications arising from NaP preparations.[98] Despite the low incidence of APN, the potential for severe renal injury prompted the FDA to issue a boxed warning in 2008 stating that potential risk factors for APN include advanced age, renal disease, decreased intravascular volumes, and the use of drugs that affect renal perfusion or function.[78] NaP preparations have also been shown to alter both macroscopic and microscopic features of intestinal mucosa[99–101] including aphthous erosions similar to those seen in inflammatory bowel disease.

Oral sodium sulfate preparations have not been associated with kidney injury but the number of published studies on OSS is few. In normal volunteers, the use of OSS was found to be less likely than NaP-induced catharsis to favor calcium salt deposition in renal tubules.[102]

Subclinical, but significant, transient shifts in serum magnesium, potassium, and calcium have been described with P/MC preparations.[103] In 1 large trial,[54] both NaP and sodium picosulfate induced mucosal inflammation 10-fold more frequently than PEG-E. A recent population-based retrospective cohort study from Canada examined

Table 2
Patterns of acute kidney injury after bowel preparation with oral NaP

Factor	Early Symptomatic	Late Insidious
Timing of onset after bowel preparation	<24 h	Days to months
Symptoms	Lethargy, confusion, seizure, and tetany	Asymptomatic or nonspecific
Serum phosphorus and calcium levels	Hyperphosphatemia and hypocalcemia	Normal, unless measured within 3 d of preparation
Phosphate load	Excessive	Standard
Pathology	Unknown	Nephrocalcinosis
Treatment options	Intravenous fluids, oral PO_4 binder, intravenous Ca^{2+}, and/or hemodialysis	None
Outcomes	Recovery, chronic kidney disease, or death	Chronic kidney disease

From Lien YH. Is bowel preparation before colonoscopy a risky business for the kidney? Nat Clin Pract Nephrol 2008;4:606–14; with permission.

the incidence of serious events (defined as a composite of nonelective hospitalization, emergency department visit, or death within 7 days of the colonoscopy) in 50,660 patients, older than 66 years of age, who received either PEG-E or P/MC for outpatient colonoscopy. The overall serious event rate was 24 per 1000 procedures and was 28 per 1000 procedures among high-risk patients, defined as those with cardiac or renal disease, long-term care residents or patients receiving concurrent diuretic therapy. The rates of serious events were similar for PEG-E and P/MC.[104] As discussed previously, the potential for selection bias in this study, with a lower probability of being treated with P/MC in higher-risk patients, cannot be excluded.

IMPACT OF PATIENT EDUCATION ON QUALITY OF BOWEL PREPARATION

Several patients' characteristics have been associated with poor bowel preparation including inpatient status, history of constipation, use of antidepressants, timing of purgative ingestion, and noncompliance with cleansing instructions.[6] It is likely that even the most effective regimens can be further enhanced through efforts to maximize patient compliance during the preparation period. Proper patient education before colonoscopy is important to ensure adherence and, as a consequence, the quality of the bowel preparation. Evidence supporting the efficacy of such education is, however, sparse and inconsistent. One randomized controlled trial showed that a preendoscopy education program has numerous psychological benefits, and resulted in apparent increase in patient compliance.[105] Another study showed that an educational pamphlet lowers anxiety levels before colonoscopy and leads to better colon preparation.[106] On the other hand, a different study failed to prove the efficacy of patient education before colonoscopy on the quality of the bowel preparation.[107] Spiegel and colleagues[108] presented in their study the development and validation of a novel booklet aimed at addressing patient knowledge, attitude, and belief barriers to colonoscopy preparation. They found that patients receiving the booklet, in a randomized controlled trial of single-dose purgatives, achieved better bowel preparation quality compared with controls receiving the usual instructions, independent of the specific purgative prescribed. Recently, a Korean study demonstrated that patients receiving a cartoon visual educational instruction for colonoscopy exhibited better bowel preparation than those receiving the traditional verbal and written instructions for colonoscopy.[109] Proper patient education about the preparation details is clearly important although studies have shown that less than 20% of patients with inadequate preparation report failure to adequately follow instructions.[110] Other measures that may improve the quality of bowel preparation include simple walking exercises. One randomized controlled trial showed that walking exercise provides a significantly better quality of colon cleansing and seems to be a useful and effective means of improving colonic cleansing, without additional discomfort, in ambulatory outpatients who are scheduled for elective colonoscopy.[111]

HOW TO OPTIMIZE THE BOWEL PREPARATION

Despite all the evidence, it remains difficult to select outright the best modern bowel preparation. **Fig. 2** depicts the efficacy of currently available bowel preparations based on data extracted from recent clinical trials with more than 100 participants. These trials were not head-to-head studies, and may not be comparable regarding diet, bowel-cleansing scales, assessment for interobserver and intraobserver variability or the burden on quality of life (such as disturbance of daily activity or sleep). In real life, physicians use many different preparations and often develop a particular preference based on personal experience. Nonetheless, such an important quality

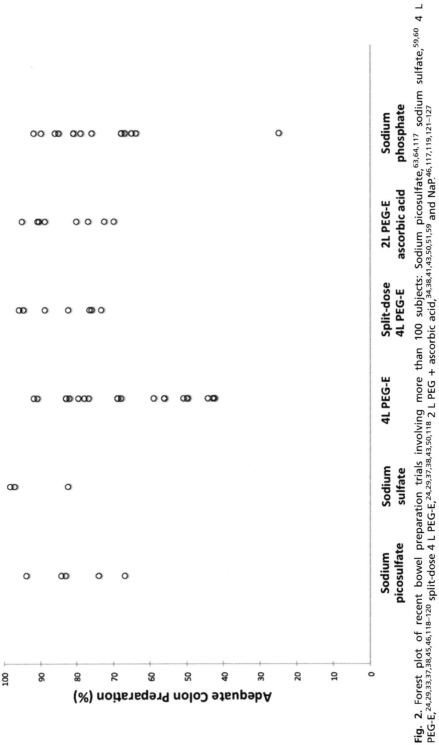

Fig. 2. Forest plot of recent bowel preparation trials involving more than 100 subjects: Sodium picosulfate, [63,64,117] sodium sulfate, [59,60] 4 L PEG-E, [24,29,33,37,38,45,46,118–120] split-dose 4 L PEG-E, [24,29,37,38,41,43,50,118] 2 L PEG + ascorbic acid, [34,38,41,43,50,51,59] 2 L PEG-E ascorbic acid, [63,64,117] and NaP. [46,117,119,121–127]

variable should be a central component of every performance improvement program in colonoscopy. Known independent predictors of inadequate colon preparation include a later colonoscopy starting time (in the absence of a second split dose with timely administration), failure to follow preparation instructions, inpatient status, procedural indication of constipation, male gender, use of tricyclic antidepressants, a history of cirrhosis, stroke, or dementia,[110] and a previous history of inadequate preparation. A personalized approach involving more stringent or extended dietary restrictions, proper patient education with reinforced need for adherence, and the additional use of stimulant laxatives, such as bisacodyl or senna, may be necessary in such situations. Few trials have examined the addition of prokinetics such as tegaserod[24] or mosapride[112] to the standard preparation regimens showing a modest improvement in quality. The adjunct use of such medications is, however, off-label and should be discouraged because of added cost and possible adverse effects. In a recent randomized controlled trial using commercially available sugar-free mentholyptus candy drops (Halls, Cadbury Adams, NJ), Sharara and colleagues[36] reported significant reduction in nausea and improvement in palatability and efficacy of split-dose PEG-E. Good or excellent preparation was achieved in 91.8% of patients using the mentholyptus drops versus 82% of controls. In addition, 92% of the mentholyptus users were willing to repeat the same preparation in the future if required versus 80% of controls. The addition of simethicone to the bowel preparation solution has been shown to improve visibility by reducing the amount of bubbles in the colon.[113]

Regardless of the regimen used, and for reasons that are not necessarily predictable,[114] there will always be patients who end up with inadequate preparation. In practice, however, physicians should strive for a minimum rate of success of 85% to 90%. As discussed previously, patients with poor preparation and residual solid or thick liquid stools should be rescheduled. Those with a fair preparation and residual thin liquid stools may benefit from washing and suctioning during colonoscopy as well as repositioning during examination[115] in an effort to achieve examination of more than 95% of the colonic mucosa. A new system for intracolonic cleansing, consisting of a disposable catheter device inserted through the working channel of a standard colonoscope coupled to an irrigation unit, has been developed to disintegrate and help remove residual stool under predefined pressure and flow rate using compressed CO_2 and minimal amounts of water. This system was recently shown to be superior to standard syringe irrigation at improving segmental colonic cleansing in a randomized trial of 42 patients with suboptimal bowel preparation.[116]

SUMMARY

Adequate bowel preparation is essential for optimal colonoscopy. The down sides of a poor or suboptimal examination are many and may be serious and costly. There are several effective formulations with good safety profile and these may be used interchangeably in patients without significant comorbidities depending on the patient profile and physician preference. PEG-E is the preferred regimen in patients with cardiac, renal, and liver disease because of limited effect on plasma volume and electrolyte homeostasis. Regardless of choice, split dosing is an important and established concept that should be implemented whenever possible in an effort to enhance tolerance and adherence, and improve mucosal visibility and overall quality of the examination. The burden of the preparation on patients, including dietary modifications and disturbance of daily routine and sleep, should be taken into consideration. Proper patient education regarding the different steps of the proposed preparation and the need for compliance and adherence are essential.

REFERENCES

1. Burke CA, Church JM. Enhancing the quality of colonoscopy: the importance of bowel purgatives. Gastrointest Endosc 2007;66:565–73.
2. Dykes C, Cash BD. Key safety issues of bowel preparations for colonoscopy and importance of adequate hydration. Gastroenterol Nurs 2008;31:30–5 [quiz: 36–7].
3. Lichtenstein GR, Cohen LB, Uribarri J. Review article: bowel preparation for colonoscopy–the importance of adequate hydration. Aliment Pharmacol Ther 2007;26:633–41.
4. Rex DK, Petrini JL, Baron TH, et al. Quality indicators for colonoscopy. Gastrointest Endosc 2006;63:S16–28.
5. Sherer EA, Imler TD, Imperiale TF. The effect of colonoscopy preparation quality on adenoma detection rates. Gastrointest Endosc 2012;75:545–53.
6. Froehlich F, Wietlisbach V, Gonvers JJ, et al. Impact of colonic cleansing on quality and diagnostic yield of colonoscopy: the European Panel of Appropriateness of Gastrointestinal Endoscopy European multicenter study. Gastrointest Endosc 2005;61:378–84.
7. Harewood GC, Sharma VK, de Garmo P. Impact of colonoscopy preparation quality on detection of suspected colonic neoplasia. Gastrointest Endosc 2003;58:76–9.
8. Chokshi RV, Hovis CE, Hollander T, et al. Prevalence of missed adenomas in patients with inadequate bowel preparation on screening colonoscopy. Gastrointest Endosc 2012;75:1197–203.
9. Lebwohl B, Kastrinos F, Glick M, et al. The impact of suboptimal bowel preparation on adenoma miss rates and the factors associated with early repeat colonoscopy. Gastrointest Endosc 2011;73:1207–14.
10. Rex DK, Imperiale TF, Latinovich DR, et al. Impact of bowel preparation on efficiency and cost of colonoscopy. Am J Gastroenterol 2002;97:1696–700.
11. Davis GR, Santa Ana CA, Morawski SG, et al. Development of a lavage solution associated with minimal water and electrolyte absorption or secretion. Gastroenterology 1980;78:991–5.
12. Cohen SM, Wexner SD, Binderow SR, et al. Prospective, randomized, endoscopic-blinded trial comparing precolonoscopy bowel cleansing methods. Dis Colon Rectum 1994;37:689–96.
13. DiPalma JA, Marshall JB. Comparison of a new sulfate-free polyethylene glycol electrolyte lavage solution versus a standard solution for colonoscopy cleansing. Gastrointest Endosc 1990;36:285–9.
14. Froehlich F, Fried M, Schnegg JF, et al. Palatability of a new solution compared with standard polyethylene glycol solution for gastrointestinal lavage. Gastrointest Endosc 1991;37:325–8.
15. Froehlich F, Fried M, Schnegg JF, et al. Low sodium solution for colonic cleansing: a double-blind, controlled, randomized prospective study. Gastrointest Endosc 1992;38:579–81.
16. Frommer D. Cleansing ability and tolerance of three bowel preparations for colonoscopy. Dis Colon Rectum 1997;40:100–4.
17. Hookey LC, Depew WT, Vanner S. The safety profile of oral sodium phosphate for colonic cleansing before colonoscopy in adults. Gastrointest Endosc 2002;56:895–902.
18. Hsu CW, Imperiale TF. Meta-analysis and cost comparison of polyethylene glycol lavage versus sodium phosphate for colonoscopy preparation. Gastrointest Endosc 1998;48:276–82.

19. Raymond JM, Beyssac R, Capdenat E, et al. Tolerance, effectiveness, and acceptability of sulfate-free electrolyte lavage solution for colon cleaning before colonoscopy. Endoscopy 1996;28:555–8.

20. Clarkston WK, Tsen TN, Dies DF, et al. Oral sodium phosphate versus sulfate-free polyethylene glycol electrolyte lavage solution in outpatient preparation for colonoscopy: a prospective comparison. Gastrointest Endosc 1996;43:42–8.

21. Henderson JM, Barnett JL, Turgeon DK, et al. Single-day, divided-dose oral sodium phosphate laxative versus intestinal lavage as preparation for colonoscopy: efficacy and patient tolerance. Gastrointest Endosc 1995;42:238–43.

22. Linden TB, Waye JD. Sodium phosphate preparation for colonoscopy: onset and duration of bowel activity. Gastrointest Endosc 1999;50:811–3.

23. Young CJ, Simpson RR, King DW, et al. Oral sodium phosphate solution is a superior colonoscopy preparation to polyethylene glycol with bisacodyl. Dis Colon Rectum 2000;43:1568–71.

24. Abdul-Baki H, Hashash JG, Elhajj II, et al. A randomized, controlled, double-blind trial of the adjunct use of tegaserod in whole-dose or split-dose polyethylene glycol electrolyte solution for colonoscopy preparation. Gastrointest Endosc 2008;68:294–300 [quiz: 334, 336].

25. Harewood GC, Wright CA, Baron TH. Assessment of patients' perceptions of bowel preparation quality at colonoscopy. Am J Gastroenterol 2004;99:839–43.

26. Fatima H, Johnson CS, Rex DK. Patients' description of rectal effluent and quality of bowel preparation at colonoscopy. Gastrointest Endosc 2010;71:1244–52.e2.

27. Rostom A, Jolicoeur E. Validation of a new scale for the assessment of bowel preparation quality. Gastrointest Endosc 2004;59:482–6.

28. El-Dika S, Mahl T, Mehboob S, et al. Is blinding the endoscopists to bowel preparations in randomized-controlled trials a reality? Cancer Detect Prev 2006;30:552–9.

29. Aoun E, Abdul-Baki H, Azar C, et al. A randomized single-blind trial of split-dose PEG-electrolyte solution without dietary restriction compared with whole dose PEG-electrolyte solution with dietary restriction for colonoscopy preparation. Gastrointest Endosc 2005;62:213–8.

30. Park DI, Park SH, Lee SK, et al. Efficacy of prepackaged, low residual test meals with 4L polyethylene glycol versus a clear liquid diet with 4L polyethylene glycol bowel preparation: a randomized trial. J Gastroenterol Hepatol 2009;24:988–91.

31. Soweid AM, Kobeissy AA, Jamali FR, et al. A randomized single-blind trial of standard diet versus fiber-free diet with polyethylene glycol electrolyte solution for colonoscopy preparation. Endoscopy 2010;42:633–8.

32. Scott SR, Raymond PL, Thompson WO, et al. Efficacy and tolerance of sodium phosphates oral solution after diet liberalization. Gastroenterol Nurs 2005;28:133–9.

33. Rapier R, Houston C. A prospective study to assess the efficacy and patient tolerance of three bowel preparations for colonoscopy. Gastroenterol Nurs 2006;29:305–8.

34. Repici A, Cestari R, Annese V, et al. Randomised clinical trial: low-volume bowel preparation for colonoscopy - a comparison between two different PEG-based formulations. Aliment Pharmacol Ther 2012;36:717–24.

35. Wu KL, Rayner CK, Chuah SK, et al. Impact of low-residue diet on bowel preparation for colonoscopy. Dis Colon Rectum 2011;54:107–12.

36. Sharara AI, El-Halabi MM, Abou Fadel CG, et al. Sugar-Free Mentholyptus Drops improve the Palatability and Bowel Cleansing Effect of PEG-Electrolyte Solution. Gastrointest Endosc 2013, in press.

37. El Sayed AM, Kanafani ZA, Mourad FH, et al. A randomized single-blind trial of whole versus split-dose polyethylene glycol-electrolyte solution for colonoscopy preparation. Gastrointest Endosc 2003;58:36–40.
38. Marmo R, Rotondano G, Riccio G, et al. Effective bowel cleansing before colonoscopy: a randomized study of split-dosage versus non-split dosage regimens of high-volume versus low-volume polyethylene glycol solutions. Gastrointest Endosc 2010;72:313–20.
39. Adams WJ, Meagher AP, Lubowski DZ, et al. Bisacodyl reduces the volume of polyethylene glycol solution required for bowel preparation. Dis Colon Rectum 1994;37:229–33 [discussion: 233–4].
40. Borkje B, Pedersen R, Lund GM, et al. Effectiveness and acceptability of three bowel cleansing regimens. Scand J Gastroenterol 1991;26:162–6.
41. Cohen LB, Sanyal SM, Von Althann C, et al. Clinical trial: 2-L polyethylene glycol-based lavage solutions for colonoscopy preparation - a randomized, single-blind study of two formulations. Aliment Pharmacol Ther 2010;32:637–44.
42. DiPalma JA, Wolff BG, Meagher A, et al. Comparison of reduced volume versus four liters sulfate-free electrolyte lavage solutions for colonoscopy colon cleansing. Am J Gastroenterol 2003;98:2187–91.
43. Ell C, Fischbach W, Bronisch HJ, et al. Randomized trial of low-volume PEG solution versus standard PEG + electrolytes for bowel cleansing before colonoscopy. Am J Gastroenterol 2008;103:883–93.
44. Hangartner PJ, Munch R, Meier J, et al. Comparison of three colon cleansing methods: evaluation of a randomized clinical trial with 300 ambulatory patients. Endoscopy 1989;21:272–5.
45. Hookey LC, Depew WT, Vanner SJ. Combined low volume polyethylene glycol solution plus stimulant laxatives versus standard volume polyethylene glycol solution: a prospective, randomized study of colon cleansing before colonoscopy. Can J Gastroenterol 2006;20:101–5.
46. Huppertz-Hauss G, Bretthauer M, Sauar J, et al. Polyethylene glycol versus sodium phosphate in bowel cleansing for colonoscopy: a randomized trial. Endoscopy 2005;37:537–41.
47. Sharma VK, Chockalingham SK, Ugheoke EA, et al. Prospective, randomized, controlled comparison of the use of polyethylene glycol electrolyte lavage solution in four-liter versus two-liter volumes and pretreatment with either magnesium citrate or bisacodyl for colonoscopy preparation. Gastrointest Endosc 1998;47: 167–71.
48. Kilgore TW, Abdinoor AA, Szary NM, et al. Bowel preparation with split-dose polyethylene glycol before colonoscopy: a meta-analysis of randomized controlled trials. Gastrointest Endosc 2011;73:1240–5.
49. Enestvedt BK, Tofani C, Laine LA, et al. 4-Liter split-dose polyethylene glycol is superior to other bowel preparations, based on systematic review and meta-analysis. Clin Gastroenterol Hepatol 2012;10:1225–31.
50. Corporaal S, Kleibeuker JH, Koornstra JJ. Low-volume PEG plus ascorbic acid versus high-volume PEG as bowel preparation for colonoscopy. Scand J Gastroenterol 2010;45:1380–6.
51. Bitoun A, Ponchon T, Barthet M, et al. Results of a prospective randomised multicentre controlled trial comparing a new 2-L ascorbic acid plus polyethylene glycol and electrolyte solution vs. sodium phosphate solution in patients undergoing elective colonoscopy. Aliment Pharmacol Ther 2006;24:1631–42.
52. Worthington J, Thyssen M, Chapman G, et al. A randomised controlled trial of a new 2 litre polyethylene glycol solution versus sodium picosulphate +

magnesium citrate solution for bowel cleansing prior to colonoscopy. Curr Med Res Opin 2008;24:481–8.

53. Tan JJ, Tjandra JJ. Which is the optimal bowel preparation for colonoscopy - a meta-analysis. Colorectal Dis 2006;8:247–58.

54. Lawrance IC, Willert RP, Murray K. Bowel cleansing for colonoscopy: prospective randomized assessment of efficacy and of induced mucosal abnormality with three preparation agents. Endoscopy 2011;43:412–8.

55. Seo EH, Kim TO, Kim TG, et al. Efficacy and tolerability of split-dose PEG compared with split-dose aqueous sodium phosphate for outpatient colonoscopy: a randomized, controlled trial. Dig Dis Sci 2011;56:2963–71.

56. Kastenberg D, Chasen R, Choudhary C, et al. Efficacy and safety of sodium phosphate tablets compared with PEG solution in colon cleansing: two identically designed, randomized, controlled, parallel group, multicenter phase III trials. Gastrointest Endosc 2001;54:705–13.

57. Rex DK, Chasen R, Pochapin MB. Safety and efficacy of two reduced dosing regimens of sodium phosphate tablets for preparation prior to colonoscopy. Aliment Pharmacol Ther 2002;16:937–44.

58. Khashab M, Rex DK. Efficacy and tolerability of a new formulation of sodium phosphate tablets (INKP-101), and a reduced sodium phosphate dose, in colon cleansing: a single-center open-label pilot trial. Aliment Pharmacol Ther 2005; 21:465–8.

59. Di Palma JA, Rodriguez R, McGowan J, et al. A randomized clinical study evaluating the safety and efficacy of a new, reduced-volume, oral sulfate colon-cleansing preparation for colonoscopy. Am J Gastroenterol 2009;104: 2275–84.

60. Rex DK, Di Palma JA, Rodriguez R, et al. A randomized clinical study comparing reduced-volume oral sulfate solution with standard 4-liter sulfate-free electrolyte lavage solution as preparation for colonoscopy. Gastrointest Endosc 2010;72:328–36.

61. Hamilton D, Mulcahy D, Walsh D, et al. Sodium picosulphate compared with polyethylene glycol solution for large bowel lavage: a prospective randomised trial. Br J Clin Pract 1996;50:73–5.

62. Renaut AJ, Raniga S, Frizelle FA, et al. A randomized controlled trial comparing the efficacy and acceptability of phospo-soda buffered saline (Fleet) with sodium picosulphate/magnesium citrate (Picoprep) in the preparation of patients for colonoscopy. Colorectal Dis 2008;10:503–5.

63. Flemming JA, Vanner SJ, Hookey LC. Split-dose picosulfate, magnesium oxide, and citric acid solution markedly enhances colon cleansing before colonoscopy: a randomized, controlled trial. Gastrointest Endosc 2012;75:537–44.

64. Katz PO, Rex DK, Epstein M, et al. A dual-action, low-volume bowel cleanser administered the day before colonoscopy: results from the SEE CLEAR II study. Am J Gastroenterol 2013;108:401–9.

65. Hjelkrem M, Stengel J, Liu M, et al. MiraLAX is not as effective as GoLytely in bowel cleansing before screening colonoscopies. Clin Gastroenterol Hepatol 2011;9:326–32.e1.

66. Enestvedt BK, Fennerty MB, Eisen GM. Randomised clinical trial: MiraLAX vs. Golytely - a controlled study of efficacy and patient tolerability in bowel preparation for colonoscopy. Aliment Pharmacol Ther 2011;33:33–40.

67. Samarasena JB, Muthusamy VR, Jamal MM. Split-dosed MiraLAX/Gatorade is an effective, safe, and tolerable option for bowel preparation in low-risk patients: a randomized controlled study. Am J Gastroenterol 2012;107:1036–42.

68. Church JM. Effectiveness of polyethylene glycol antegrade gut lavage bowel preparation for colonoscopy–timing is the key! Dis Colon Rectum 1998;41:1223–5.

69. Johanson JF, Popp JW Jr, Cohen LB, et al. A randomized, multicenter study comparing the safety and efficacy of sodium phosphate tablets with 2L polyethylene glycol solution plus bisacodyl tablets for colon cleansing. Am J Gastroenterol 2007;102:2238–46.

70. Parra-Blanco A, Nicolas-Perez D, Gimeno-Garcia A, et al. The timing of bowel preparation before colonoscopy determines the quality of cleansing, and is a significant factor contributing to the detection of flat lesions: a randomized study. World J Gastroenterol 2006;12:6161–6.

71. Seo EH, Kim TO, Park MJ, et al. Optimal preparation-to-colonoscopy interval in split-dose PEG bowel preparation determines satisfactory bowel preparation quality: an observational prospective study. Gastrointest Endosc 2012;75:583–90.

72. Longcroft-Wheaton G, Bhandari P. Same-day bowel cleansing regimen is superior to a split-dose regimen over 2 days for afternoon colonoscopy: results from a large prospective series. J Clin Gastroenterol 2012;46:57–61.

73. Greenfield SM, Webster GJ, Brar AS, et al. Assessment of residual gastric volume and thirst in patients who drink before gastroscopy. Gut 1996;39:360–2.

74. Webster GJ, Bowling TE, Greenfield SM, et al. Drinking before endoscopy: milk or water? Gastrointest Endosc 1997;45:406–8.

75. Lichtenstein DR, Jagannath S, Baron TH, et al. Sedation and anesthesia in GI endoscopy. Gastrointest Endosc 2008;68:815–26.

76. Cohen K, Mount S. Current issues in optimal bowel preparation: excerpts from a roundtable discussion among colon-cleansing experts. Gastroenterol Hepatol 2009;5:3–11.

77. Khan MA, Wasiuddin N, Brown MD. Patient acceptance, convenience and efficacy of one-day versus two-day colonoscopy bowel preparation [abstract]. Gastrointest Endosc 2008;67:A246.

78. Wexner SD, Beck DE, Baron TH, et al. A consensus document on bowel preparation before colonoscopy: prepared by a task force from the American Society of Colon and Rectal Surgeons (ASCRS), the American Society for Gastrointestinal Endoscopy (ASGE), and the Society of American Gastrointestinal and Endoscopic Surgeons (SAGES). Gastrointest Endosc 2006;63:894–909.

79. Rex DK, Johnson DA, Anderson JC, et al. American College of Gastroenterology guidelines for colorectal cancer screening 2009 [corrected]. Am J Gastroenterol 2009;104:739–50.

80. Ayus JC, Levine R, Arieff AI. Fatal dysnatraemia caused by elective colonoscopy. BMJ 2003;326:382–4.

81. Frizelle FA, Colls BM. Hyponatremia and seizures after bowel preparation: report of three cases. Dis Colon Rectum 2005;48:393–6.

82. Nagler J, Poppers D, Turetz M. Severe hyponatremia and seizure following a polyethylene glycol-based bowel preparation for colonoscopy. J Clin Gastroenterol 2006;40:558–9.

83. Cohen CD, Keuneke C, Schiemann U, et al. Hyponatraemia as a complication of colonoscopy. Lancet 2001;357:282–3.

84. Dillon CE, Laher MS. The rapid development of hyponatraemia and seizures in an elderly patient following sodium picosulfate/magnesium citrate (Picolax). Age Ageing 2009;38:487.

85. Aasebo W, Scott H, Ganss R. Kidney biopsies taken before and after oral sodium phosphate bowel cleansing. Nephrol Dial Transplant 2007;22:920–2.

86. Desmeules S, Bergeron MJ, Isenring P. Acute phosphate nephropathy and renal failure. N Engl J Med 2003;349:1006–7.
87. Gonlusen G, Akgun H, Ertan A, et al. Renal failure and nephrocalcinosis associated with oral sodium phosphate bowel cleansing: clinical patterns and renal biopsy findings. Arch Pathol Lab Med 2006;130:101–6.
88. Markowitz GS, Stokes MB, Radhakrishnan J, et al. Acute phosphate nephropathy following oral sodium phosphate bowel purgative: an underrecognized cause of chronic renal failure. J Am Soc Nephrol 2005;16:3389–96.
89. Lieberman DA, Ghormley J, Flora K. Effect of oral sodium phosphate colon preparation on serum electrolytes in patients with normal serum creatinine. Gastrointest Endosc 1996;43:467–9.
90. Ehrenpreis ED. Increased serum phosphate levels and calcium fluxes are seen in smaller individuals after a single dose of sodium phosphate colon cleansing solution: a pharmacokinetic analysis. Aliment Pharmacol Ther 2009;29:1202–11.
91. Holte K, Nielsen KG, Madsen JL, et al. Physiologic effects of bowel preparation. Dis Colon Rectum 2004;47:1397–402.
92. Beloosesky Y, Grinblat J, Weiss A, et al. Electrolyte disorders following oral sodium phosphate administration for bowel cleansing in elderly patients. Arch Intern Med 2003;163:803–8.
93. Caswell M, Thompson WO, Kanapka JA, et al. The time course and effect on serum electrolytes of oral sodium phosphates solution in healthy male and female volunteers. Can J Clin Pharmacol 2007;14:e260–74.
94. Russmann S, Lamerato L, Marfatia A, et al. Risk of impaired renal function after colonoscopy: a cohort study in patients receiving either oral sodium phosphate or polyethylene glycol. Am J Gastroenterol 2007;102:2655–63.
95. Zuccaro G Jr, Connor JT, Schreiber M Jr. Colonoscopy preparation: are our patients at risk? Am J Gastroenterol 2007;102:2664–6.
96. Hurst FP, Bohen EM, Osgard EM, et al. Association of oral sodium phosphate purgative use with acute kidney injury. J Am Soc Nephrol 2007;18:3192–8.
97. Lien YH. Is bowel preparation before colonoscopy a risky business for the kidney? Nat Clin Pract Nephrol 2008;4:606–14.
98. Rex DK. Dosing considerations in the use of sodium phosphate bowel preparations for colonoscopy. Ann Pharmacother 2007;41:1466–75.
99. Hixson LJ. Colorectal ulcers associated with sodium phosphate catharsis. Gastrointest Endosc 1995;42:101–2.
100. Rejchrt S, Bures J, Siroky M, et al. A prospective, observational study of colonic mucosal abnormalities associated with orally administered sodium phosphate for colon cleansing before colonoscopy. Gastrointest Endosc 2004;59:651–4.
101. Zwas FR, Cirillo NW, el-Serag HB, et al. Colonic mucosal abnormalities associated with oral sodium phosphate solution. Gastrointest Endosc 1996;43:463–6.
102. Patel V, Nicar M, Emmett M, et al. Intestinal and renal effects of low-volume phosphate and sulfate cathartic solutions designed for cleansing the colon: pathophysiological studies in five normal subjects. Am J Gastroenterol 2009;104:953–65.
103. Rahman A, Vanner SJ, Baranchuk A, et al. Serial monitoring of the physiological effects of the standard Pico-Salax(R) regimen for colon cleansing in healthy volunteers. Can J Gastroenterol 2012;26:424–8.
104. Ho JM, Gruneir A, Fischer HD, et al. Serious events in older Ontario residents receiving bowel preparations for outpatient colonoscopy with various

comorbidity profiles: a descriptive, population-based study. Can J Gastroenterol 2012;26:436–40.

105. Abuksis G, Mor M, Segal N, et al. A patient education program is cost-effective for preventing failure of endoscopic procedures in a gastroenterology department. Am J Gastroenterol 2001;96:1786–90.

106. Shaikh AA, Hussain SM, Rahn S, et al. Effect of an educational pamphlet on colon cancer screening: a randomized, prospective trial. Eur J Gastroenterol Hepatol 2010;22:444–9.

107. Modi C, Depasquale JR, Digiacomo WS, et al. Impact of patient education on quality of bowel preparation in outpatient colonoscopies. Qual Prim Care 2009;17:397–404.

108. Spiegel BM, Talley J, Shekelle P, et al. Development and validation of a novel patient educational booklet to enhance colonoscopy preparation. Am J Gastroenterol 2011;106:875–83.

109. Tae JW, Lee JC, Hong SJ, et al. Impact of patient education with cartoon visual aids on the quality of bowel preparation for colonoscopy. Gastrointest Endosc 2012;76:804–11.

110. Ness RM, Manam R, Hoen H, et al. Predictors of inadequate bowel preparation for colonoscopy. Am J Gastroenterol 2001;96:1797–802.

111. Kim HS, Park DH, Kim JW, et al. Effectiveness of walking exercise as a bowel preparation for colonoscopy: a randomized controlled trial. Am J Gastroenterol 2005;100:1964–9.

112. Tajika M, Niwa Y, Bhatia V, et al. Efficacy of mosapride citrate with polyethylene glycol solution for colonoscopy preparation. World J Gastroenterol 2012;18: 2517–25.

113. Sudduth RH, DeAngelis S, Sherman KE, et al. The effectiveness of simethicone in improving visibility during colonoscopy when given with a sodium phosphate solution: a double-blind randomized study. Gastrointest Endosc 1995;42:413–5.

114. Hassan C, Fuccio L, Bruno M, et al. A predictive model identifies patients most likely to have inadequate bowel preparation for colonoscopy. Clin Gastroenterol Hepatol 2012;10:501–6.

115. East JE, Suzuki N, Arebi N, et al. Position changes improve visibility during colonoscope withdrawal: a randomized, blinded, crossover trial. Gastrointest Endosc 2007;65:263–9.

116. Rigaux J, Juriens I, Deviere J. A novel system for the improvement of colonic cleansing during colonoscopy. Endoscopy 2012;44:703–6.

117. Yoshioka K, Connolly AB, Ogunbiyi OA, et al. Randomized trial of oral sodium phosphate compared with oral sodium picosulphate (Picolax) for elective colorectal surgery and colonoscopy. Dig Surg 2000;17:66–70.

118. Park SS, Sinn DH, Kim YH, et al. Efficacy and tolerability of split-dose magnesium citrate: low-volume (2 liters) polyethylene glycol vs. single- or split-dose polyethylene glycol bowel preparation for morning colonoscopy. Am J Gastroenterol 2010;105:1319–26.

119. Aronchick CA, Lipshutz WH, Wright SH, et al. A novel tableted purgative for colonoscopic preparation: efficacy and safety comparisons with Colyte and Fleet Phospho-Soda. Gastrointest Endosc 2000;52:346–52.

120. Szojda MM, Kuik DJ, Mulder CJ, et al. Colonic lavage with two polyethylene glycol solutions prior to colonoscopy makes no difference: a prospective randomized controlled trial. Scand J Gastroenterol 2008;43:622–6.

121. Arezzo A. Prospective randomized trial comparing bowel cleaning preparations for colonoscopy. Surg Laparosc Endosc Percutan Tech 2000;10:215–7.

122. Ell C, Fischbach W, Keller R, et al. A randomized, blinded, prospective trial to compare the safety and efficacy of three bowel-cleansing solutions for colonoscopy (HSG-01*). Endoscopy 2003;35:300–4.

123. Hookey LC, Depew WT, Vanner SJ. A prospective randomized trial comparing low-dose oral sodium phosphate plus stimulant laxatives with large volume polyethylene glycol solution for colon cleansing. Am J Gastroenterol 2004;99: 2217–22.

124. Hwang KL, Chen WT, Hsiao KH, et al. Prospective randomized comparison of oral sodium phosphate and polyethylene glycol lavage for colonoscopy preparation. World J Gastroenterol 2005;11:7486–93.

125. Law WL, Choi HK, Chu KW, et al. Bowel preparation for colonoscopy: a randomized controlled trial comparing polyethylene glycol solution, one dose and two doses of oral sodium phosphate solution. Asian J Surg 2004;27:120–4.

126. Seinela L, Pehkonen E, Laasanen T, et al. Bowel preparation for colonoscopy in very old patients: a randomized prospective trial comparing oral sodium phosphate and polyethylene glycol electrolyte lavage solution. Scand J Gastroenterol 2003;38:216–20.

127. Bektas H, Bilsel Y, Yamaner S, et al. Comparison of sodium phosphate, polyethylene glycol and senna solutions in bowel preparation: a prospective, randomized controlled clinical study. Dig Endosc 2005;17:290–6.

Colonoscopy Quality
Metrics and Implementation

Audrey H. Calderwood, MD*, Brian C. Jacobson, MD, MPH

KEYWORDS

- Colonoscopy • Quality • Metrics • Quality improvement

KEY POINTS

- Quality in colonoscopy is essential to maintaining the trust of patients and the public.
- Several metrics have been suggested as quality indicators, including appropriate screening/surveillance intervals, adenoma detection rates, cecal intubation rates, and appropriate documentation.
- Implementation of quality improvement projects requires identification of a problem and outcome for measurement and development of an intervention followed by frequent short-term assessments and adjustments.
- The electronic health records and other registries facilitate quality reporting and measurement.

INTRODUCTION TO QUALITY

Keen interest in quality within medicine began after the Institute of Medicine's report on medical errors was published in 2000.[1] This report described the landscape of medicine at the time in the United States and revealed, for example, that 44,000 to 98,000 Americans die each year from medical errors. This report, along with public opinion regarding current care in the United States, led to a national call for reform within medicine. The report listed the major quality domains as safety, practice consistent with present medical knowledge, and customization.

Many parties have a stake in the measurement and reporting of quality. Stakeholders include patients, providers, professional societies, payors, regulatory bodies and accrediting organizations, the National Quality Forum, and the Centers for Medicare and Medicaid Services. Most stakeholders agree that the goal is to improve outcomes and avoid unintended consequences. There are financial incentives for providers to report quality measures and, as of 2015, there will be financial penalties for failing to report within Medicare.

The authors have no financial or other conflicts of interest to disclose.

Section of Gastroenterology, Boston University School of Medicine, 85 East Concord Street, Boston, MA 02118, USA

* Corresponding author.

E-mail address: audrey.calderwood@bmc.org

Given this landscape, colonoscopy is an excellent area for quality improvement work for several reasons. First, colonoscopy is the most common endoscopic procedure in United States[2,3] and there is significant associated risk and expense. Second, standardized reporting of colonoscopies has been advocated,[4] but evidence exists that performance of colonoscopy varies and this variation may affect effectiveness.[5–7] Publication of the joint American Society for Gastrointestinal Endoscopy/American College of Gastroenterology "Quality Indicators for Colonoscopy" in 2006 highlighted the importance of quality issues within colonoscopy and provided tangible benchmarks for achievement.[8] The importance of ensuring the highest quality in colonoscopy is further promoted by several recent studies questioning the effectiveness of colonoscopy in reducing colorectal cancer (CRC) mortality, especially from right-sided lesions.[9–11]

Before discussing quality in colonoscopy, it is important to emphasize the distinction between clinical guidelines and quality indicators. The former relates to recommendations for clinical care often related to a specific condition or work-up of a particular symptom. Guidelines may be supported by varying degrees of evidence, ranging from randomized controlled trials to expert opinion. In contrast, quality indicators are concrete, measurable items related either to the process of care in which the receipt of medical services is tracked[12] (eg, whether the cecum was reached and photodocumented with landmarks) or outcome measures (eg, whether a cancer was diagnosed within 3 years of colonoscopy), which in part reflect the results of medical care.[12]

QUALITY IN COLONOSCOPY

When quality metrics are developed, consideration is given to the end point by which the metric(s) can be monitored and validated. What is the best end point for validation of quality metrics in colonoscopy? CRC incidence and mortality are arguably the most relevant and important outcome in performance of colonoscopy and, as such, ideally would be the end point by which to validate metrics. However, these end points are difficult to measure and, because of low incidence, require many person-years of follow-up to yield meaningful results. Years of data collection are not often feasible in the quality work in which data collection, results, and adjustments are made more rapidly than in classic clinical research. Another end point is the incidence of so-called interval cancers, which are CRCs that arise within a certain time frame after colonoscopy. These interval cancers may arise from missed or incompletely removed lesions at initial colonoscopy, but may also be caused by biologically aggressive tumors that arise de novo. Interval CRCs can be measured in 2 different ways.[13,14] One is a prospective evaluation after colonoscopy with removal of polyps of patients who are enrolled in a surveillance program and return for a follow-up colonoscopy. A second way uses a case-control design in which patients with CRC are identified and assessed for whether or not they had a prior colonoscopy within 3 years of diagnosis. Because of the resources, time, and large numbers necessary to measure interval CRCs, a more readily accessible metric is the adenoma detection rate (ADR). ADR has gained international acceptance as a quality indicator and is discussed in detail later. In addition, patient satisfaction is also an important metric for consideration, but may be challenging to interpret because of variation in patient population and other factors difficult to control for at the endoscopist level.

COLONOSCOPY QUALITY METRICS

Most colonoscopy quality metrics are process measures rather than outcome measures and occur at the level of the endoscopist rather than the endoscopy unit or hospital. The American Society of Gastrointestinal Endoscopy/American College of Gastroenterology Task Force on Quality Indicators for Colonoscopy proposed 14 quality metrics that occur at the preprocedure, intraprocedure, and postprocedure phases of colonoscopy (**Table 1**).[8] Only 2 measures have strong recommendations (appropriate indication and use of recommended postpolypectomy and postcancer resection surveillance intervals) and 4 have intermediate recommendations (cecal intubation rates, ADR, inflammatory bowel disease [IBD] surveillance biopsies, and endoscopic management of postpolypectomy bleeding). This article highlights several of these indicators in decreasing order of strength of recommendation and provides background information on the measure, including whether the literature supports its association with improved outcomes.

Screening/Surveillance Intervals

The use of recommended screening intervals for normal colonoscopies and recommended postpolypectomy and postcancer surveillance intervals for those with neoplasia is important to minimize risks of excessive procedures and maximize cost-effectiveness of population-based screening.[8] Ample literature suggests that patients are told to return more frequently than is dictated by guidelines.[15–17] However,

Table 1
Proposed quality indicators for colonoscopy (ASGE/ACG 2006)

Quality Indicator	Grade of Recommendation
Preprocedure Indicators	
Appropriate indication	1C+
Informed consent including discussion of risks	3
Use of postpolypectomy and postcancer resection surveillance intervals	1A
Use of IBD disease surveillance intervals	2C
Documentation of quality of bowel preparation in note	2C
Intraprocedure Indicators	
Cecal intubation rates including photographic documentation of landmark in note	1C
Adenoma detection during screening	1C
Withdrawal time: mean >6 min in normal examinations	2C
Biopsy specimens in patients with chronic diarrhea	2C
Number and distribution of biopsy specimens in IBD surveillance	1C
Endoscopic resection attempted for pedunculated polyps and sessile polyps <2 cm	3
Postprocedure Indicator	
Incidence of perforation	2C
Incidence of postpolypectomy bleeding	2C
Postpolypectomy bleeding managed nonoperatively	1C

1A = Strong: clear benefit, supported by randomized trials without important limitations. 1C+ = Strong: clear benefit, supported by overwhelming evidence from observational studies. 1C = Intermediate: clear benefit, supported by observational studies. 2C = Very weak: unclear benefit, supported by observational studies. 3 = Weak: unclear benefit, expert opinion only.

Adapted from Rex DK, Petrini JL, Baron TH, et al. Quality indicators for colonoscopy. Am J Gastroenterol 101:873–85, copyright 2006, Macmillan Publishers Ltd; with permission.

those who are deemed high risk who do not return for surveillance also indicate poor-quality care. In one study, 34% of those with polyps greater than 1 cm did not return for surveillance.[18] In another study of patients with adenomas or CRC, 35% had no follow-up and 38% had their follow-up delayed.[19]

The importance of appropriate polyp surveillance and avoidance of inappropriate use has been recognized at the national level with the endorsement of colonoscopy interval quality measures by the National Quality Forum and their adoption by the Physician Quality Reporting System (PQRS). PQRS was initiated in 2007 by the Centers for Medicare and Medicaid Services (CMS) as a reporting program that uses "a combination of incentive payments and payment adjustments to promote reporting of quality information by eligible professionals."[20] Those who report satisfactorily on the measure receive incentive payments based on their Medicare Part B fee charges. Starting in 2015, there will also be a payment penalty for those who do not satisfactorily report data on quality measures for covered professional services.

Of the 190 measures included in the 2011 PQRS measurements, only 1 pertained to colonoscopy. Measure 185, "Endoscopy & Polyp Surveillance: Colonoscopy Interval for Patients with a History of Adenomatous Polyps – Avoidance of Inappropriate Use" specifies reporting of the percentage of patients aged 18 years and older receiving a surveillance colonoscopy and a history of colonic polyp(s) in a previous colonoscopy who had a follow-up interval of 3 or more years since their last colonoscopy documented in the colonoscopy report. Detailed measure specifications can be found at http://www.cms.gov/Medicare/Quality-Initiatives-Patient-Assessment-Instruments/PQRS/downloads/2011_physqualrptg_measurespecificationsmanual_033111.pdf.

There is no performance threshold yet set for this measure, and providers receive credit simply for reporting their performance scores.

ADR

Detecting and removing adenomas is a fundamental goal of screening colonoscopy. Missed lesions are a potential cause of interval cancers and perhaps the lower than expected protection rate from colonoscopy. Despite its importance, there are large disparities in the detection rates of practicing endoscopists,[21] which has been shown in studies of tandem colonoscopy,[22,23] small group practices,[6,7,24,25] missed neoplasia,[26–28] and computed tomography colonography.[29] The target rate for ADR is greater than or equal to 25% in men and greater than or equal to 15% in women more than 50 years old presenting for average-risk screening based on observed prevalence rates of neoplasia in the United States.[8]

Measurement of ADR should be a priority. The most accepted method for measurement is calculation of the number of screening colonoscopies in which at least 1 adenoma was found divided by the total number of screening colonoscopies performed. Others have suggested the mean number of adenomas per patient as another calculation that may add additional information.[30–32] To calculate mean adenomas per patient, the total number of adenomas is divided by the total number of colonoscopies performed. Although mean adenoma per patient may prove to be a good measure of adenoma detection, current data are insufficient to establish compliance rate benchmarks for its use as a quality metric.

The type of examinations and the time period or volume over which ADR should be calculated has not been confirmed. For now, ADR should be limited to screening colonoscopy examinations, although, as more data emerge on adenoma rates in surveillance colonoscopy, surveillance may be monitored as well, whether in combination with screening or independently. The time period or number of cases over which ADR is calculated is not specified, which may cause difficulty in interpreting results, especially for low-volume endoscopists. One study highlights the importance of the number of procedures over which this measure is calculated because low numbers may not accurately represent the ADR (**Table 2**). At least 500 procedures need to be included in the calculation to have a reliable point estimate of ADR and a 95% confidence interval can account for uncertainty and should be used in the setting of lower numbers of procedures to help interpret endoscopist performance.[32]

There is some debate over whether a polyp detection rate (PDR) or polypectomy rate can be used reliably as a surrogate for ADR. The benefit would be ease of calculation by avoiding linking with pathology results facilitating tracking given the logistical hurdles when using a registry to determine ADR.[33] PDR is highly correlated with ADR, with proposed benchmarks of 40% in men and 30% in women.[34,35] If there is concern over gaming the system, in which endoscopists report and/or remove polyps of which few are adenomas, sporadic audits with pathology reports could help prevent this.[35] In the Clinical Outcomes Research Initiative registry, the use of polyps greater than 9 mm as a surrogate for advanced neoplasia is 84% specific,[36] suggesting that surrogate markers might facilitate calculation of metrics within registries. In addition, novel algorithms may help facilitate linking pathology with endoscopy reports,[33] especially in the setting of electronic health records.

Robust data support that ADR is a valid predictor of CRC. In a large study of more than 45,000 patients in a national CRC screening program in Poland, ADR and patient age were the only predictors of interval CRC, defined as CRC before the next surveillance examination was due (<5 years).[37] Patient sex, doctor specialty, and cecal intubation rates were not associated with interval cancer. This study highlighted that measurement of ADR should have a role in continuous quality improvement programs for CRC screening. Some hypothesize that ADR may be a proxy for a more thorough examination of the colon. In a large German study, ADR was associated with endoscopist continuing medical education attendance and colonoscope instrument model, but not endoscopist procedural volume or withdrawal times.[38]

Numerous studies have attempted to address whether or not ADR can be improved. A systematic review that included 7 studies and 10 abstracts found that improving ADR is difficult.[39] This is exemplified by a study of 5 ambulatory endoscopy centers in Minnesota in which they attempted to systematically evaluate variability in ADR over time after application of specific quality improvement programs.[40] None of the interventions (blinded and unblinded review of individual ADR, education about colonoscopy quality literature highlighting ADR goals and importance of withdrawal time, discussion between practice leaders and poor performing endoscopists, and financial consequences for withdrawal time <6 minutes) resulted in a significant improvement in ADR, which was associated only with patient factors (age, sex, and bowel prep quality). More research needs to be conducted to determine methods for improving ADR among low performers.

Table 2
ADR and confidence intervals

# of Colonoscopies	ADR					
	15%	20%	25%	30%	35%	40%
100	8–22	12–28	17–33	21–39	26–44	30–50
500	12–18	16–24	21–29	26–34	31–39	36–44
1000	13–17	18–22	22–28	27–33	32–38	37–43

In addition, although ADR is typically calculated from traditional adenomas, the importance of serrated lesions is apparent.[41,42] Whether serrated lesions should be included in the measurement of ADR or whether they merit their own metric remains to be determined.

Cecal Intubation Rates

Complete colonoscopy to the cecum is necessary for detection of a substantial fraction of proximal colon lesions.[43] Quality indicators encourage documentation of cecal intubation with naming of the identified cecal landmarks (appendiceal orifice and ileocecal valve) and photographs.[8] Intubation of the cecum should be achieved in greater than or equal to 95% of healthy subjects and greater than or equal to 90% of all colonoscopies. Cecal intubation rates are associated with postcolonoscopy CRC. In a large database study from Canada, higher cecal intubation rates were associated with protection from CRC in the right side. In a study in the UK, higher cecal intubation rates were similarly associated with higher ADRs.[30,44]

Withdrawal Times

Withdrawal time, defined as the time from the colonoscope reaching the cecum to removal of the instrument from the patient, is considered a quality indicator in colonoscopy. Expert opinion suggests that the mean withdrawal time should be greater than or equal to 6 minutes in colonoscopies with normal results performed in patients with intact colons.[8] This recommendation was qualified by the statement that, for those with adequate ADR, secondary measures such as withdrawal time are of less importance.[8] Withdrawal time should not be applied to individual patient cases but must be averaged over many cases for an individual endoscopist.

The importance of withdrawal time and establishment of a threshold of 6 minutes came after publication of a study of 12 gastroenterologists in a community-based practice.[6] The investigators compared the differences in ADR between endoscopists with greater than or equal to 6 minutes and less than 6 minutes withdrawal times. They found a strong correlation between mean withdrawal time on cases without polypectomy and detection of lesions (Spearman rank correlation coefficient $[r_s]$ = 0.90, $P<.001$). Endoscopists with mean withdrawal time greater than or equal to 6 minutes also detected more advanced lesions (6.4% vs 2.3%, P = .005).

However, adopting a minimum withdrawal time alone is not likely to result in a substantially improved ADR.[45] Simply recording withdrawal time did not improve ADR in one study.[45] After the institution of using a cecal time stamp to record withdrawal time, PDR did not change significantly. Another study in Peru found that adopting a 6-minute or longer withdrawal time minimum did not change PDR.[46] This study should be interpreted with caution because of overall low rates of PDR, in the range of 15% to 16%. Confidential feedback on withdrawal time with follow-up monitoring resulted in an increase in withdrawal time and in PDR, but not ADR. Mean withdrawal time without polyps went from 6.6 minutes to 8.1 minutes ($P<.0001$), PDR went from 33% to 38% (P = .04), without a significant change in ADR (20%–23%, P = .17).[47] In a study of 42 endoscopists at an academic medical center, an institution-wide policy requiring a minimum of 7 minutes withdrawal time per case increased the proportion of examinations with mean withdrawal time of 7 minutes (65%–100%), but did not affect PDR.[48] In addition, a study of a large German colonoscopy registry found that withdrawal time was not associated with ADR.[38]

Withdrawal time is a surrogate marker for ADR and thus has limited value if endoscopists are already performing careful inspections. However, for those with low

ADR, withdrawal time should be measured to see if short inspection time might be a modifiable factor for improvement.

Bowel Preparation Quality

The diagnostic accuracy of colonoscopy depends on the cleanliness of the colon and ability to visualize lesions. Poor preparation leads not only to missed lesions but also prolonged duration of procedure, repeated examinations at earlier intervals, increased complications, and excessive costs.[49–52] The quality of bowel preparation should be documented in every procedure note.[8] Qualitative descriptives (excellent, good, fair, poor) used in clinical practice lack standardized definitions and the Quality Assurance Task Force and Multi-Society Task Force on CRC advocate the use of "Inadequate to exclude polyps >5 mm in size" as a cutoff for repeating colonoscopy.[4] The Ottawa and Aronchick bowel preparation rating scales were created as potential standardized bowel preparation scales, but were limited by lack of extensive validation and reliability testing. Furthermore, the Ottawa scale is complex, limiting practical use, and the Aronchick scale relies on global assessments that do not address individual colonic segments.[53,54] The Boston Bowel Preparation Scale has been shown to be reliable and was validated prospectively, showing correlation with important outcomes like polyp detection, and has been incorporated in the Clinical Outcomes Research Initiative (CORI) and ProVation endowriters.[55,56] However, there are no rating scales that receive universal acceptance as a gold standard.

If bowel preparation is inadequate in more than 10% of examinations, this may reflect quality-control issues and special attention may need to be given to patient education and type of preparation.[4] Bowel preparation considerations are covered by Sharara and colleagues in more detail elsewhere in this issue.

Complications

Of the known complications of colonoscopy,[57] only the incidences of perforation and postpolypectomy bleeding are proposed as quality measures.[8] A benchmark has been set such that, if perforation rates are greater than 1 in 500 for all colonoscopies or 1 in 1000 for screening colonoscopies, evaluation should be pursued.[8] Bleeding rates greater than 1% should prompt evaluation of whether inappropriate practices are taking place.[8] Some data suggest that perforation rates may be higher among low-volume endoscopists.[58] In an administrative database study of more than 97,000 patients undergoing outpatient colonoscopy in Canada, older age, male sex, having a polypectomy, and having the colonoscopy performed by a low-volume endoscopist (<300/y) were associated with increased odds of bleeding or perforation.[58]

The performance benchmarks established by the Joint American Society of Gastrointestinal Endoscopy/American College of Gastroenterology Task Force on Quality Indicators for Colonoscopy were based on available literature; however, without proper documentation or systems for capturing delayed complications, rates may be underreported,[59,60] rendering the rate of acceptable complications inaccurate. A structured assessment tool was used to survey patients who had undergone colonoscopy in the Netherlands to determine major adverse events (hospital visit required), minor adverse events, and days missed from work. Adverse events were further categorized as definite, possible, or unrelated adverse events. The rate of definite major and minor events was 1% and 29% respsectively.[61] Development of a proper lexicon for reporting complications should also help promote the consistent and accurate classification of adverse events.[62]

Colonoscopy-related complications are covered in detail elsewhere in this issue.

Documentation

Although proper documentation may not at seem to affect patient outcomes related to colonoscopy, it plays an essential role in the ability to track indicators and develop benchmarks for performance. The absence of key information hinders communication with other physicians and may impede appropriate follow-up, whether too soon or delayed.

In the past, there has been variability in the quality of colonoscopy reports and documentation. A study of colonoscopy reports as part of a statewide screening program in Maryland analyzed 25 data elements and found that 27% of reports did not document bowel preparation quality, 18% did not use specific cecal landmarks, and, in cases with polyps, size and morphology were missing 13% and 47% of the time, respectively.[63] A different study of 4800 colonoscopies by 116 Dutch endoscopists also found considerable variability in documentation of the quality of bowel prep and cecal landmarks.[64] A study of 135 reports from the US community setting also showed low completeness rates.[65]

Even with the use of a computer-generated standardized endoscopy report within the CORI network, 13.9% did not include bowel preparation quality, and cecal landmarks were not recorded in 14%. In addition, 10% did not include comorbidity classification, and key polyp descriptors were often missing.[66]

This variability in reporting led to the development of the standardized Colonoscopy Reporting and Data System (CO-RADS) in 2007.[4] CO-RADS suggests key areas for documentation (**Box 1**). The literature suggests that colonoscopy reporting has improved since CO-RADS, whether because of the publication or temporal trends. A quality audit of 250 colonoscopy reports in 2009 showed improvement in quality of reporting, with 100% listing indication and informed consent, 99.6% prep quality, 78.8% cecal landmarks, 67% photographic documentation of the cecum, and 65.8% and 62.2% polyp size and morphology, respectively.[67] Targeted modifications to electronic colonoscopic reporting systems can improve the quality of reports. Changes to software such as drop-down menus and visual cues to optimize completion of required fields have helped improve reporting.[68]

Box 1
CO-RADS to improve the quality of colonoscopy

Key subject areas for colonoscopy report

Patient demographics and history

Assessment of patient risk and comorbidity

Procedure indication(s)

Procedure: technical description

Colonoscopic findings

Assessment

Interventions/unplanned events

Follow-up plan

Pathology

From Lieberman D, Nadel M, Smith RA, et al. Standardized colonoscopy reporting and data system: report of the Quality Assurance Task Group of the National Colorectal Cancer Roundtable. Gastrointest Endosc 2007;65:75; with permission.

DATABASES AND REGISTRIES

Measurement of quality is facilitated by use of electronic health records (EHRs), administrative data, and quality-oriented registries. When using such data, it is important to accurately identify the denominator of reference for the metric being assessed. Inclusion of cases in the denominator of a measure that do not accurately represent the condition being measured can result in a falsely low quality score and, conversely, exclusion of cases from the denominator that do represent the condition being measured can result in a falsely high score. Understanding the source of data and their potential inherent biases can help in interpreting results.[69]

EHR

The EHR can be used to enhance quality.[70–73] The main advantages are that the data are already collected and represent the full spectrum of care without limitations. The disadvantages are that the data content or format may not meet standards necessary for other uses because of imprecise terminology or missing or inconsistent data, or may be difficult to extract from narrative text. If specific data elements can be captured from well-defined, discrete, coded fields then the EHR can be useful for secondary purposes like quality research and reporting. Using the EHR has the additional advantage of allowing for discovery of better quality measures that reflect differing degrees of disease severity.[69]

Administrative Data

Administrative data collected from insurance companies, billing records, or national databases are another source of data that can be used for evaluating quality in colonoscopy. These data are already collected and typically are inexpensive to use. Large numbers of events provide sufficient power for statistical analyses, and there is the unique ability to measure samples of geographically dispersed patients. It is also potentially possible to assemble longitudinal records across providers and settings (eg, inpatient vs outpatient care). One disadvantage of administrative data is that they are not collected specifically for the purpose of measuring quality and may be of questionable validity depending on the outcomes and variables being measured. Coding for a specific condition may not be specific or sensitive enough to meet the standards for quality measurement, with resultant underdetection, and there may be incomplete physician documentation.

An example of using administrative data for CRC screening comes from The National Healthcare Quality Report (NHQR) from the Agency for Healthcare Research and Quality (AHRQ), which was developed in coordination with the Department of Health and Human Services.[12] The project drew on more than 33 databases to report on process and outcome measures at the national and state levels. Reports were based on recommendations from the Institute of Medicine's *Future Directions for the National Healthcare Quality and Disparities Reports*.[74] The NHQR evaluated 3 core measures, of which prevention of CRC was one. The overall percentage of adults age 50 years and older who reported having received colorectal cancer screening significantly increased from 52% in 2005 to 56% in 2008, with some disparities noted (eg, higher screening rates in adults in large fringe metropolitan areas than in large central metropolitan areas). The 5 states with the highest rates of screening reached a benchmark of 67%.

Performance measures related to colonoscopy can be measured from administrative data. A study of the Ontario Cancer Registry from 2000 to 2005 analyzed data from patients who underwent colonoscopy 7 to 36 months before diagnosis of CRC.[44]

Endoscopist specialty (gastrointestinal [GI] vs other), setting (hospital vs non hospital), procedure completion rates ($\geq$95% vs <80%), and polypectomy rates ($\geq$30% vs <10%), but not volume, were associated with postcolonoscopy CRC.

Electronic Reporting Software

The CORI is a network of practice-based endoscopists who use a standardized endoscopic reporting software program to generate reports. Data from these reports are uploaded to a central repository, where they can be used to measure and enhance quality. Data from multiple practices can also be pooled for benchmarking. Although quality can be measured in such an electronic setting, even with this structured reporting system, clinicians may omit important quality data. In a study of 430,000 colonoscopy reports from 74 practice sites, many quality metrics were incomplete.[66] For example, 14% failed to report cecal landmarks and 14% failed to report quality of bowel preparation.

Registries

Registries are repositories of data derived specifically for the disease registry itself or from a health survey. A registry can be specifically designed for research and quality reporting and, as such, can avoid many of the biases of administrative data. One disadvantage is that it requires significant investment from participants for data collection and quality control. If there is automated data extraction, for example directly from electronic reporting software, there may be an initial up-front investment in time and money and systematic errors may occur throughout. Manual abstraction has ongoing costs caused by time and expense and can lead to random errors at any point.

The balance between the burden of data collection and the benefits of participation is delicate. AHRQ has a handbook for registries performing outcomes and quality research.[75] This handbook addresses topics in registry methodology and relevant legislative issues.

States may develop their own registries to help with quality improvement. For example, New Hampshire has its own colonoscopy registry that is supported by federal funding. Such registries are not usually available for participation outside that state.[33]

Two gastroenterology-specific registries have been developed for monitoring of endoscopy quality. The GI Quality Improvement Consortium, Ltd (GIQuIC; http:// giquic.gi.org) is a national registry for individual physicians and groups to determine performance on selected quality measures and to benchmark against other participants.[76] This registry was created by a nonprofit partnership between American College of Gastroenterology and American Society for Gastrointestinal Endoscopy. Reports can be submitted manually to the registry Web site or automatically from certain electronic reporting software programs. Endowriters certified with GIQuIC include Amkai, CORI, eMerge Health Solutions, Endosoft, gMed, MD Reports, Olympus (version 7.4), Pentax (endoPRO iQ), and ProVation (version 5.0). There are 84 data fields and 10 quality measures benchmarked, including rate of cecal intubation, ADR, prep assessment, and appropriate indications for procedure. Participants can submit any individual PQRS measure to GIQuIC's CMS-certified registry partner, Outcome Sciences. **Fig. 1** shows a sample report on ADR generated by GIQuIC.

The American Gastroenterology Association (AGA) Digestive Health Outcomes Registry (AGA Registry) has been certified by CMS as an official PQRS registry (http:// www.gastro.org/practice/digestive-health-outcomes-registry). The AGA Registry requires a clinical profile, office location profile, data entry either online or via her, and patient sampling for CRC prevention or IBD. It currently supports gMED's Gastro v4

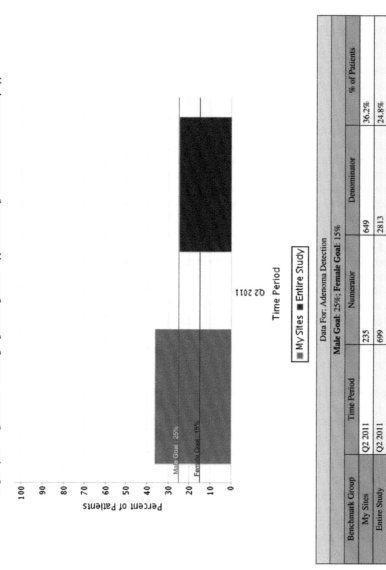

Adenoma Detection

Percentage of patients age 50 and over undergoing screening colonoscopy with a finding of at least one adenomatous polyp.

Percent of Patients (axis: 0, 10, 20, 30, 40, 50, 60, 70, 80, 90, 100)

Male Goal : 25%
Female Goal : 15%

Time Period — Q2 2011

My Sites ■ Entire Study

Data For: Adenoma Detection				
Male Goal: 25%; Female Goal: 15%				
Benchmark Group	Time Period	Numerator	Denominator	% of Patients
My Sites	Q2 2011	235	649	36.2%
Entire Study	Q2 2011	699	2813	24.8%

Fig. 1. A sample report on the ADR for an individual site generated within the GIQuIC registry. The metric for the individual site is compared with all sites within GIQuIC and national benchmarks are indicated. (*Courtesy of* the GI Quality Improvement Consortium, Ltd, 2013; with permission.)

or custom integration with FIGMD's Quality Measurement and Improvement Solution Platform. AGA Registry monitors 6 colorectal cancer prevention measures: identification of CRC risk, endoscopic examination interval, use of anesthesia professionals, procedure-related complications, colonoscopy assessment, and ADR. In April 2012, AGA Registry developed a collaboration with United Healthcare for quality reporting. **Fig. 2** shows a sample report on appropriate endoscopic examination intervals.

QUALITY IMPROVEMENT INITIATIVES

Unlike traditional biomedical research, in which a protocol is designed and data collection occurs over years before analysis or results, quality improvement work involves rapid assessments and implementation of changes on an iterative basis.

Implementation

The first step in implementing a quality improvement project is to select an outcome for the intervention. This outcome should be clearly defined with strict parameters. For example, to improve ADR, it must first be decided which colonoscopies to include in the measurement. This typically includes screening procedures only, but should first-time screenings or a repeat screening 10 years after an initial colonoscopy be included? Should all patients be included, or should those with a strong family history of CRC and/or partial colectomies be excluded? If an outcome is to be compared with national benchmarks, published quality measure guidelines should be followed for the criteria for inclusion of cases in the measure calculation's numerator and denominator. However, if clinicians seek simply to improve their own ADRs, consistency in their measurement algorithms over time may be more important than matching national standards for which cases to include.

The next step is to collect measurements to determine the baseline starting point. At this stage, the quality may already be high, such as a near-100% cecal intubation rate. If there is little room for improvement, there is no reason to focus on that quality measure. This stage is also where the method for data measurement may need refinement. Was it too cumbersome or time consuming? Is there a way to automate the process? Is there variation in how providers are reporting the key information?

Once the data collection methods are developed, clinicians must consider how to improve compliance with the quality measure. If it is ADR, they could consider being even more meticulous in inspection of the colonic mucosa. Are bowel preparations adequate? Perhaps purchasing an automated water pump for improved flushing during procedures could be considered. In quality improvement projects, it is not necessary to collect data for extended periods of time before analyzing results. One method is the Plan-Do-Study-Act (PDSA) process, which is part of the Institute for Healthcare Improvement Model for Improvement.[77] In a PDSA cycle, the intervention is planned and rolled out, the outcomes are studied for a brief period (eg, 1 month), and results are noted (**Fig. 3**). During the study phase, clinicians are looking for any problems in implementation (which may include lack of provider buy-in) or unintended consequences. For example, if 30 minutes are being spent on the withdrawal phase of procedures, are patients backing up in the waiting room? After the study phase, some changes may be identified that are needed in the protocol. This process leads to the act phase in which clinicians consider how to alter the quality improvement project to try to address any shortcomings. They then plan how to roll out these changes as they begin the next PDSA cycle.

It may be wise to limit the first few PDSA cycles to a few providers, endoscopy rooms, or nursing staff. This limitation helps resolve problems and allows quality

Digestive Health
Outcomes Registry

Performance Metric Detail
CRC-P 2: Endoscopic Examination Interval

Powered By MEDASSURANT™

Practice Name:	MedAssurant Internal Practice
Practice ID:	101090
Report Date/Time:	1/5/2011 12:31
Metric Description:	CRC-P 2 Endoscopic Examination Interval

This measure is designed to assess what the endoscopist has determined to be the appropriate follow up interval for colonoscopy by post-procedure risk classification. This measure will take into consideration the physician's determination of CRC-P risk factors following the endoscopic examination based on the examination findings, the examination type (ex. flex sig, colonoscopy) and presenting characteristics, such as current CRC risk classification; family history of CRC; other bowel conditions; bleeding; and or genetic syndromes associated with high incidence of CRC. This measure will assist with the evaluation of national, regional, and local endoscopic utilization trends and assist in the identification of possible over and under-utilization of endoscopy in the process of CRC prevention.

Numerator:	0
Denominator:	4
Metric Rate:	N/A

Report Parameters

Sex:	All
Age:	
Report Begin Date:	06/01/2010
Report End Date:	01/05/2011
Responsible Clinician:	All Clinicians
Report Details:	All Colonoscopies (i.e. both included and excluded from Rate Calculation)

Fig. 2. A sample report on appropriate endoscopic examination intervals for an individual site generated within the AGA Digestive Health Outcomes Registry (AGA Registry). (*Courtesy of* the American Gastroenterology Association, 2013; with permission.)

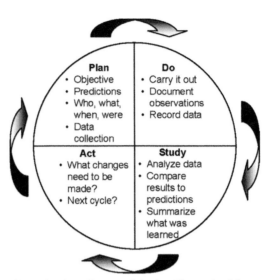

Fig. 3. The PDSA cycle, a simple and powerful scientific method for quality improvement whereby a team plans a test or observation, carries it out on a small scale, studies the results, and refines the change.

improvement projects to be optimized before exposing a large group to the new protocol. There are often providers or nurses who are reluctant to adopt change. Launching a full-scale quality improvement project while there are still obstacles to work through emboldens nay-sayers and makes it difficult to continue. However, once those in a pilot project begin to see progress, their enthusiasm and empirical observations can often help encourage all parties to get involved.

Colonoscopy-specific Initiatives

Quality improvement for colonoscopy can span the continuum of care, from access and use,[78] patient education regarding the preprocedure[79,80] or postprocedure times, patient recall systems,[81] bowel preparation,[82,83] sedation/monitoring, and adverse events recognition and reporting. Whether or not specific interventions can improve performance or outcomes related to colonoscopy is variable; documentation, minimum standard requirements, education, and other forms of monitoring with videotaping have been tried. A few of many studies in the literature are discussed later.

Withdrawal time

A study compared historical data on 2053 screening colonoscopies with 2325 screening colonoscopies using a minimum 8-minute withdrawal time.[48] The intervention was a timer beeping every 2 minutes to alert the endoscopist of the passage of time. Postintervention patients had higher rates of neoplasia (35% vs 24%, $P<.0001$) and endoscopists with mean withdrawal times greater than or equal to 8 minutes had higher ADRs (38% vs 23%, $P<.0001$).

Documentation

An educational initiative was undertaken to improve documentation in an unstructured dictation system for colonoscopy reporting.[84] The intervention included lectures sharing baseline quality indicator compliance for recommended quality indicators. Individual compliance rates were also shared directly with endoscopists. An email was sent to remind endoscopists about documentation and an educational poster was displayed in each procedure room. In addition, a standardized procedure data sheet was developed to help with dictations. The investigators noted a significant improvement in quality measures. Bowel preparation documentation increased from 64% to 83%, identification of the appendiceal orifice increased from 53% to 68%, photography of the cecum increased from 20% to 63%, and documentation of polyp morphology increased from 17% to 54%. Whether these improvements were sustainable remains unknown.

Complications

To better manage perforations after endoscopy, one center formed a multidisciplinary team (GI, surgery, and radiology) to review the existing literature and data from the previous 10 years at their site.[85] They then developed an algorithm for management of endoscopic perforations. Implementation of the algorithm and monitoring of its impact on outcomes is ongoing.

SUMMARY

Quality in colonoscopy is essential to maintaining the trust of patients and the public. There is a need to continually define and refine quality metrics that can help improve the care of patients and optimize outcomes. Measurement and reporting of quality, as well as achieving performance benchmarks, will become increasingly relevant as more financial incentives and penalties surrounding particular metrics from organizations and payors emerge. Endoscopy unit–level quality measures will likely become increasingly important as well. Future research should focus on bolstering evidence to support how particular metrics correlate with clinically relevant outcomes, as well as on identifying types of interventions that improve these metrics (eg, how can ADR be improved? How can inappropriate use of surveillance colonoscopy be reduced?). Further adoption of EHRs will make registry reporting easier and will permit greater automation of quality measurement.

REFERENCES

1. Kohn LT, Corrigan JM, Donaldson MS, editors. Committee on Quality of Health Care in America, Institute of Medicine. To err is human: building a safer health system. Washington, DC: The National Academies Press; 2000.
2. Everhart JE, Ruhl CE. Burden of digestive diseases in the United States part II: lower gastrointestinal diseases. Gastroenterology 2009;136:741–54.
3. Seeff LC, Richards TB, Shapiro JA, et al. How many endoscopies are performed for colorectal cancer screening? Results from CDC's survey of endoscopic capacity. Gastroenterology 2004;127:1670–7.
4. Lieberman D, Nadel M, Smith RA, et al. Standardized colonoscopy reporting and data system: report of the Quality Assurance Task Group of the National Colorectal Cancer Roundtable. Gastrointest Endosc 2007;65:757–66.
5. Cotton PB, Connor P, McGee D, et al. Colonoscopy: practice variation among 69 hospital-based endoscopists. Gastrointest Endosc 2003;57:352–7.
6. Barclay RL, Vicari JJ, Doughty AS, et al. Colonoscopic withdrawal times and adenoma detection during screening colonoscopy. N Engl J Med 2006;355: 2533–41.
7. Chen SC, Rex DK. Endoscopist can be more powerful than age and male gender in predicting adenoma detection at colonoscopy. Am J Gastroenterol 2007;102:856–61.

8. Rex DK, Petrini JL, Baron TH, et al. Quality indicators for colonoscopy. Am J Gastroenterol 2006;101:873–85.

9. Baxter NN, Goldwasser MA, Paszat LF, et al. Association of colonoscopy and death from colorectal cancer. Ann Intern Med 2009;150:1–8.

10. Brenner H, Hoffmeister M, Arndt V, et al. Protection from right- and left-sided colorectal neoplasms after colonoscopy: population-based study. J Natl Cancer Inst 2009;102:89–95.

11. Singh H, Nugent Z, Demers AA, et al. The reduction in colorectal cancer mortality after colonoscopy varies by site of the cancer. Gastroenterology 2010;139: 1128–37.

12. National healthcare quality report 2010. AHRQ Publication No. 11-0004. Rockville (MD): Agency for Healthcare Research and Quality; 2011.

13. Lieberman D. Progress and challenges in colorectal cancer screening and surveillance. Gastroenterology 2010;138:2115–26.

14. Lieberman D. How good is your dentist? How good is your endoscopist? The quality imperative. Gastroenterology 2012;142:194–6.

15. Saini SD, Nayak RS, Kuhn L, et al. Why don't gastroenterologists follow colon polyp surveillance guidelines?: results of a national survey. J Clin Gastroenterol 2009;43:554–8.

16. Mysliwiec PA, Brown ML, Klabunde CN, et al. Are physicians doing too much colonoscopy? A national survey of colorectal surveillance after polypectomy. Ann Intern Med 2004;141:264–71.

17. Schoen RE, Pinsky PF, Weissfeld JL, et al. Utilization of surveillance colonoscopy in community practice. Gastroenterology 2010;138:73–81.

18. Brueckl WM, Fritsche B, Seifert B, et al. Non-compliance in surveillance for patients with previous resection of large (> or = 1 cm) colorectal adenomas. World J Gastroenterol 2006;12:7313–8.

19. Mulder SA, Van Leerdam ME, Ouwendijk RJ, et al. Attendance at surveillance endoscopy of patients with adenoma or colorectal cancer. Scand J Gastroenterol 2007;42:66–71.

20. Physicians quality reporting system (PQRS). Woodlawn (MD): US Department of Health & Human Services, Centers for Medicare and Medicaid Services; 2012. Available at: http://www.cms.gov/Medicare/Quality-Initiatives-Patient-Assessment-Instruments/PQRS/index.html?redirect=/pqri. Accessed November 23, 2012.

21. Rex DK, Hewett DG, Snover DC. Editorial: detection targets for colonoscopy: from variable detection to validation. Am J Gastroenterol 2010;105:2665–9.

22. van Rijn JC, Reitsma JB, Stoker J, et al. Polyp miss rate determined by tandem colonoscopy: a systematic review. Am J Gastroenterol 2006;101:343–50.

23. Rex DK, Cutler CS, Lemmel GT, et al. Colonoscopic miss rates of adenomas determined by back-to-back colonoscopies. Gastroenterology 1997;112:24–8.

24. Atkin W, Rogers P, Cardwell C, et al. Wide variation in adenoma detection rates at screening flexible sigmoidoscopy. Gastroenterology 2004;126:1247–56.

25. Bretthauer M, Skovlund E, Grotmol T, et al. Inter-endoscopist variation in polyp and neoplasia pick-up rates in flexible sigmoidoscopy screening for colorectal cancer. Scand J Gastroenterol 2003;38:1268–74.

26. Hosokawa O, Shirasaki S, Kaizaki Y, et al. Invasive colorectal cancer detected up to 3 years after a colonoscopy negative for cancer. Endoscopy 2003;35: 506–10.

27. Leaper M, Johnston MJ, Barclay M, et al. Reasons for failure to diagnose colorectal carcinoma at colonoscopy. Endoscopy 2004;36:499–503.

28. Schoen RE, Pinsky PF, Weissfeld JL, et al. Results of repeat sigmoidoscopy 3 years after a negative examination. JAMA 2003;290:41–8.

29. Pickhardt PJ, Nugent PA, Mysliwiec PA, et al. Location of adenomas missed by optical colonoscopy. Ann Intern Med 2004;141:352–9.

30. Lee TJ, Rutter MD, Blanks RG, et al. Colonoscopy quality measures: experience from the NHS Bowel Cancer Screening Programme. Gut 2012;61:1050–7.

31. Denis B, Sauleau EA, Gendre I, et al. Measurement of adenoma detection and discrimination during colonoscopy in routine practice: an exploratory study. Gastrointest Endosc 2011;74:1325–36.

32. Do A, Weinberg J, Kakkar A, et al. Reliability of adenoma detection rate is based on procedural volume. Gastrointest Endosc 2013;77(3):376–80.

33. Greene MA, Butterly LF, Goodrich M, et al. Matching colonoscopy and pathology data in population-based registries: development of a novel algorithm and the initial experience of the New Hampshire Colonoscopy Registry. Gastrointest Endosc 2011;74:334–40.

34. Williams JE, Holub JL, Faigel DO. Polypectomy rate is a valid quality measure for colonoscopy: results from a national endoscopy database. Gastrointest Endosc 2012;75:576–82.

35. Williams JE, Le TD, Faigel DO. Polypectomy rate as a quality measure for colonoscopy. Gastrointest Endosc 2011;73:498–506.

36. Lieberman DA, Holub JL, Moravec MD, et al. Prevalence of colon polyps detected by colonoscopy screening in asymptomatic black and white patients. JAMA 2008;300:1417–22.

37. Kaminski MF, Regula J, Kraszewska E, et al. Quality indicators for colonoscopy and the risk of interval cancer. N Engl J Med 2010;362:1795–803.

38. Adler A, Wegscheider K, Lieberman D, et al. Factors determining the quality of screening colonoscopy: a prospective study on adenoma detection rates, from 12 134 examinations (Berlin colonoscopy project 3, BECOP-3). Gut 2013;62(2):236–41.

39. Corley DA, Jensen CD, Marks AR. Can we improve adenoma detection rates? A systematic review of intervention studies. Gastrointest Endosc 2011;74:656–65.

40. Shaukat A, Oancea C, Bond JH, et al. Variation in detection of adenomas and polyps by colonoscopy and change over time with a performance improvement program. Clin Gastroenterol Hepatol 2009;7:1335–40.

41. Kahi CJ, Hewett DG, Norton DL, et al. Prevalence and variable detection of proximal colon serrated polyps during screening colonoscopy. Clin Gastroenterol Hepatol 2011;9:42–6.

42. Kahi CJ, Li X, Eckert GJ, et al. High colonoscopic prevalence of proximal colon serrated polyps in average-risk men and women. Gastrointest Endosc 2011;75:515–20.

43. Rabeneck L, Souchek J, El-Serag HB. Survival of colorectal cancer patients hospitalized in the Veterans Affairs Health Care System. Am J Gastroenterol 2003;98:1186–92.

44. Baxter NN, Sutradhar R, Forbes SS, et al. Analysis of administrative data finds endoscopist quality measures associated with postcolonoscopy colorectal cancer. Gastroenterology 2011;140:65–72.

45. Taber A, Romagnuolo J. Effect of simply recording colonoscopy withdrawal time on polyp and adenoma detection rates. Gastrointest Endosc 2010;71:782–6.

46. Velasquez J, Espinoza-Rios J, Huerta-Mercado J, et al. Impact assessment of increasing the time of withdrawal of colonoscopy in the detection rate of polyps in our midst. Rev Gastroenterol Peru 2009;29:321–5.

47. Lin OS, Kozarek RA, Arai A, et al. The effect of periodic monitoring and feedback on screening colonoscopy withdrawal times, polyp detection rates, and patient satisfaction scores. Gastrointest Endosc 2010;71:1253–9.

48. Barclay RL, Vicari JJ, Greenlaw RL. Effect of a time-dependent colonoscopic withdrawal protocol on adenoma detection during screening colonoscopy. Clin Gastroenterol Hepatol 2008;6:1091–8.

49. Burke CA, Church JM. Enhancing the quality of colonoscopy: the importance of bowel purgatives. Gastrointest Endosc 2007;66:565–73.

50. Froehlich F, Wietlisbach V, Gonvers JJ, et al. Impact of colonic cleansing on quality and diagnostic yield of colonoscopy: the European Panel of Appropriateness of Gastrointestinal Endoscopy European multicenter study. Gastrointest Endosc 2005;61:378–84.

51. Harewood GC, Sharma VK, de Garmo P. Impact of colonoscopy preparation quality on detection of suspected colonic neoplasia. Gastrointest Endosc 2003;58:76–9.

52. Thomas-Gibson S, Rogers P, Cooper S, et al. Judgement of the quality of bowel preparation at screening flexible sigmoidoscopy is associated with variability in adenoma detection rates. Endoscopy 2006;38:456–60.

53. Rostom A, Jolicoeur E. Validation of a new scale for the assessment of bowel preparation quality. Gastrointest Endosc 2004;59:482–6.

54. Aronchick CA, Lipshutz WH, Wright SH, et al. A novel tableted purgative for colonoscopic preparation: efficacy and safety comparisons with Colyte and Fleet Phospho-Soda. Gastrointest Endosc 2000;52:346–52.

55. Calderwood AH, Jacobson BC. Comprehensive validation of the Boston Bowel Preparation Scale. Gastrointest Endosc 2010;72:686–92.

56. Lai EJ, Calderwood AH, Doros G, et al. The Boston Bowel Preparation Scale: a valid and reliable instrument for colonoscopy-oriented research. Gastrointest Endosc 2009;69:620–5.

57. Fisher DA, Maple JT, Ben-Menachem T, et al. Complications of colonoscopy. Gastrointest Endosc 2011;74:745–52.

58. Rabeneck L, Paszat LF, Hilsden RJ, et al. Bleeding and perforation after outpatient colonoscopy and their risk factors in usual clinical practice. Gastroenterology 2008;135:1899–906, 1906.e1.

59. Warren JL, Klabunde CN, Mariotto AB, et al. Adverse events after outpatient colonoscopy in the Medicare population. Ann Intern Med 2009;150:849–57 W152.

60. Ko CW, Riffle S, Michaels L, et al. Serious complications within 30 days of screening and surveillance colonoscopy are uncommon. Clin Gastroenterol Hepatol 2009;8:166–73.

61. de Jonge V, Sint Nicolaas J, van Baalen O, et al. The incidence of 30-day adverse events after colonoscopy among outpatients in the Netherlands. Am J Gastroenterol 2011;107:878–84.

62. Cotton PB, Eisen GM, Aabakken L, et al. A lexicon for endoscopic adverse events: report of an ASGE workshop. Gastrointest Endosc 2010;71:446–54.

63. Li J, Nadel MR, Poppell CF, et al. Quality assessment of colonoscopy reporting: results from a statewide cancer screening program. Diagn Ther Endosc 2010; 2010. pii:419796.

64. de Jonge V, Sint Nicolaas J, Cahen DL, et al. Quality evaluation of colonoscopy reporting and colonoscopy performance in daily clinical practice. Gastrointest Endosc 2012;75:98–106.

65. Palmer LB, Abbott DH, Hamilton N, et al. Quality of colonoscopy reporting in community practice. Gastrointest Endosc 2010;72:321–7, 327.e1.

66. Lieberman DA, Faigel DO, Logan JR, et al. Assessment of the quality of colonoscopy reports: results from a multicenter consortium. Gastrointest Endosc 2009;69:645–53.

67. Beaulieu D, Barkun A, Martel M. Quality audit of colonoscopy reports amongst patients screened or surveilled for colorectal neoplasia. World J Gastroenterol 2012;18:3551–7.

68. Beaulieu D, Martel M, Barkun AN. A prospective intervention study of colonoscopy reporting among patients screened or surveilled for colorectal neoplasia. Can J Gastroenterol 2012;26:718–22.

69. Logan JR, Lieberman DA. The use of databases and registries to enhance colonoscopy quality. Gastrointest Endosc Clin N Am 2010;20:717–34.

70. Einbinder JS, Scully K. Using a clinical data repository to estimate the frequency and costs of adverse drug events. Proc AMIA Symp 2001;154–8.

71. McDonald CJ, Overhage JM, Dexter P, et al. A framework for capturing clinical data sets from computerized sources. Ann Intern Med 1997;127:675–82.

72. Owen RR, Thrush CR, Cannon D, et al. Use of electronic medical record data for quality improvement in schizophrenia treatment. J Am Med Inform Assoc 2004; 11:351–7.

73. Tang PC, Ralston M, Arrigotti MF, et al. Comparison of methodologies for calculating quality measures based on administrative data versus clinical data from an electronic health record system: implications for performance measures. J Am Med Inform Assoc 2007;14:10–5.

74. National Research Council. Future directions for the national healthcare quality and disparities reports. Washington, DC: The National Academies Press; 2010.

75. Gliklich RE, Dreyer NA, editors. Registries for evaluating patient outcomes: a user's guide. 2nd edition. Rockville (MD); 2010 (Prepared by Outcome DEcIDE Center [Outcome Sciences, Inc dba Outcome] under Contract No. HHSA290200500035I TO1.).

76. Deas T, Pike IM. Benchmarking to Excellence: Using quality indicators to improve performance. EndoEconomics, Spring 2010;19–20.

77. Langley GL, Nolan KM, Nolan TW, et al. The improvement guide: a practical approach to enhancing organizational performance. 2nd edition. San Francisco (CA): Jossey-Bass Publishers; 2009.

78. Christie J, Itzkowitz S, Lihau-Nkanza I, et al. A randomized controlled trial using patient navigation to increase colonoscopy screening among low-income minorities. J Natl Med Assoc 2008;100:278–84.

79. Shaw MJ, Beebe TJ, Tomshine PA, et al. A randomized, controlled trial of interactive, multimedia software for patient colonoscopy education. J Clin Gastroenterol 2001;32:142–7.

80. Friedman M, Borum ML. Colorectal cancer screening of African Americans by internal medicine resident physicians can be improved with focused educational efforts. J Natl Med Assoc 2007;99:1010–2.

81. Leffler DA, Neeman N, Rabb JM, et al. An alerting system improves adherence to follow-up recommendations from colonoscopy examinations. Gastroenterology 2011;140:1166–73.e1–3.

82. Siddiqui AA, Yang K, Spechler SJ, et al. Duration of the interval between the completion of bowel preparation and the start of colonoscopy predicts bowel-preparation quality. Gastrointest Endosc 2009;69:700–6.

83. Calderwood AH, Lai EJ, Fix OK, et al. An endoscopist-blinded, randomized, controlled trial of a simple visual aid to improve bowel preparation for screening colonoscopy. Gastrointest Endosc 2011;73:307–14.

84. Coe SG, Panjala C, Heckman MG, et al. Quality in colonoscopy reporting: an assessment of compliance and performance improvement. Dig Liver Dis 2012;44:660–4.

85. Kowalczyk L, Forsmark CE, Ben-David K, et al. Algorithm for the management of endoscopic perforations: a quality improvement project. Am J Gastroenterol 2011;106:1022–7.

Colonoscopy and Colorectal Cancer Incidence and Mortality

Nirav Thosani, MD, MHA[a], Sushovan Guha, MD, PhD[a],
Harminder Singh, MD, MPH[b,c],*

KEYWORDS

- Colonoscopy • Colorectal cancer incidence • Colorectal cancer mortality
- Right colon

KEY POINTS

- Although the 3 large randomized controlled trials assessing efficacy of colonoscopy were initiated only recently, there is already substantial indirect evidence for the effectiveness of colonoscopy in reducing colorectal cancer incidence and mortality.
- However, several recently published observational studies suggest that colonoscopy has had a lower magnitude of benefit in reducing right-sided colorectal cancer incidence and mortality than that of left-sided colorectal cancers. This finding has raised questions on the magnitude of incremental benefit of colonoscopy compared with flexible sigmoidoscopy.
- The reports of variation in performance and outcomes after colonoscopy by different groups of endoscopy physicians, especially for the right-sided colorectal cancers, suggests that the recent quality assurance and enhancement efforts and technical advances in colonoscopy should lead to improvements in outcomes after colonoscopy.
- Because colonoscopy is an essential initial, intermediate, or final test for colon cancer screening and detection, improvements in outcomes after colonoscopy will benefit all undergoing colorectal cancer screening or detection, irrespective of the initial choice of the screening test.

INTRODUCTION

Colorectal cancer (CRC) is the second leading cause of cancer-related deaths in the United States.[1] It is estimated that up to 52,000 deaths will be attributed to CRC in the

---

Grant Support: None.
Disclosures: None.
[a] Department of Gastroenterology, Hepatology and Nutrition, The University of Texas Medical School at Houston, 6431 Fannin Street, Houston, TX 77030, USA; [b] Department of Internal Medicine, IBD Clinical and Research Centre, University of Manitoba, 715 McDermot Avenue, Winnipeg, Manitoba R3E 3P4, Canada; [c] Department of Community Health Sciences, IBD Clinical and Research Centre, University of Manitoba, 715 McDermot Avenue, Winnipeg, Manitoba R3E 3P4, Canada
* Corresponding author. Departments of Internal Medicine and Community Health Sciences, IBD Clinical and Research Centre, University of Manitoba, Winnipeg, Manitoba, Canada.
E-mail address: harminder.singh@med.umanitoba.ca

United States in 2012.[1] There has been a steady decline in age-adjusted incidence rates of CRC in the US over the last 3 decades.[1,2] A substantial recent decline in CRC incidence has been attributed to the removal of premalignant polyps detected on screening.[1,3] In addition, the removal of the adenomatous colon polyps and early-stage detection of CRC by screening have been shown to lead to reduction in CRC mortality.[4–6]

CRC screening with fecal occult blood testing (FOBT) or flexible sigmoidoscopy (FS) has been shown in randomized controlled trials (RCTs) to lead to reduction in CRC mortality.[6–10] However, the benefits of primary screening colonoscopy for CRC have not yet been established in an RCT of colonoscopy, and there is indirect evidence for the role of colonoscopy in CRC screening. Three RCTs of primary screening colonoscopy have recently been launched to address the unresolved issues.

In the United States, colonoscopy has become the most commonly used modality for CRC screening.[11] A recent survey found that, in the United States, 95% of primary care physicians recommend colonoscopy as the preferred CRC screening modality.[12] Compared with FOBT, which primarily detects CRC and not adenomas, and FS, which mainly reduces distal CRC incidence and mortality, colonoscopy has the theoretic advantage of providing complete colonic examination and detecting and removing adenomas in both sides of the colon at the same time.[4–6,9,13–17] In average-risk screening populations, colonoscopy has extremely low risk of serious adverse side effects.[18,19] However, it is an invasive procedure and it has to be done at long intervals to maintain a risk/benefit ratio that is acceptable for a screening test.

This article discusses the effect of colonoscopy on CRC incidence and mortality. However, it first discusses the importance of evaluating CRC incidence and mortality as highlighted by the limitations of assessing surrogate markers such as detection of advanced adenomas and improved survival after detection of CRC on screening.

COLONOSCOPY AND DETECTION OF ADVANCED ADENOMAS

Colonoscopy has dominated in the United States since Medicare's decision to cover screening colonoscopy in average-risk persons in 2001, and similar decisions by other third-party payers.[20–22] Endorsements by celebrities and heightened media attention have helped to increase public acceptance and demand for screening colonoscopy.[23,24] These developments followed the landmark US Department of Veterans Affairs (VA) and Eli Lilly cohort studies published in 2000, which established that colonoscopy detects higher proportions of advanced adenomas than could be detected by FS or FOBT.[13,25] In the VA cohort study, Lieberman and colleagues[13] examined the role of colonoscopic screening to identify advanced colonic neoplasia in asymptomatic adults at 13 VA medical centers across the country. Advanced colonic neoplasia was defined as an adenoma that was 10 mm or more in diameter, a villous adenoma, an adenoma with high-grade dysplasia, or invasive cancer.[13] The study concluded that colonoscopy found advanced colonic neoplasia in 37.5% of asymptomatic adults.[13] Imperiale and colleagues[25] showed that asymptomatic adults 50 years of age or older who have polyps in the distal colon are more likely to have advanced proximal colon neoplasia than are adults without a distal colon polyp. In addition, 46% of asymptomatic adults with proximal colonic neoplasia did not have any distal polyps.[25] Both studies showed that screening colonoscopy can identify additional advanced colonic neoplasia in asymptomatic adults, which would have not been detected by FOBT or FS. Because advanced adenomas are the precursor lesions for most CRCs, it is intuitive that higher detection rates of advanced adenomas will lead to greater reductions in CRC incidence and mortality. However, only a minority of advanced adenomas are estimated to develop into CRC[26] and hence the magnitude of reduction in CRC incidence and mortality, due to higher detection rate of right-sided advanced adenomas at colonoscopy is not known. The modeling studies used to estimate the benefits of colonoscopy depend on the model assumptions and often do not model the natural history of right-sided adenomas separately. There are biological differences between right-sided and left-sided CRCs and the natural history of right-sided polyps (adenomatous and serrated) may also be different.

SURVIVAL AFTER DETECTION OF CRC ON SCREENING

There are powerful biases such as lead-time bias, length-biased sampling, and over-diagnosis that can be associated with observational studies of screening tests and can confound assessment of screening-test efficacy.[27] Early detection of cancer advances the date of diagnosis and adds apparent survival time compared with symptomatic detection. However, early detection of the disease, if it does not translate into an overall longer lifespan for a given individual, introduces lead-time bias. Lead-time bias has important implications for the use of 5-year survival as an indicator for screening effectiveness.[27] Improved 5-year overall survival rate, without accompanying improvement in cause-specific mortality, is likely caused by lead-time bias or length-biased sampling. Screening tests tend to discover less aggressive, slow-growing lesions compared with cancers discovered as a result of symptoms (length-biased sampling).[27] Individuals found to have less aggressive cancers have longer 5 year survival after cancer diagnosis than those with more aggressive cancers, which are more likely to be detected at the symptomatic stage. Overdiagnosis is an extreme form of length-bias sampling in which, despite its pathologic appearance, the cancer either has no malignant potential or is so indolent that it cannot alter the remaining lifespan because the person will die of another cause first.[27]

CURRENT EVIDENCE FOR CRC INCIDENCE AND MORTALITY AFTER COLONOSCOPY

Most of the current knowledge regarding effectiveness of screening colonoscopy is derived from follow-up of the cohorts in the National Polyp Study, Minnesota FOBT study, observational studies, and from the assumed extension of benefit with FS screening shown in several randomized trials.[6,9,10,28]

National Polyp Study

The National Polyp Study (NPS) was an RCT designed to evaluate the appropriate timing of surveillance colonoscopy for the patients found to have one or more colorectal adenoma.[29] The NPS cohort consisted of 3778 patients who underwent polypectomy.[29] Of these, 2632 patients had one or more adenomatous polyps. After exclusions, 2602 patients with adenomas and 773 patients without adenoma were identified.[29] Of the 2602 patients with adenoma, 1418 patients were randomized to surveillance colonoscopy at varying intervals (1 year vs 3 years).[14,29] All of these patients subsequently underwent a second colonoscopy during an average follow-up of 5.9 years.[14] The study also compared incidence of CRC with 3 reference groups, including 2 polyp bearing cohorts (Mayo Clinic in Rochester,[26] and St Mark's Hospital in London, United Kingdom[30]) and 1 general population registry (Surveillance, Epidemiology, and End Results [SEER] registry).[14] During follow-up colonoscopy, 5 asymptomatic early-stage CRCs were detected; 3 at 3 years, 1 at 6 years, and 1 at 7 years.[14] The observed incidence of CRC per 1000 person-years was 0.6 in the study cohort, whereas the expected incidence was 5.7 per Mayo Clinic data, 5.2 per the St Mark's data, and 2.5 per the SEER data.[14] The standardized incidence ratio (SIR) for CRC in the NPS cohort was 0.10 (95% confidence interval [CI], 0.03–0.24) compared with the Mayo Clinic group, 0.12 (95% CI, 0.04–0.27) compared with the St Mark's group, and 0.24 (95% CI, 0.08–0.56) compared with the SEER group, suggesting a 76% to 90% reduction in CRC incidence after colonoscopic polypectomy.[14] The cohort component of this study was the first to show that colonoscopic polypectomy resulted in a lower-than-expected incidence of CRC and supported the practice of searching for and removing adenomatous polyps to prevent CRC.[14] Most recently, the NPS investigators examined the long-term risk of CRC mortality in 3 groups of patients: (1) NPS patients who had adenoma (n = 2602), (2) NPS patients who did not have adenoma (n = 773), and (3) the general US population using data from SEER registry.[31] The investigators used the National Death Index (NDI) to identify deaths and determine the cause of death, and compared the CRC mortality in each of the two study groups with that expected from the SEER registry.[31] Median follow-up period for the study was 16 years, with maximum follow-up as long as 23 years.[31] In the adenoma cohort (n = 2602), 12 patients died of CRC compared with 25.4 expected CRC deaths based on SEER registry data, suggesting 53% reduction in CRC mortality (standardized mortality ratio [SMR], 0.47; 95% CI, 0.26–0.80) with colonoscopic polypectomy.[31] In the nonadenoma cohort (n = 773), only 1 patient died of CRC at 7.7 years after index colonoscopy.[31] These findings support the hypothesis that colonoscopic removal of adenomatous polyps prevents death from CRC.[31]

Minnesota FOBT Study

Mandel and colleagues[4] evaluated the efficacy of CRC screening by FOBT in a randomized trial. They randomly assigned 46,551 participants who were 50 to 80 years of age to screening for CRC once a year, or twice a year using FOBT, or to a control group.[4] Participants who tested positive for FOBT underwent further diagnostic evaluation including colonoscopy.[4] Over a 13-year follow-up period, cumulative mortality per 1000 from CRC was 5.88 (95% CI, 4.61–7.15) in the annually screened group, 8.33 (95% CI, 6.82–9.84) in the biennially screened group, and 8.83 (95% CI, 7.26–10.40) in the control group.[4] The annual FOBT decreased the 13-year cumulative mortality from CRC by 33%.[4] In addition to reduction in mortality, improved survival in those with CRC and a shift in detecting an earlier stage of cancer were noted in the annually screened group.[4] Among the screening group with positive FOBT, more than 96% of those examined underwent colonoscopy at the University of Minnesota Hospital and a total of 12,246 colonoscopies were performed.[4] Overall, 38% of the individuals undergoing FOBT annually had at least 1 colonoscopy during the course of the study, which resulted in a 20% reduction in CRC incidence after a follow-up of 18 years.[5] This is the only FOBT trial that has shown a reduction in CRC incidence after FOBT screening. This reduction in CRC incidence (and higher reduction in CRC mortality than in any other FOBT trial) has been attributed to the high proportion of individuals undergoing colonoscopy after FOBT testing in the Minnesota study,[32] which was much higher than in any of the other FOBT trials, a difference attributed to the high positive rates of rehydrated FOBT used in the trial leading to higher colonoscopy use. Although the primary focus of the study was to evaluate the reduced mortality from CRC with use of FOBT, the higher reduction in CRC mortality and the reduction in CRC incidence in this trial provided an early hint of the effectiveness of colonoscopy in CRC screening.

Observational Studies of the Effectiveness of Screening Colonoscopy

Incidence and risk of occurrence of CRC after colonoscopy

Müller and colleagues[33] performed a case-control study of 32,702 veterans in the United States (**Table 1**). They identified 8722 cases of colon cancer; 7629 cases of rectal cancer; and age-matched, sex-matched, and race-matched controls for each case. Exposure to endoscopic procedures including FS, colonoscopy, and polypectomy before development of CRC was evaluated.[33] Compared with controls, patients with CRC were less likely to have undergone colonoscopy before being diagnosed with colon cancer (odds ratio [OR] 0.47; 95% CI, 0.37–0.58) or rectal cancer (OR, 0.61; 95% CI, 0.48–0.77).[33] Kahi and colleagues[34] assessed CRC incidence and mortality in a group of asymptomatic average-risk patients who underwent screening colonoscopy between 1989 and 1993 at a university hospital. Using the SIRs and SMRs, they compared the observed CRC rates with the expected rates from the SEER data.[34] They found 12 cases of CRC in the cohort of 715 patients with 10,492 patient-years of follow-up.[34] In their cohort, the SIR for CRC was 0.33 (95% CI, 0.10–0.62).[34] Compared with SEER data, relative risk reduction for CRC incidence was 67%.[34] Singh and colleagues[35] performed a cohort study using an administrative claims database. After negative colonoscopy, they found an overall low incidence of CRC in men (SIR, 0.59; 95% CI, 0.50–0.70) and women (SIR, 0.71; 95% CI, 0.61–0.83).[35] Brenner and colleagues[36] compared a total of 1688 patients with CRC with 1932 control participants aged 50 years or older in a population-based case-control study in Germany. In this study, colonoscopy in the preceding 10 years was associated with strong risk reduction (OR, 0.23; 95% CI, 0.19–0.27) for CRC.[36] The same group of investigators evaluated the risk of CRC after detection and removal of at least 1 adenoma at colonoscopy in 2582 cases of CRC against 1798 matched controls.[37] Colonoscopy with polypectomy was associated with a strong risk reduction of CRC up to less than 3 years (OR, 0.2; 95% CI, 0.2–0.3) and 3 to 5 years (OR, 0.4; 95% CI, 0.3–0.6), even after detection and removal of high-risk polyps.[37]

CRC mortality after colonoscopy

Müller and Sonnenberg[38] showed that colonoscopy reduced the mortality from CRC (OR, 0.45; 95% CI, 0.30–0.66) for the comparison with living control patients in a case-control study among veterans (**Table 2**). Kahi and colleagues[34] found 3 deaths from CRC in a cohort of 715 patients with 10,492 patient-years of follow-up. Compared with SEER data, they found 65% relative risk reduction in CRC mortality (SMR, 0.35; 95% CI, 0.0–1.06).[34] Baxter and colleagues[39] performed a population-based case-control study in Ontario, Canada. They evaluated prior exposure to complete colonoscopy in 10,292 cases of CRC and 51,460 controls matched by age, sex, geographic location, and socioeconomic status.[39] Compared with controls, cases were less likely to have undergone complete colonoscopy (OR, 0.63; 95% CI, 0.57–0.69).[39] Complete colonoscopy was strongly associated with fewer deaths from left-sided CRC (OR, 0.33; 95% CI, 0.28–0.39) but not from right-sided CRC (OR, 0.99; 95% CI, 0.86–1.14).[39] Singh and colleagues[40] showed a 29% reduction in overall CRC mortality (SMR, 0.71; 95% CI, 0.61–0.82) with the use of colonoscopy compared with the general population. Once again, colonoscopy was associated with fewer deaths from left-sided CRC (SMR, 0.53; 95% CI, 0.42–0.67) but not from right-sided CRC (SMR, 0.94; 95% CI, 0.77–1.17). Baxter and colleagues[41] performed another case-control study using the SEER-Medicare data. They identified patients diagnosed with CRC (aged 70–89 years) who died as a result of CRC, and selected 3 matched controls without cancer for each case.[41] They identified prior exposure to colonoscopy up to 6 months before the diagnosis of CRC in the case group and to the referent date of CRC in the control group.[41] Overall, 11.3% of cases and 23.7% of controls underwent colonoscopy more than 6 months before the diagnosis.[41] Compared with the controls, cases were less likely to have undergone colonoscopy (OR, 0.40; 95% CI,

Table 1
Colonoscopy and subsequent risk of CRC: case-control and cohort studies

Source	Location and Study Type	Study Database	Study Period	Number (N)	Follow-up (y)	CRC Risk		Other Details in the Study
Müller et al,[33] 1995	United States Case control	VA	1988–1993	16,351 with CRC vs general veterans population; exposure to endoscopic procedures including FS, colonoscopy and polypectomy	10	OR 0.47 (0.37–0.58) Colon cancer OR 0.61 (0.48–0.77) rectal cancer		Flexible sigmoidoscopy OR 0.56 (0.46–0.67) colon cancer OR 0.61 (0.49–0.75) rectal cancer
Singh et al,[67] 2006	Canada Cohort	Administrative claims data in Manitoba, Canada	1989–2003	35,975 with negative colonoscopy compared with expected CRC rates in general population	>10	Incidence SIR >6 mo >1 y >2 y >5 y >10 y	0.69 (0.59–0.81) 0.66 (0.56–0.78) 0.59 (0.48–0.72) 0.55 (0.41–0.73) 0.28 (0.09–0.65)	The proportion of CRC located in the right side of the colon was significantly higher in the colonoscopy cohort than the rate in the Manitoba population (47% vs 28%; $P<.001$)
Lakoff et al,[42] 2008	Canada Cohort	Administrative claims data in Ontario, Canada	1992–1997	110,402 with negative colonoscopy compared with rates in population	Up to 14	Incidence RR Year 2 Year 3 Year 5 Year 10 Year 14	0.80 (0.66–0.93) 0.65 (0.54–0.77) 0.56 (0.46–0.67) 0.45 (0.34–0.55) 0.25 (0.12–0.37)	Consistent reduction in risk of proximal CRC seen only from 10 to 14 y of follow-up
Kahi et al,[34] 2009	United States Cohort	University Hospital Screening Colonoscopy Database vs SEER Registry	1989–1993	715 patients with 10,492 patient-years follow-up	Up to 18	SIR 0.33 (0.10–0.62)		—

						SIR (Men)	SIR (Women)	
Singh et al,[35] 2010	Canada	Manitoba's provincial physician's billing claims database	1989–2006	45,985 with negative colonoscopy compared with expected rates of CRC in population	>10	—		Proximal vs distal CRC in men and women: There was no reduction in the risk of proximal CRC among men or women in the first 5 y following the index colonoscopy. Distal CRC risk was reduced in all of the follow-up time among both men and women.
	Cohort					6–12 mo 0.53 (0.25–0.98)	1.27 (0.81–1.89)	Risk factors for early CRC (6–36 mo after index colonoscopy) included proximal site of CRC and specialty of endoscopist
						13–24 mo 0.64 (0.40–0.97)	0.97 (0.67–1.36)	
						25–36 mo 0.71 (0.44–1.08)	0.84 (0.55–1.23)	
						3–5 y 0.59 (0.38–0.89)	0.53 (0.35–0.77)	
						5–10 y 0.55 (0.39–0.76)	0.60 (0.45–0.80)	
						>10 y 0.53 (0.28–0.90)	0.51 (0.28–0.83)	

(continued on next page)

Table 1
(continued)

Source	Location and Study Type	Study Database	Study Period	Number (N)	Follow-up (y)	CRC Risk		Other Details in the Study
Brenner et al,[68] 2011	Germany Case control	Rhine-Neckar region population registry	2003–2007	1945 CRC vs 2399 controls	Up to 20	Incidence OR 1–2 y 3–4 y 5–9 y 10–19 y 20+ y	0.14 (0.10–0.20) 0.12 (0.08–0.19) 0.26 (0.18–0.39) 0.28 (0.17–0.45) 0.40 (0.24–0.66)	Also examined the risk in smokers and men and women
Brenner et al,[36] 2011	Germany Case control	Rhine-Neckar region population registry	2003–2004	1688 CRC vs 1932 controls aged more than 50 y	10	OR 0.23 (0.19–0.27)		Proximal CRC OR 0.44 (0.35–0.55) Distal CRC OR 0.16 (0.12–0.20)

Abbreviations: OR, odds ratio; RR, relative risk; SEER, Surveillance, Epidemiology, and End Results.

Table 2
Colonoscopy and CRC mortality: case-control and cohort studies

Source	Location and Study Type	Study Database	Study Period[a]	Number (N)	Follow-up (y)	CRC Risk	Other Details in the Study
Müller et al,[38] 1995	United States Case control	VA Patient Treatment File	1998–1992	4411 CRC vs 16,531 living controls	Mean: 6.4 cases 8.3 controls	OR 0.45 (0.30–0.66)	—
Baxter et al,[39] 2009	Canada Case control	Administrative claims data in Ontario, Canada	1996–2001	10,292 CRC vs 51,460 controls	7.8 (median)	OR 0.69 (0.63–0.74) —	Proximal CRC OR 0.99 (0.86–1.14) Distal CRC OR 0.33 (0.28–0.39)
Kahi et al,[34] 2009	United States Cohort	University Hospital Screening Colonoscopy database vs SEER Registry	1989–1993	715 patients with 10,492 patient-years follow-up	Up to 18	SMR 0.35 (0.0–1.06) —	—
Singh et al,[40] 2010	Canada Cohort	Administrative claims data in Manitoba, Canada	1987–2007	54,803 individuals with 310,718 person-years of follow-up	>10	SMR 0.71 (0.61–0.82)	Proximal CRC SMR 0.94 (0.77–1.17) Distal CRC SMR 0.53 (0.42–0.67)
Baxter et al,[41] 2012	United States Case control	SEER-Medicare	2002–2007	9458 CRC cases vs 27,641 controls; measured exposure to colonoscopy	—	OR 0.40 (0.37–0.43)	Proximal CRC OR 0.58 (0.53–0.64) Distal CRC OR 0.24 (0.21–0.27)

Abbreviation: SEER, Surveillance, Epidemiology and End Results.
[a] Study period for performance of colonoscopy in the cohort studies or for identification of CRC cases in the case-control studies.

0.37–0.43).[41] The association was stronger for distal (OR, 0.24; 95% CI, 0.21–0.27) than proximal (OR, 0.58; 95% CI, 0.53–0.64) CRC.[41]

Efficacy of FS Screening

In intention-to-screen analysis, 3 of the 4 RCTs of FS screening for CRC have recently reported significant reduction in CRC incidence and the 2 larger trials a significant reduction in CRC mortality. The follow-up in the trial (Norwegian Colorectal Cancer Prevention [NORCAAP]) with no reduction in CRC incidence was shorter than in the other trials (because it has only reported early interim findings so far) making the effect of prevalent cancer harvesting more pronounced. The estimates for CRC mortality reduction in the smaller trials (Screening for Colon Rectum [SCORE], NORCAAP) with nonsignificant results were similar to those of the larger trials (UK FS, and Prostate, Lung, Colorectal, and Ovarian Cancer screening [PLCO] trial).

The NORCAAP study found no significant difference in the 7-year cumulative incidence of CRC between the screening and control groups.[28] In intention-to-screen analysis, a trend toward reduced risk of CRC mortality (hazard ratio [HR] 0.73; 95% CI, 0.47–1.13) was found.[28] The UK FS trial subsequently showed significant mortality benefit with the use of FS screening.[9] CRC mortality was reduced by 31% (HR, 0.69; 95% CI, 0.59–0.82) in intention-to-treat analyses.[9] The SCORE trial in Italy showed substantial reduction in CRC incidence and mortality.[6] The CRC incidence was reduced by 18% (relative risk [RR] 0.82; 95% CI, 0.69–0.96) and the CRC mortality was reduced by 22% (RR, 0.78; 95% CI, 0.56–1.08).[6] The PLCO trial showed that, in addition to reduction in distal CRC incidence, there was significant reduction in proximal CRC incidence (RR, 0.86; 95% CI, 0.76–0.97) among the FS screening group.[10] This trial also showed reduction in mortality from distal CRC (RR, 0.50; 95% CI, 0.38–0.64) but not from proximal CRC (RR, 0.97; 95% CI, 0.77–1.22).[10] The significant reduction in the proximal CRC incidence in the PLCO trial may be caused by the higher colonoscopy use in the trial: 21.9% of the FS in the PLCO trial led to colonoscopy,[10] compared with, for example, 5.2% in the UK FS trial.[9] However, there was no significant reduction in the incidence of the stage IV proximal CRC in the PLCO trial.[10]

COLONOSCOPY AND RIGHT-SIDED CRC INCIDENCE AND MORTALITY

Several recent studies have suggested that colonoscopy may lead to lower reductions in right-sided CRC incidence and mortality than that for left-sided CRC. These studies have raised questions on the magnitude of incremental benefit of colonoscopy compared with FS when colonoscopy is performed in the usual clinical practice.[35,39,40,42,43] In a cross-sectional study from Germany, Brenner and colleagues[43] showed that prevalence of left-sided advanced colorectal neoplasms (OR, 0.33; 95% CI, 0.21–0.53), but not right-sided advanced neoplasms (OR, 1.05; 95% CI, 0.63–1.76), was strongly reduced within a 10-year period after colonoscopy. The same group of investigators also reported that colonoscopy was associated with strong risk reduction for all stages of CRC for all different age groups, except right-sided CRC in persons aged 50 to 59 years (OR, 0.74; 95% CI, 0.37–1.46).[36] Using SMR, Singh and colleagues[40] compared the CRC mortality in a cohort of 54,803 individuals after index colonoscopy with the general population in Manitoba, Canada. They found a 29% reduction in overall CRC mortality (SMR, 0.71; 95% CI, 0.61–0.82).[40] There was a 47% reduction in mortality from distal CRC (SMR, 0.53; 95% CI, 0.42–0.67), but no reduction in mortality from proximal CRC (SMR, 0.94; 95% CI, 0.77–1.17).[40] Another population-based study in Ontario, Canada, showed that complete colonoscopy was strongly associated with fewer deaths from left-sided

CRC (OR, 0.33; 95% CI, 028 to 0.39) but not from right-sided CRC (OR, 0.99; 95% CI, 0.86–1.14).[39]

The limited effectiveness of colonoscopy in usual clinical practice for right-sided CRC is likely caused by an interplay of the biology of the tumors and technical performance of colonoscopy. Potential endoscopic reasons for a higher miss rate of proximal CRC include worse bowel preparation in the proximal colon and incomplete colonoscopies.[40,44] Lesions in the right colon are more often endoscopically subtle and therefore may not be detected by some endoscopists, especially those who have a lower rate of reaching the end of the right side of the colon.[45] Flat-appearing lesions are more common in the proximal colon and are more likely to be missed.[46,47] Also, polyps with advanced neoplasia, high-grade dysplasia, or adenocarcinoma tend to be smaller in the right colon compared with the left colon.[48] A recent pathology study showed that advanced polyps were 5-fold more likely to be less than 6 mm in size in the right colon compared with those in the left colon (OR, 5.27; 95% CI, 4.06–6.82).[48] There are also important differences in tumor biology between proximal and distal CRC, with proximal CRC carrying a worse prognosis.[49,50] A higher proportion of proximal CRCs and interval CRCs (ie, CRC detected after colonoscopies on which no CRCs were reported) are likely to arise from the more recently described alternate pathway for CRC pathogenesis involving serrated colon polyps.[51] Serrated colon polyps, especially those in the right colon, are often subtle, slightly raised lesions with indistinct margins and overlying mucus caps that are yellow, green, or rust-colored in white light or red in narrow band imaging, which leads to marked variation in detection of these lesions.[52,53] A future strategy to prevent right-sided CRC will require more accurate detection of flat, subtle, and small polyps in the right colon.

THE SPECIALTY OF ENDOSCOPY AND OUTCOMES FOLLOWING COLONOSCOPY

One of the most disconcerting new findings in CRC screening is the wide variation in performance of colonoscopy by different operators. Gastroenterologists receive more extensive colonoscopy training during fellowship than physicians with other specialty training. Given that colonoscopy is a complex skill with a long learning curve,[54,55] the quality of gastroenterologist-provided colonoscopy may be higher on average than colonoscopy by other providers, although at the individual level there are poor-quality performers who are gastroenterologists and high-quality performers who are not gastroenterologists.[41] In a study of the US Medicare population, colonoscopy performed by a gastroenterologist was more likely to result in polyp detection and removal: compared with gastroenterologists, the RR for polyp detection was 0.93 (95% CI, 0.89–0.98) for internists and 0.80 (95% CI, 0.77–0.83) for general surgeons.[56] Another US study done at 20 Indiana hospitals found that colonoscopy performed by a gastroenterologist was more sensitive (97.3%) for cancer detection than colonoscopy performed by a nongastroenterologist (87%), with an OR of 5.36 (95% CI, 2.94–9.77) for missed cancer by a nongastroenterologist compared with a gastroenterologist.[57]

A population-based study in Manitoba, Canada, found that performance of index colonoscopy by nongastroenterologists was an independent predictor of early/missed CRC (cancers occurring within 3 years) after negative colonoscopy.[35] Compared with gastroenterologists, the HR for early CRC after negative colonoscopy was 1.68 (95% CI, 1.03–2.74) for urban surgeons, 2.09 (95% CI, 1.09–4.02) for internists, 2.92 (95% CI, 1.29–6.60) for family practice physicians, and 3.34 (95% CI, 1.69–6.61) for rural surgeons.[35] Another cohort study examined residents aged 50 to 80 years old in Ontario, Canada, who had negative complete colonoscopy examination.[58] This cohort consisted of 110,402 individuals without history of CRC, inflammatory bowel disease, or recent history of colonic resection.[58] During a 15-year follow-up period, 1596 (14.5%) developed CRC. On multivariate analysis, residents who had colonoscopy performed by nongastroenterologists were at significantly increased risk of developing CRC.[58]

QUALITY OF COLONOSCOPY

Irrespective of the initial test, colonoscopy is a vital test for CRC screening, and so there is a renewed focus now to improve the performance of colonoscopy in usual practice. Quality of the baseline endoscopy is associated with the risk of interval cancer.[59] Since 2002, various quality indicators for reporting and performance, such as cecal intubation rate and adenoma detection rate, have been published and adopted by various societies.[59–62] Kaminski and colleagues[63] evaluated the influence of cecal intubation rate and adenoma detection rate on interval CRC. They found that an adenoma detection rate of less than 20% in the initial screening examination was associated with significantly higher risk of interval cancer in next 5 years.[63] Baxter and colleagues[64] compared endoscopist with high and low polyp detection rates (estimated from the rates of polypectomy) and found that interval cancers were less likely when the colonoscopy was performed by an endoscopist with high polyp detection rate. They also compared endoscopist with high (>95%) and low (<80%) cecal intubation rates, and postcolonoscopy interval cancers in proximal colon were less common (OR, 0.72; 95% CI, 0.53–0.97) in patients who had colonoscopy performed by an endoscopist with high cecal intubation rate.[64]

The current wide variation in performance of colonoscopy and improved outcomes when the colonoscopy is performed by well-trained physicians suggests that there is a large potential for improvement in outcomes after performance of colonoscopy in usual clinical practice with the recent focus on quality of colonoscopy.

DURATION OF REDUCED RISK AFTER NEGATIVE COLONOSCOPY

Within the last decade, the literature on risk of interval advanced adenomas and CRC after colonoscopy examination has grown. Imperiale and colleagues[65] examined the 5-year risk of colorectal neoplasia after negative screening colonoscopy (see **Table 1**). Of 1256 persons rescreened at 5 years, 201 (16%) persons had 1 or more adenoma.[65] In a logistic regression model adjusting for age, sex, and baseline findings as independent variables, adjusted ORs for any adenoma and advanced adenoma were 1.92 (95% CI, 1.49–2.47) and 3.17 (95% CI, 0.88–11.33), respectively.[65] Lieberman and colleagues[66] evaluated 5-year colon surveillance after screening colonoscopy and included 895 patients with neoplasia and 298 patients without neoplasia at baseline who underwent repeat colonoscopy at 5 years. Of 298 patients with no neoplasia at baseline, 7 (2.4%) had advanced neoplasia at the 5-year examination. Both of the studies focused on advanced adenoma, a surrogate marker for CRC, and showed that after negative colonoscopy there is a low risk of advanced adenoma at 5 years.

Lakoff and colleagues[42] identified a cohort of 110,402 individuals with negative colonoscopy in Ontario, Canada, and evaluated the RR for CRC against the general population. Negative colonoscopy was associated with an RR of 0.65 (95% CI, 0.54–0.77) at 3 years, 0.56 (95% CI, 0.46–0.67) at 5 years, 0.45 (95% CI, 0.34–0.55) at 10 years, and 0.25 (95% CI, 0.12–0.37) at 14 years.[42] Singh and colleagues[67] performed a population-based retrospective analysis of 35,975 individuals residing in Manitoba, Canada, whose baseline colonoscopy examinations were negative. They examined the duration and magnitude of the risk of CRC following a negative colonoscopy by calculating the SIRs and comparing the CRC incidence in their cohort with CRC incidence in the provincial population.[67] Negative colonoscopy was associated with SIRs of 0.60 (95% CI, 0.59–0.81) for follow-up beyond 6 months, 0.55 (95% CI, 0.41–0.73) beyond 5 years, and 0.28 (95% CI, 0.09–0.65) for follow-up of more than 10 years.[67] Brenner and colleagues[68] evaluated long-term risk of CRC after negative colonoscopy in 1945 patients with CRC and 2399 population controls in Germany. Negative colonoscopy was associated with reduced risk of CRC with OR of 0.14 (95% CI, 0.10–0.20) at 1–2 years, 0.12 (95% CI, 0.08–0.19) at 3–4 years, 0.26 (95% CI, 0.18–0.39) at 5–9 years, 0.28 (95% CI, 0.17–0.45) at 10–19 years, and 0.40 (95% CI, 0.24–0.66) at 20 or more years.[68] Low risks even beyond 10 years after negative colonoscopy were observed for both right-sided and left-sided CRC and in all risk groups assessed except current smokers.[68]

These studies as well as the FS trials suggest that the risk stratification effect of negative endoscopy extends beyond 10 years, limiting the need to repeat colonoscopy for asymptomatic individuals with negative colonoscopy.

THE FUTURE

Randomized trials are the method of choice to establish efficacy of screening tests. For screening colonoscopy, 3 randomized trials are ongoing, 1 trial comparing screening colonoscopy with no screening for CRC,[69] and the other 2 trials comparing screening colonoscopy with fecal immunochemical testing (**Table 3**).[70,71] The Nordic-European Initiative on Colorectal Cancer (NordICC) study has recently been initiated in several European countries.[69] The study design is focused on men and women aged 55 to 64 years, randomly assigned to either once-only colonoscopy screening with removal of all detected lesions, or no screening (standard of care in trial regions).[69] The study is aiming for inclusion of 45,600 participants in the control arm and 22,800 participants in the colonoscopy group using a 2:1 randomization.[69] The primary end point of the study is effect of colonoscopy on CRC incidence and mortality.[69] The study is currently recruiting and the results will be available at least 10 years after the completion of recruitment. The Colorectal cancer screening in the average-risk population: a pragmatic, multicentre, randomised, controlled trial comparing colonoscopy and faecal immunochemical testing (COLONPREV study) is another randomized, controlled, non inferiority trial conducted in 8 Spanish regions comparing colonoscopy with faecal immunochemical test (FIT) in CRC screening.[70] This trial included asymptomatic adults 50 to 69 years of age and compared one-time colonoscopy in 26,703 subjects with FIT every 2 years in 26,599 subjects.[70] The primary outcome of the study is morality from CRC at 10 years.[70] The interim report describing rate of participation, diagnostic findings, and occurrence of major complications at completion of baseline screening have been published.[70] The Colonoscopy Versus Fecal Immunochemical Test in Reducing Mortality from Colorectal Cancer (CONFIRM) study is a randomized trial examining colonoscopy versus FIT in reducing mortality from CRC.[71] This study is sponsored by the VA and was recently initiated in 42 different locations in the United States. The study plans to include 50,000 individuals between 50 and 75 years of age and randomized either to screening colonoscopy or annual FIT screening using a 1:1 randomization.

The results of these trials are likely to provide strong insight into mortality benefits using colonoscopy screening. However, these results will only be available 10 to 15 years from now. There has been significant progress in colonoscopy technology and quality over the last decade and, with expected ongoing progress, results of these trials may pertain to technology that may be outdated by the time of the publication of their results.[72] For example, newer technology/devices like the wide-angle lens

Table 3
Design of ongoing RCTs assessing efficacy of colonoscopy in reducing CRC incidence and mortality

	NordICC[64]	COLONPREV[65]	CONFIRM[67]
Study			
Country/continent	Europe	Spain	United States
Lead investigator/s	Bretthauer, M	Quintero, E and Castells, A	Dominitz, JA and Robertson, DJ
Recruitment period	2010 (ongoing)	2009–2011	2011 (ongoing)
Population			
Number randomized/ estimated enrollment	68,400	57,404	50,000
Setting	Several European countries	Eight Spanish regions: Aragón, Basque Country, Canarias, Catalonia, Galicia, Madrid, and Valencia	42 VA hospital in United States
Source	Population registry	Community health registry	Veterans eligible for VA care
Age (y)	55–64	50–69	50–75
Study Groups			
Randomization	Before invitation	Before invitation	After invitation
Study arms	1. One-time colonoscopy 2. No screening	1. One-time colonoscopy 2. Biennial FIT	1. Colonoscopy 2. Annual FIT
Power Calculation Assumptions			
Screening arm (n)	22,800 colonoscopy	27,749	25,000
Control arm (n)	45,600	27,749	25,000
Compliance with colonoscopy (%)	50	30	NA
CRC mortality reduction (intent to treat) (%)	25	75 for colonoscopy and 51 for FIT	40 between the 2 groups
Follow-up mortality (y)	15	10	10
Significance level (%)	5 (2-sided)	2.5 (1-sided)	5 (2-sided)
Power (%)	90	80	82

colonoscope, transparent detachable plastic cap, and through-the-scope retrograde viewing device have recently been investigated against standard colonoscopy.[73] Initial results show a positive trend toward lower adenoma miss rates and increased adenoma detection rates.[73] In addition, colonoscopy and sigmoidoscopy are increasingly used for both screening and diagnostic purposes in the United States and some European countries, and prevalence of lower gastrointestinal endoscopy has become so high in the target population of screening that randomized trials in those populations would be affected by contamination of the control group and limitation of enrolment to a select group of individuals who do not undergo routine screening.[72,74,75]

Even though the trials have adjusted their sample sizes and will adjust their statistical analyses for the possibility of contamination, higher than anticipated rates of contamination may affect the interpretation of the trial results. Further, randomized trials are able to evaluate screening efficacy under standardized trial conditions, but they are unable to completely evaluate the effectiveness of colonoscopy screening in routine practice.[72] Comparative evaluation of different options, like effect of different screening or surveillance intervals, will not be possible with the current ongoing randomized trials.[72] Therefore, current and future recommendations and decisions on colonoscopy screening for CRC will need to be based on evidence gained from both the carefully conducted observational studies that evaluate the effectiveness of colonoscopy in routine practice and results from ongoing randomized trials.

SUMMARY

Although RCTs for evaluating the efficacy of colonoscopy on CRC incidence and mortality have been initiated only in the last few years, there is substantial indirect evidence for effectiveness of colonoscopy in reducing CRC incidence and mortality. There is an urgent need to develop and adopt measures to improve effectiveness of colonoscopy in reducing the incidence and mortality of right-sided CRC and to ensure that colonoscopy provides incremental benefit compared with FS. Variation of performance and outcomes among endoscopy providers suggests that quality assurance and enhancement programs could lead to improvement in outcomes after colonoscopy.

REFERENCES

1. Siegel R, Naishadham D, Jemal A. Cancer statistics, 2012. CA Cancer J Clin 2012;62(1):10–29.
2. Rabeneck L, El-Serag HB, Davila JA, et al. Outcomes of colorectal cancer in the United States: no change in survival (1986-1997). Am J Gastroenterol 2003; 98(2):471–7.
3. Edwards BK, Ward E, Kohler BA, et al. Annual report to the nation on the status of cancer, 1975-2006, featuring colorectal cancer trends and impact of interventions (risk factors, screening, and treatment) to reduce future rates. Cancer 2010;116(3):544–73.
4. Mandel JS, Bond JH, Church TR, et al. Reducing mortality from colorectal cancer by screening for fecal occult blood. Minnesota Colon Cancer Control Study. N Engl J Med 1993;328(19):1365–71.
5. Mandel JS, Church TR, Bond JH, et al. The effect of fecal occult-blood screening on the incidence of colorectal cancer. N Engl J Med 2000;343(22): 1603–7.
6. Segnan N, Armaroli P, Bonelli L, et al. Once-only sigmoidoscopy in colorectal cancer screening: follow-up findings of the Italian Randomized Controlled Trial–SCORE. J Natl Cancer Inst 2011;103(17):1310–22.
7. Scholefield JH, Moss S, Sufi F, et al. Effect of faecal occult blood screening on mortality from colorectal cancer: results from a randomised controlled trial. Gut 2002;50(6):840–4.
8. Hardcastle JD, Chamberlain JO, Robinson MH, et al. Randomised controlled trial of faecal-occult-blood screening for colorectal cancer. Lancet 1996; 348(9040):1472–7.
9. Atkin WS, Edwards R, Kralj-Hans I, et al. Once-only flexible sigmoidoscopy screening in prevention of colorectal cancer: a multicentre randomised controlled trial. Lancet 2010;375(9726):1624–33.

10. Schoen RE, Pinsky PF, Weissfeld JL, et al. Colorectal-cancer incidence and mortality with screening flexible sigmoidoscopy. N Engl J Med 2012;366(25): 2345–57.

11. Meissner HI, Breen N, Klabunde CN, et al. Patterns of colorectal cancer screening uptake among men and women in the United States. Cancer Epidemiol Biomarkers Prev 2006;15(2):389–94.

12. Klabunde CN, Lanier D, Nadel MR, et al. Colorectal cancer screening by primary care physicians: recommendations and practices, 2006-2007. Am J Prev Med 2009;37(1):8–16.

13. Lieberman DA, Weiss DG, Bond JH, et al. Use of colonoscopy to screen asymptomatic adults for colorectal cancer. Veterans Affairs Cooperative Study Group 380. N Engl J Med 2000;343(3):162–8.

14. Winawer SJ, Zauber AG, Ho MN, et al. Prevention of colorectal cancer by colonoscopic polypectomy. The National Polyp Study Workgroup. N Engl J Med 1993;329(27):1977–81.

15. Lin OS, Kozarek RA, Schembre DB, et al. Screening colonoscopy in very elderly patients: prevalence of neoplasia and estimated impact on life expectancy. JAMA 2006;295(20):2357–65.

16. Regula J, Rupinski M, Kraszewska E, et al. Colonoscopy in colorectal-cancer screening for detection of advanced neoplasia. N Engl J Med 2006;355(18): 1863–72.

17. Schoenfeld P, Cash B, Flood A, et al. Colonoscopic screening of average-risk women for colorectal neoplasia. N Engl J Med 2005;352(20):2061–8.

18. Kim DH, Pickhardt PJ, Taylor AJ, et al. CT colonography versus colonoscopy for the detection of advanced neoplasia. N Engl J Med 2007;357(14): 1403–12.

19. Ko CW, Riffle S, Michaels L, et al. Serious complications within 30 days of screening and surveillance colonoscopy are uncommon. Clin Gastroenterol Hepatol 2010;8(2):166–73.

20. Harewood GC, Wiersema MJ, Melton LJ 3rd. A prospective, controlled assessment of factors influencing acceptance of screening colonoscopy. Am J Gastroenterol 2002;97(12):3186–94.

21. Harewood GC, Lieberman DA. Colonoscopy practice patterns since introduction of Medicare coverage for average-risk screening. Clin Gastroenterol Hepatol 2004;2(1):72–7.

22. Robertson RH, Burkhardt JH, Powell MP, et al. Trends in colon cancer screening procedures in the US Medicare and Tricare populations: 1999-2001. Prev Med 2006;42(6):460–2.

23. Cram P, Fendrick AM, Inadomi J, et al. The impact of a celebrity promotional campaign on the use of colon cancer screening: the Katie Couric effect. Arch Intern Med 2003;163(13):1601–5.

24. Prajapati DN, Saeian K, Binion DG, et al. Volume and yield of screening colonoscopy at a tertiary medical center after change in Medicare reimbursement. Am J Gastroenterol 2003;98(1):194–9.

25. Imperiale TF, Wagner DR, Lin CY, et al. Risk of advanced proximal neoplasms in asymptomatic adults according to the distal colorectal findings. N Engl J Med 2000;343(3):169–74.

26. Stryker SJ, Wolff BG, Culp CE, et al. Natural history of untreated colonic polyps. Gastroenterology 1987;93(5):1009–13.

27. Kramer BS, Croswell JM. Cancer screening: the clash of science and intuition. Annu Rev Med 2009;60:125–37.

28. Hoff G, Grotmol T, Skovlund E, et al. Risk of colorectal cancer seven years after flexible sigmoidoscopy screening: randomised controlled trial. BMJ 2009;338: b1846.
29. Winawer SJ, Zauber AG, O'Brien MJ, et al. The National Polyp Study. Design, methods, and characteristics of patients with newly diagnosed polyps. The National Polyp Study Workgroup. Cancer 1992;70(Suppl 5):1236–45.
30. Atkin WS, Morson BC, Cuzick J. Long-term risk of colorectal cancer after excision of rectosigmoid adenomas. N Engl J Med 1992;326(10):658–62.
31. Zauber AG, Winawer SJ, O'Brien MJ, et al. Colonoscopic polypectomy and long-term prevention of colorectal-cancer deaths. N Engl J Med 2012;366(8): 687–96.
32. Lang CA, Ransohoff DF. Fecal occult blood screening for colorectal cancer. Is mortality reduced by chance selection for screening colonoscopy? JAMA 1994;271(13):1011–3.
33. Muller AD, Sonnenberg A. Prevention of colorectal cancer by flexible endoscopy and polypectomy. A case-control study of 32,702 veterans. Ann Intern Med 1995;123(12):904–10.
34. Kahi CJ, Imperiale TF, Juliar BE, et al. Effect of screening colonoscopy on colorectal cancer incidence and mortality. Clin Gastroenterol Hepatol 2009;7(7): 770–5 [quiz: 711].
35. Singh H, Nugent Z, Mahmud SM, et al. Predictors of colorectal cancer after negative colonoscopy: a population-based study. Am J Gastroenterol 2010; 105(3):663–73 [quiz: 674].
36. Brenner H, Chang-Claude J, Seiler CM, et al. Protection from colorectal cancer after colonoscopy: a population-based, case-control study. Ann Intern Med 2011;154(1):22–30.
37. Brenner H, Chang-Claude J, Rickert A, et al. Risk of colorectal cancer after detection and removal of adenomas at colonoscopy: population-based case-control study. J Clin Oncol 2012;30(24):2969–76.
38. Muller AD, Sonnenberg A. Protection by endoscopy against death from colorectal cancer. A case-control study among veterans. Arch Intern Med 1995; 155(16):1741–8.
39. Baxter NN, Goldwasser MA, Paszat LF, et al. Association of colonoscopy and death from colorectal cancer. Ann Intern Med 2009;150(1):1–8.
40. Singh H, Nugent Z, Demers AA, et al. The reduction in colorectal cancer mortality after colonoscopy varies by site of the cancer. Gastroenterology 2010;139(4): 1128–37.
41. Baxter NN, Warren JL, Barrett MJ, et al. Association between colonoscopy and colorectal cancer mortality in a US cohort according to site of cancer and colonoscopist specialty. J Clin Oncol 2012;30(21):2664–9.
42. Lakoff J, Paszat LF, Saskin R, et al. Risk of developing proximal versus distal colorectal cancer after a negative colonoscopy: a population-based study. Clin Gastroenterol Hepatol 2008;6(10):1117–21 [quiz: 1064].
43. Brenner H, Hoffmeister M, Arndt V, et al. Protection from right- and left-sided colorectal neoplasms after colonoscopy: population-based study. J Natl Cancer Inst 2010;102(2):89–95.
44. Rex DK, Eid E. Considerations regarding the present and future roles of colonoscopy in colorectal cancer prevention. Clin Gastroenterol Hepatol 2008; 6(5):506–14.
45. Rex DK. Preventing colorectal cancer and cancer mortality with colonoscopy: what we know and what we don't know. Endoscopy 2010;42(4):320–3.

46. Soetikno RM, Kaltenbach T, Rouse RV, et al. Prevalence of nonpolypoid (flat and depressed) colorectal neoplasms in asymptomatic and symptomatic adults. JAMA 2008;299(9):1027–35.

47. Park DH, Kim HS, Kim WH, et al. Clinicopathologic characteristics and malignant potential of colorectal flat neoplasia compared with that of polypoid neoplasia. Dis Colon Rectum 2008;51(1):43–9 [discussion: 49].

48. Gupta S, Balasubramanian BA, Fu T, et al. Polyps with advanced neoplasia are smaller in the right than in the left colon: implications for colorectal cancer screening. Clin Gastroenterol Hepatol 2012;10(12):1395–401.e2.

49. Meguid RA, Slidell MB, Wolfgang CL, et al. Is there a difference in survival between right- versus left-sided colon cancers? Ann Surg Oncol 2008;15(9): 2388–94.

50. Benedix F, Kube R, Meyer F, et al. Comparison of 17,641 patients with right- and left-sided colon cancer: differences in epidemiology, perioperative course, histology, and survival. Dis Colon Rectum 2010;53(1):57–64.

51. Snover DC. Update on the serrated pathway to colorectal carcinoma. Hum Pathol 2011;42(1):1–10.

52. Kahi CJ, Hewett DG, Norton DL, et al. Prevalence and variable detection of proximal colon serrated polyps during screening colonoscopy. Clin Gastroenterol Hepatol 2011;9(1):42–6.

53. Rex DK, Ahnen DJ, Baron JA, et al. Serrated lesions of the colorectum: review and recommendations from an expert panel. Am J Gastroenterol 2012;107(9): 1315–29 [quiz: 1314, 1330].

54. Spier BJ, Durkin ET, Walker AJ, et al. Surgical resident's training in colonoscopy: numbers, competency, and perceptions. Surg Endosc 2010;24(10): 2556–61.

55. Spier BJ, Benson M, Pfau PR, et al. Colonoscopy training in gastroenterology fellowships: determining competence. Gastrointest Endosc 2010;71(2):319–24.

56. Ko CW, Dominitz JA, Green P, et al. Specialty differences in polyp detection, removal, and biopsy during colonoscopy. Am J Med 2010;123(6):528–35.

57. Rex DK, Rahmani EY, Haseman JH, et al. Relative sensitivity of colonoscopy and barium enema for detection of colorectal cancer in clinical practice. Gastroenterology 1997;112(1):17–23.

58. Rabeneck L, Paszat LF, Saskin R. Endoscopist specialty is associated with incident colorectal cancer after a negative colonoscopy. Clin Gastroenterol Hepatol 2010;8(3):275–9.

59. Lieberman DA, Rex DK, Winawer SJ, et al. Guidelines for colonoscopy surveillance after screening and polypectomy: a consensus update by the US Multi-Society Task Force on Colorectal Cancer. Gastroenterology 2012;143(3): 844–57.

60. Rex DK, Bond JH, Winawer S, et al. Quality in the technical performance of colonoscopy and the continuous quality improvement process for colonoscopy: recommendations of the U.S. Multi-Society Task Force on Colorectal Cancer. Am J Gastroenterol 2002;97(6):1296–308.

61. Rex DK, Petrini JL, Baron TH, et al. Quality indicators for colonoscopy. Am J Gastroenterol 2006;101(4):873–85.

62. Lieberman D, Nadel M, Smith RA, et al. Standardized colonoscopy reporting and data system: report of the Quality Assurance Task Group of the National Colorectal Cancer Roundtable. Gastrointest Endosc 2007;65(6):757–66.

63. Kaminski MF, Regula J, Kraszewska E, et al. Quality indicators for colonoscopy and the risk of interval cancer. N Engl J Med 2010;362(19):1795–803.

64. Baxter NN, Sutradhar R, Forbes SS, et al. Analysis of administrative data finds endoscopist quality measures associated with postcolonoscopy colorectal cancer. Gastroenterology 2011;140(1):65–72.

65. Imperiale TF, Glowinski EA, Lin-Cooper C, et al. Five-year risk of colorectal neoplasia after negative screening colonoscopy. N Engl J Med 2008;359(12): 1218–24.

66. Lieberman DA, Weiss DG, Harford WV, et al. Five-year colon surveillance after screening colonoscopy. Gastroenterology 2007;133(4):1077–85.

67. Singh H, Turner D, Xue L, et al. Risk of developing colorectal cancer following a negative colonoscopy examination: evidence for a 10-year interval between colonoscopies. JAMA 2006;295(20):2366–73.

68. Brenner H, Chang-Claude J, Seiler CM, et al. Long-term risk of colorectal cancer after negative colonoscopy. J Clin Oncol 2011;29(28):3761–7.

69. Kaminski MF, Bretthauer M, Zauber AG, et al. The NordICC Study: rationale and design of a randomized trial on colonoscopy screening for colorectal cancer. Endoscopy 2012;44(7):695–702.

70. Quintero E, Castells A, Bujanda L, et al. Colonoscopy versus fecal immuno-chemical testing in colorectal-cancer screening. N Engl J Med 2012;366(8): 697–706.

71. Colonoscopy Versus Fecal Immunochemical Test in Reducing Mortality From Colorectal Cancer (CONFIRM). 2012. Available at: http://clinicaltrials.gov/ct2/show/study/NCT01239082. Accessed December 1, 2012.

72. Ausk KJ, Dominitz JA. Colonoscopy prevents colorectal cancer in both the right and left colon. Gastroenterology 2011;141(1):393–6 [discussion: 396].

73. Mamula P, Tierney WM, Banerjee S, et al. Devices to improve colon polyp detection. Gastrointest Endosc 2011;73(6):1092–7.

74. Stock C, Knudsen AB, Lansdorp-Vogelaar I, et al. Colorectal cancer mortality prevented by use and attributable to nonuse of colonoscopy. Gastrointest Endosc 2011;73(3):435–443.e5.

75. Stock C, Brenner H. Utilization of lower gastrointestinal endoscopy and fecal occult blood test in 11 European countries: evidence from the Survey of Health, Aging and Retirement in Europe (SHARE). Endoscopy 2010;42(7):546–56.

Complications of Colonoscopy

James Church, MB, ChB, FRACS

KEYWORDS

- Colonoscopy • Colonoscopy complications • Colorectal disease
- Colorectal cancer screening

KEY POINTS

- Colonoscopy is a complex process that offers several opportunities for misadventures and complications.
- The continuing increase in demand for colonoscopy as a way of screening for colorectal cancer, diagnosing colorectal disease, and treating colorectal mucosal lesions means that complications are certain to occur with increasing frequency.
- An awareness of common complications, a routine to minimize or prevent them, and a familiarity with the treatment options and how to apply them is an essential part of every colonoscopist's practice.

INTRODUCTION

In the context of medical practice, a complication is an unfavorable outcome related to some form of procedure or therapy. Whereas the procedure or therapy is intended for good, it causes harm. Consideration of a procedure or therapy always involves a calculation of the likelihood of complications, and balances this against the likelihood of a benefit to the patient. In general terms, every procedure and therapy has a literature from which estimates of the risk of complications are drawn. There are usually multiple studies that show factors contributing to high risk, and what must be done to minimize risk. Colonoscopy is a good example of this.

Colonoscopy is a difficult procedure to master. It involves passing a flexible scope retrograde up a tortuous length of bowel that contains at least 4 right-angle (or more acute) bends in 1 dimension, and a number of extra angles in other dimensions. The colonoscope naturally tends to form loops, and adherent bowel can be difficult to straighten. Patients vary in their ability to tolerate the procedure when under conscious sedation, and endoscopists vary in the skill with which they use the colonoscope. This article describes the complications of colonoscopy, and their incidence, presentation, diagnosis, and treatment. Prevention of complications is an inherent part of this discussion.

Department of Colorectal Surgery, Digestive Diseases Institute, Cleveland Clinic, Desk A30, 9500 Euclid Avenue, Cleveland, OH 44195, USA
E-mail address: church@ccf.org

Gastroenterol Clin N Am 42 (2013) 639–657
http://dx.doi.org/10.1016/j.gtc.2013.05.003
0889-8553/13/$ – see front matter © 2013 Elsevier Inc. All rights reserved.

gastro.theclinics.com

THREE PRINCIPLES

Before discussing specific complications, there are 3 principles affecting the discussion that must be emphasized.

Risk Management

Risk management means defining the risks that apply to each patient for any procedure, and considering the benefits to be achieved by that procedure in the light of those risks. This is the essence of informed consent, a process that is applied to any invasive procedure. Accurate risk assessment on the basis of a careful history and examination allows minimization of risk by adapting the colonoscopy to the patient; adjusting the bowel preparation, changing sedation practices, and managing anticoagulation. For example, colonoscopic perforation can be lethal in patients with American Society of Anesthesiologists Physical Status Classification System Scores (ASA) 3 and 4, particularly in those older than 80 years.[1] The benefits offered by an examination in these high-risk, elderly patients must be particularly high to counterbalance the risks.

Teaching

Learning colonoscopy is essentially a practical exercise in which trainees must do the examination themselves to acquire the skills and "feel" required to become expert. There is therefore no way to avoid supervised patient experience for fellows in training. Complication rates of colonoscopy are inversely related to the experience of the examiner,[2,3] and teaching colonoscopy calls for a balance between the teaching experience and patient safety, a balance that can be achieved by careful patient selection and judicious supervision.[4]

Putting the Literature into Perspective

There is an extensive literature on colonoscopy complications, but the reports should be read with care. The range and quality of endoscopic technology is constantly changing, the effectiveness of bowel preparation, sedation, and analgesia is improving and the average experience level in endoscopy units is increasing. Furthermore, the outcome of complications has improved as advances in antibiotics, anesthesia technique, and surgical options (ie, laparoscopy) have made treatment more effective and less risky. This means that older studies may not be relevant to today.

Correct interpretation of reports by study design is important. Case reports may be interesting and illustrative, but do not allow generalizations based on a single patient or two. Retrospective review studies are prone to errors of selection and definition, but will show the range of severity of a complication, whereas a single endoscopist or single unit study will usually report overoptimistic results. Published studies generally represent the best of experiences at high-volume, expert centers. They therefore tend to underestimate the true incidence of complications and overestimate the quality of outcomes.

Colonoscopy can be considered in 3 phases: preparation, examination, and recovery. Complications can occur during preparation and examination, but often present during recovery.

COMPLICATIONS OF PREPARATION
Attendance

For colonoscopy to be effective, the patient must actually show up. Rates of nonattendance are not well documented but represent a significant complication of the appointment-making process. One study reported nonattendance rates of 38% to 42% for patients with colonoscopy appointments.[5] The outcome of the planned examination is poor because the colon is not examined, the lost appointment prevents another patient from being examined, and the opportunity cost of the empty spot on the schedule is high. Preprocedure phone calls are effective in reducing nonattendance and should be routine.[6] They also can help resolve issues related to the bowel preparation.[5,7]

Bowel Preparation

A clean colon is essential for a thorough, safe, and comfortable colonoscopy. Although retrograde flushes are possible, there is no practical alternative to an antegrade flush. Sodium phosphate preparations were commonly used 10 years ago and had the advantage of being low volume or in pill form. However, the risk of nephrocalcinosis and renal failure has resulted in their removal as an option.[8] Patients most commonly receive a polyethylene-glycol (PEG)-based antegrade gut lavage. PEG lavage is unpleasant but safe, although aspiration has been described in elderly patients[9] and vomiting is common.[10,11] Sometimes metoclopramide is given to improve passage of the liquid, although this is not always effective.[12] Laxatives given before the preparation may reduce the amount to drink and there is increased compliance found with the smaller-volume preparations.[13] Sometimes a lack of tolerance of lavage solutions can be a sign of upper gastrointestinal pathology.[14] Poor bowel preparation means solid or semisolid stool and results in inadequate inspection of the mucosa, excess air insufflation during attempts at insertion, potentially risky polypectomy, and significantly worse consequences should a perforation occur. Practices should aim for fewer than 10% of patients with poor bowel preparation, but barriers to achieving this include poorly written instructions, a lack of understanding of the importance of following instructions, noncompliance with dietary restrictions, and trouble tolerating the purgative.[15] Bowel preparation is discussed in detail in the article by Sharara and colleagues, elsewhere in this issue.

Sedation

Most colonoscopies are performed in sedated patients who have been given either a combination of a benzodiazepine and a narcotic, or an anesthetic agent, such as propofol. Oversedation can impair respirations, initially seen as hypoxia, and can also produce hypotension. Patients with cardiac conditions may be susceptible to hypotension and hypoxia and rare serious complications can occur. There is a temptation to be liberal with sedative and analgesic, partly because many patients are anxious about the examination, sometimes because of a bad personal experience or that of a friend or acquaintance, sometimes because of fear of what may be found, and sometimes because of an underlying anxious personality. High doses of sedation can also "hide" a suboptimal technique. In fact, with good technique, colonoscopy is associated with severe pain in only about 10% of examinations.[16] Severe pain is usually attributable to an irreducible loop, which stretches the colonic mesentery. Irreducibility in a loop is normally caused by adhesions. Patients particularly at risk for a painful examination are women who have had a hysterectomy,[17] or slim patients with an unzygosed colon and no fat to cushion the colonic flexures.[18,19] So, despite the demand to be "put out completely," many patients can tolerate colonoscopy with light or even no sedation/analgesia. Other techniques, such as warm water irrigation, can help.[20] Low-dose sedation minimizes the chances of complications, and allows for a quick recovery and resumption of activity.

Recently, there has been an increasing use of propofol for colonoscopy. This is effective, short acting, and generally safe, and recent consensus statements support its use as a routine way of facilitating colonoscopy in average-risk patients. These statements also comment that endoscopist-administered and endoscopy nurse–administered propofol is safe in ASA 1 and 2 patients.[21,22]

COMPLICATIONS OF THE EXAMINATION
Perforation

Causes
Perforation is the most serious common complication of colonoscopy, happening in 0.016% to 0.8% of diagnostic examinations and up to 5% of therapeutic colonoscopies.[23,24] Diagnostic perforation usually occurs during intubation because of direct scope trauma, splitting of the bowel at a stricture, by the sideways pressure of a loop, or pneumatic dilatation.[25] Most diagnostic perforations occur in the sigmoid colon, probably as a result of a tear in a fixed loop. Pushing the end of the scope through the bowel wall is uncommon, especially in healthy bowel. However, unhealthy bowel, especially affected by deep ulcers or chronic ischemia, is prone to rupture on repeated intubation. Perforation can sometimes occur after cold biopsy, especially in elderly patients in whom the bowel wall (especially the cecum) can become extremely thin.[26] Biopsy of an unrecognized diverticulum can also cause a perforation, and, in general, biopsies should be done on a muscular fold in a collapsed section of colon.

Postpolypectomy perforation occurs because coagulation used for polypectomy causes full-thickness necrosis of the colonic wall. This may be because too much electrocautery is used (check the settings), because cutting current is used, or because the colonic wall is unusually thin. Bad technique (including normal bowel wall in the snare) and misdiagnosis (trying to snare the ileocecal valve or an inverted diverticulum) can also lead to perforation.

Although diagnostic perforation happens on intubation and is often clinically obvious immediately, postpolypectomy perforation can occur either immediately after polypectomy or later, when a necrotic patch of colon sloughs out. This makes a difference in its management.

Prevention
Traumatic perforation Colonoscope insertion should be gentle, unhurried, and efficient, using an economy of action and minimizing loops.[27] "Pushing through" or "sliding by" are high-risk maneuvers and should be avoided. If insertion is painful, it should stop and other approaches tried. Some reports of traumatic complications of colonoscopy describe the examination as "uneventful" or "easy," yet there is colonic perforation, or some other catastrophe. Perhaps the colon wall is unusually brittle in these cases or the definition of "uneventful" or "easy" needs to be reworked.

Colonoscopists need to have a better acceptance of an incomplete examination. Because completeness is commonly used to measure colonoscopic expertise, there is a tendency to get there "at all costs." Sometimes the cost may be a perforation.

There are some situations in which the risk of perforation is increased over baseline:

i. Severe diverticulosis with muscular hypertrophy and a narrow sigmoid
    If the colonoscope becomes impacted in the sigmoid, a proximal pneumatic blowout is possible. Options are to use CO_2 as an insufflating gas,[28] to avoid fellows or trainees as examiners, to use a pediatric colonoscope, or finally to abandon the examination.

ii. Severe Crohn colitis, acute-on-chronic ischemia, acute (sealed) diverticulitis, and deeply invasive cancer may significantly weaken the colonic wall. Colonoscopists should avoid using "slide by" in a diseased colon, use a pediatric colonoscope, avoid loops, avoid repeated examinations, and may be justified in abandoning the examination.

iii. Intraoperative colonoscopy, or any colonoscopy done under general anesthetic, is generally safe, although the anesthetized patient cannot complain of pain.[29] Insertion techniques should still be as gentle as possible, and pushing through loops should be avoided. Immediate postcolectomy colonoscopy is also safe if done gently.[30]

Postpolypectomy perforations Postpolypectomy perforations can be minimized by accurate placement of the snare, allowing the mucosa to be lifted away from the underlying muscle. Limiting the amount of sessile polyp enclosed in the snare to 2 cm is important, and correct endoscopic diagnosis in avoiding lipomas and cancers is critical. Cancers have invaded the colonic submucosa and sometimes the muscle, making polypectomy attempts prone to causing full-thickness injury. Use of pure coagulation current applied intermittently in short bursts prevents inadvertent damage to the colonic wall. Special care is needed in elderly patients with cecal polyps. The cecal wall can be very thin and prone to perforation with standard amounts of current. Saline or adrenalin infiltration under polyps will raise them away from the colonic wall and make cautery safer. This also applies to treatment of arteriovenous malformations in the cecum.

Endoscopic submucosal dissection is a recently introduced technique that involves dissection of polyp at the submucosal level, first raising the lesion and expanding the bowel wall by injection of saline. When performed in the right colon, this technique is associated with a relatively high rate of perforation.[31,32] Yoshida and colleagues[32] reviewed 9 studies (mostly from Japan) with a range of perforation rates from 1.5% to 10.4%. There is no doubt that this technique requires patience and skill, and is not for the average colonoscopist.

Recognition of Perforations

Colonic perforation during colonoscopy is a problem, but if recognized is not usually a disaster. The colon is clean and prompt treatment is usually effective in preventing sepsis. Failing to recognize that a perforation has occurred may be disastrous, however, as the likelihood of fecal contamination will increase with time. Most traumatic perforations are obvious by the appearance of extracolonic fat, gaseous distention of the abdomen, or pain.[33] The examination must stop. If a perforation is suspected, an immediate abdominal radiograph may show free intraperitoneal gas, which could be due to either a perforation or a partial split of the colonic wall. A surgical consultation should be requested, and the decision for surgery is based on the likely cause of the perforation, size of the perforation, the state of the bowel (diseased vs normal), and the comorbidity present in the patient. For traumatic perforations, the threshold for surgery is low.[33]

Successful treatment of postpolypectomy perforation also depends on early diagnosis and appropriate decision making. Sometimes a perforation can be suspected at the time of polypectomy (target sign),[34] offering the opportunity for successful preventive treatment with clips.[34,35] A histologic diagnosis of a large lipoma or cancer should also arouse suspicion and trigger a call to the patient. Abdominal distension without liver dullness or delayed onset of abdominal pain warrants investigation with abdominal examination and radiograph.

Treatment of Perforations

i. Presentation during the colonoscopy

If the perforation is recognized at the time it happens, it can be treated endoscopically in a large number of cases. Suitability for endoscopic clipping depends on having a normal colon, a clean colon, and a relatively small hole. If the colon is abnormal or full of stool, or if the hole is large and ragged, surgery is necessary.

ii. Presentation after the examination

This depends on the time from the examination to the onset of symptoms, and is usually with abdominal pain. Sometimes there are signs of sepsis, such as fever, leukocytosis, and peritonitis. The presence of generalized peritonitis means that urgent laparotomy is necessary. Localized peritonitis or pain and tenderness are an indication for a computed tomography (CT) scan, whereas extraintestinal gas means there has been perforation or thinning of the colonic wall. It does not necessarily indicate surgery and in a patient without peritonitis, bowel rest and intravenous antibiotics are often effective. Perforations diagnosed early are less clinically harmful, as fecal contamination is minimal, and, at surgery, simple closure is a realistic option. Colonic perforations presenting and diagnosed late are rarely amenable to closure and usually require resection and colostomy. A decision for surgery can also be made on the basis of the presumed cause of the perforation. Postpolypectomy perforations can often resolve with conservative management because they are small and may be sealed off by adjacent structures. Traumatic perforations tend to be larger and are unlikely to heal spontaneously.

iii. Laparoscopy

Laparoscopic technique has been applied to the management of colonoscopic complications with good success and offers the advantages of less pain and shorter hospital stay.[36,37] **Figs. 1** and **2** are algorithms that illustrate approaches to colonoscopic perforations.

Extraperitoneal Perforations

Sometimes the colonic perforation is on the mesenteric side of the colon or in a part of the bowel circumference that is extraperitoneal. The escaping air passes into the mesentery or retroperitoneum, and may reach the mediastinum[38] or even the neck.[39] Pneumothorax has been reported.[40] Extraperitoneal perforations can usually be treated with intravenous antibiotics and observation.

Postpolypectomy Syndrome

When there has been a perforation that is sealed, patients sometimes present with localized pain, tenderness, and fever but without peritonitis. This occurred in 1% of polypectomies reported by Waye and colleagues,[41] with all cases resolving on antibiotic therapy. Hospitalization and treatment with intravenous antibiotics and bowel rest is usually successful in resolving such symptoms within a few days.

BLEEDING

Significant bleeding during or after diagnostic colonoscopy is very rare and usually follows biopsy.[4,42] Kavic and Basson[43] reviewed 5 studies of colonoscopic complications and found 26 cases of 101,397 diagnostic colonoscopies, most following biopsy. By contrast, there were 284 postpolypectomy hemorrhages of 14, 951 cases. Sometimes a lesion, such as a hemangioma, an arteriovenous malformation, or a

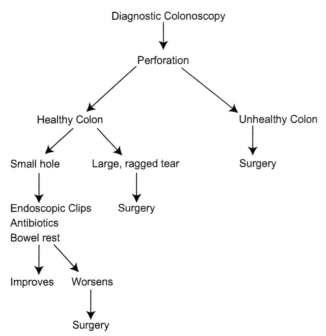

Fig. 1. Algorithm for the management of a colonic perforation caused by a diagnostic colonoscopy.

prominent mucosal vein is biopsied and bleeds, but cold biopsy forceps will rarely reach deep enough into the submucosa to damage the submucosal arteries. Care in choosing which places to biopsy is the key to avoiding this complication. An arteriovenous malformation does not need to be biopsied.

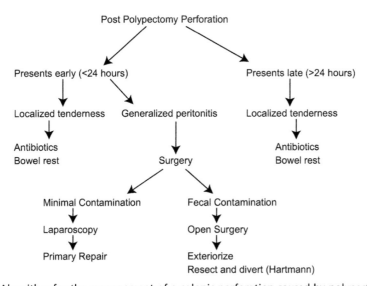

Fig. 2. Algorithm for the management of a colonic perforation caused by polypectomy.

Postpolypectomy Bleeding

Significant hemorrhage after polypectomy frightens the patient and usually leads to hospitalization. The overall incidence ranges from 0.3% to 6.1%, with individual rates varying according to the setting and definition of bleeding.[44–47] Postpolypectomy bleeding (PPB) is classically described as immediate or delayed; however, immediate bleeding could be considered as part of the polypectomy. Delayed bleeding after polypectomy is more significant, as the patient is away from the hospital and must seek urgent attention. It occurs in 0.3% to 1.2% of patients.[48–50] Management of delayed PPB often involves repeat colonoscopy and blood transfusion. Sometimes interventional radiology is used to embolize bleeding vessels, and occasionally colectomy is necessary.[51,52] Deaths have been reported, although this is very rare. Not all polyps are at an equal risk of bleeding.

Risk Factors for PPB

Location

Buddingh and colleagues[53] found that right-sided polyps had an almost fivefold increased risk for delayed PPB compared with left colon polyps. Cecal polyps were especially high risk. This predilection of right-sided polyps to bleed after polypectomy may be because the bowel wall is thinner here and submucosal arteries are closer to the snare or zone of coagulation. Submucosal arteries may be denser in the right colon, although there are no data regarding this point.

Size and shape

The incidence of bleeding after removal of large polyps (>2 cm) was summarized by Waye and colleagues[42] at 5.4%. Sawhney and colleagues[54] found a 9% increase in the risk of delayed PPB for every additional millimeter of polyp size, whereas Watabe and colleagues[48] found that polyps larger than 10 mm were at a 4.5-fold greater risk of delayed PPB than smaller ones. The incidence of delayed PPB was 0.4% for polyps smaller than 10 mm, 1.6% for those 10 to 19 mm, 3.8% in those 20 to 29 mm, and 5.3% in those larger than 29 mm. Although some studies yield conflicting results, sessile polyps have also been reported to be at increased risk of delayed PPB compared with pedunculated polyps.

Patient factors

Patients on anticoagulants, including coumadin, aspirin, and platelet-inhibiting agents, or patients with a coagulopathy are at risk of bleeding. Colonoscopy with polypectomy in these patients is a "high-risk" procedure. American Society for Gastrointestinal Endoscopy (ASGE) Guidelines[55,56] state that in patients with a high risk of thromboembolism, warfarin must be stopped 3 to 5 days before the procedure, and consideration should be given to the use of heparin while the international normalized ratio (INR) is subtherapeutic. When risk of thromboembolism is low, warfarin is stopped as before but no heparin bridge is necessary. Colonoscopists should communicate with vascular medicine or internal medicine colleagues to determine the best course of action in each patient. ASGE Guidelines also state that there is no evidence to show that aspirin and other nonsteroidal anti-inflammatory drugs (NSAIDs) increase the risk of PPB. However, when there is a large right-sided polyp, or a pedunculated polyp with a thick stalk, stopping such medications 5 days before until 5 days after polypectomy is a reasonable thing to do. Hypertension may be associated with postpolypectomy bleeding.[48]

Technique

Hot biopsy is just as likely if not more likely to cause bleeding as snaring, despite the smaller size of polyps treated in this way.[46,57] The zone of coagulation produced by hot biopsy cautery is directed downward into the submucosa, where it can damage the wall of submucosal arteries. This contrasts the cautery produced by a snare, which is directed inward, parallel to the mucosa, and will not damage submucosal arteries unless they are included in the pedicle. Risk factors for PPB are summarized in **Table 1**.

Preventing PPB

Choosing your battles

The decision about which polyp to remove and which to refer to surgery is an individual one, based on the experience and confidence of the endoscopist. Alternatives include referring a difficult polyp to a different endoscopist or referring the patient to a surgeon. When there are multiple large polyps in different locations throughout the colon, a reasonable strategy is to remove polyps in only one well-defined location, leaving the others for another time. In this way, the site of any postpolypectomy hemorrhage is easy to determine.

Stop anticoagulants

Coumadin needs to be stopped at least 5 days before polypectomy. Patients on coumadin should have a normalized INR before the procedure. The patient's cardiologist, primary physician, or vascular specialists can help determine the risks of stopping anticoagulation, and whether a heparin or low molecular weight heparin bridge is necessary. The decision on whether to stop aspirin and antiplatelet medications depends on the balance of the risk of bleeding from the lesion to be removed, and the risk of thrombotic events should the drugs be stopped.[56]

Good technique

It is wise to use pure coagulation current, interrupting the current to give the heat a chance to dissipate between applications, and closing the snare slowly. The larger the amount of tissue enclosed in the snare, the greater the chance of picking up submucosal arteries, and so piecemeal polypectomy should take pieces no bigger than 2 cm in one bite.

Use of detachable snares on pedunculated polyps with a large stalk, and/or use of clips can be effective in preventing immediate and delayed hemorrhage.[58]

Submucosal lift

Lifting a polyp on a bed of saline or other fluid increases the distance from the base of the polyp to the submucosal arteries. This is effective in minimizing the risk of bleeding and should be almost routine in large (>2 cm) cecal and ascending colon polyps. Use of epinephrine makes immediate bleeding less likely but may not prevent a secondary hemorrhage.[59,60]

Table.1 Risk factors for and prevention of post polypectomy bleeding	Polyp	Patient
Risk Factors	Size (>2cm) Shape (sessile) Location (Right colon [cecum])	Hypertensive Anticoagulant therapy
Prevention	<2cm pieces of polyp Pre-inject with saline or adrenaline Use detachable snares or clips on stalk Coagulate edges of wound with APC	

Treating PPB

Consent

Part of the consenting process is to inform patients of the possibility of postpolypec-tomy hemorrhage. This involves making sure that the patient is not planning any trip that would make urgent care inaccessible for the following 2 weeks. Patients living more than 2 hours away from the treating institution should be given a copy of the colonoscopy report with clear descriptions of the site and method of the polypectomy. If necessary, the polypectomy should be deferred.

Immediate bleeding

The options for treating immediate bleeding include injection with 1:10,000 epineph-rine, use of endoscopic clips, or thermal therapy. If the polyp is pedunculated, the stalk can be resnared and held for 10 minutes, or a detachable snare or clip placed.[61]

Delayed bleeding

Delayed postpolypectomy hemorrhage can occur from 1 to 15 days after polypec-tomy. Regardless of the precautions taken against it, postpolypectomy hemorrhage can occur in any patient, although it is more common after removal of large right-sided or rectal polyps. Passage of large amounts of blood after colonoscopic polypec-tomy must be taken seriously. The patient is admitted to the hospital, stabilized, and a coagulation profile is checked and optimized. If the bleeding continues, patients should be given a bowel preparation and recolonoscoped. If the patient is unstable, interventional radiology may embolize the bleeding vessel.[62] Very rarely, surgery is necessary. Sometimes the bleeding has stopped by the time the repeat colonoscopy is done. Nevertheless, in the presence of active bleeding or high-risk stigmata, the site can be clipped; injected with 1:10,000 epinephrine; or treated by heater probe, bipolar electrocautery, or argon plasma coagulator.[61] Once a secondary bleed has stopped, a further bleeding episode is unusual. An algorithm for the management of PPB is given in **Fig. 3**.

Extraluminal bleeding Sometimes patients undergoing colonoscopy can suffer serosal or mesenteric tears that may bleed. These occur when colonic loops pull on adhesions and avulse them. Most cases are not detected, but tears can be seen occasionally in patients who undergo laparotomy immediately after a colonoscopy.

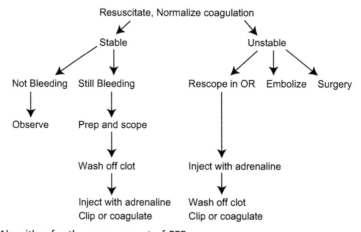

Fig. 3. Algorithm for the management of PPB.

Splenic trauma Splenic injury during colonoscopy is very rare, but is important to think about in patients whose post colonoscopy course is not smooth. It been described in several case reports and small series.[63,64] Singla and colleagues[63] reviewed 75 reports, including 102 patients; 76.5% were women. Two-thirds of the colonoscopies were apparently performed "without difficulty," which suggests that the definition of "difficulty" may be subjective and variable. Most patients presented within 24 hours of the examination and although the commonest symptom was left upper quadrant pain, presentation can be more obscure. A CT scan with intravenous contrast is the most effective diagnostic test. Surgery was performed in 73 patients, and almost all underwent splenectomy. Five patients died.

The spleen is a fragile organ, and small adhesions to adjacent organs are prone to tear a segment of the capsule. The spleen is also intimately attached to the splenic flexure of the colon, which can be the site of complex looping. Possible causes of splenic injury include traction on the spleno-colic ligament, direct trauma by a loop of colon, and excess fragility of the spleen because of splenomegaly. Splenic rupture at colonoscopy usually presents with abdominal pain developing within 24 hours of the procedure. Anemia is not always present but there is usually an increased white blood cell count. CT scan makes the diagnosis and treatment depends on the degree of blood loss and the hemodynamic stability of the patient.[64] Massive hemorrhage demands urgent surgery but a less severe bleed allows the possibility of splenic preservation or semielective splenectomy.[65] Stein and colleagues[66] describe treatment of a splenic injury with embolization.

The best way to prevent splenic trauma is to use gentle technique, minimize loops (especially in the sigmoid), and avoid the "slide-by" technique at the splenic flexure. The possibility of splenic damage is important to consider in patients complaining of significant and unrelieved postcolonoscopy abdominal pain.

Complications in other organs

There have been a few case reports describing unusual cases of rare and unusual complications, including cases of postcolonoscopy priapism,[67] small bowel obstruction,[68,69] mesenteric ischemia,[70] cecal volvulus,[71,72] acute pancreatitis,[73] appendicitis,[74,75] cholecystitis,[76] and small bowel perforation.[77] Given the millions of colonoscopies done yearly, these extremely rare cases represent the bottom of the differential list in patients with postcolonoscopy pain.

Cardiopulmonary complications

Vasovagal reaction A vasovagal reaction is a slowing of the heart rate, often accompanied by a drop in blood pressure that is reflective of abnormal vagal stimulation. It is usually associated with painful intubation of a sigmoid colon with a tight mesentery, and anxiety may predispose to it.[78,79] The bradycardia and hypotension may also be associated with sweating, pallor, and a feeling of impending fainting. Treatment of a vasovagal reaction is to stop insertion, although intravenous fluids and atropine can be given.

Isolated hypotension without bradycardia can occur during colonoscopy but is more likely to be due to dehydration, potentiated by the combination of benzodiazepines and narcotics. Hypotension caused by oversedation or dehydration can be treated with intravenous fluids and narcotic antagonists.

Hypoxia and cardiac events Cardiac events, such as arrhythmias, ST segment depression or elevation, ventricular tachycardia, and ventricular fibrillation, can happen during colonoscopy but are uncommon.[80–82] More serious problems like infarction and arrest are very rare.[83] Hypoxia, defined as an oxygen saturation below

90%, is more common and is related to the amount of sedation and analgesics given to the patient.[84] Hypoxia happens even in unsedated patients[84,85] but tends to be transitory and responds to increased breathing efforts. Holm and colleagues[86] reported that 2 of 8 patients with hypoxia had electrocardiogram evidence of myocardial ischemia and one had runs of extrasystoles, reinforcing the need for cardiac and oxygenation monitoring and close patient observation during colonoscopy. Patients within 3 weeks of a myocardial infarction usually tolerate endoscopy well, although patients with unstable angina are at particularly high risk.[87]

Patients with severe chronic obstructive pulmonary disease are at risk of hypercapnia, and may have a respiratory arrest if pain and distress levels rise. Such patients should receive sedation cautiously, and increasing distress is an indication to stop the examination.

Infectious complications of colonoscopy

Colonoscopy has been associated with bacteremia in 2% to 4% of patients.[88] The rate of infectious complications is considerably lower than this. There have been isolated cases of peritonitis in patients with cirrhosis,[89,90] but Llach and colleagues[91] have shown that colonoscopy does not induce significant bacteremia in patients with cirrhosis with or without ascites. There are only a handful of cases of endocarditis following colonoscopy[92] and prophylaxis for high-risk cardiac conditions is recommended at the endoscopist's discretion on a "case-by-case" basis.[93]

The risk of introduction of an infectious agent into a patient through a contaminated colonoscope or endoscopic instrument has been estimated as 1 in 1.8 million. Transmission of *Salmonella* species by colonoscope has been reported,[94,95] whereas *Klebsiella*, *Enterobacter*, and *Serratia* infections, and hepatitis B and hepatitis C have been described.[95] Rigorous infection control measurements are essential to maintaining a minimal infection rate.[96]

Preventing infectious complications

Cleaning, disinfecting and sterilizing Standards for the cleaning of endoscopes are widely published, involving the types of solutions, routines, and methods to be used.[96,97]

Antibiotic prophylaxis The ASGE published guidelines for antibiotic prophylaxis in endoscopy in 2008,[98] and the American Heart Association reviewed its guidelines for prophylaxis of endocarditis in 2007.[93] These guidelines state that antibiotic prophylaxis against infective endocarditis (prosthetic heart valves, prior endocarditis, surgically constructed systemic-pulmonary shunts or conduits) is not supported by evidence and is not indicated. Furthermore, ASGE found no evidence to support the use of prophylaxis before colonoscopy in an individual with a recent (within 1 year) synthetic vascular graft or an orthopedic prosthesis.

Protection of the endoscopist and endoscopy assistants Measures to avoid contact with potentially contaminated body fluids (such as gowns, gloves, goggles, and masks) and the use of plastic/nonrecapped needles is now standard in endoscopy units, and should minimize the risks of staff acquiring an infection. All patients should be treated as potential carriers of a bloodborne pathogen, and all endoscopy units need to comply with Centers for Disease Control and Prevention guidelines for precautions.

Other complications

Incarceration of the colonoscope Occasionally the colonoscope will get stuck in the colon. This has been described in 2 settings: a hernia and a tight, tortuous sigmoid colon. Koltun and Coller[99] and Leisser and colleagues[100] describe the former situation in patients with an inguinal hernia. Although the scope could not be removed by simply pulling from the anus, in Koltun and Coller's report,[99] the hernia sac was large enough to accommodate a loop of the scope, which was maintained by the examiner's fingers while the scope was removed. Incarceration in a tight sigmoid colon is more difficult to remove; time, an antispasmodic, and warm water irrigation may help resolution.

Impaction of snare in polyp If a snare enters a polyp deeply with coagulation current and the endoscopist abandons the resection, the snare may be stuck and not retrievable. The easiest way out of this situation is to cut the handle off the snare, remove the colonoscope over the snare, pass the colonoscope again and resect the polyp head piecemeal until the original snare can be retrieved. Alternatively, the patient can be admitted to hospital until the original snare falls out when the enclosed polyp sloughs off.

Inaccurate localization of significant colonic pathology This can have a disastrous effect on surgery if the wrong segment of colon is removed. When resection of a colonic lesion is to be done laparoscopically, 3-quadrant or 4-quadrant tattooing may be necessary to prevent removal of the wrong section of bowel. Even with an open resection, on-table colonoscopy may sometimes be needed to make sure the correct section of colon is removed with adequate margins.

DEATH

The worst complication of any procedure is the unexpected, unanticipated death of the patient. Risk management is important in minimizing mortality, considering whether the colonoscopy should be done at all, and whether to persist with a difficult examination in an elderly, frail patient. Selection of patients for colonoscopy should reflect such decision making. Elective examinations are contraindicated in critically ill patients, or patients with a limited life expectancy. However, even under the best circumstances, patients sometimes die from the complications of colonoscopy. In 1983, Macrae and colleagues[50] reported a mortality rate of 0.06% in a series of 5000 consecutive examinations. Most deaths occur after serious complications (perforation, hemorrhage) in patients with serious comorbidity.[101] Waye and colleagues[42] summarized 12 reports describing 165 perforations of 99,539 diagnostic colonoscopies and 76 perforations of 18,659 therapeutic colonoscopies. The overall mortality was 5 (0.006%) of 83,725. As shown in this article, death can occur from any serious complication of colonoscopy, from the electrolyte imbalance caused by sodium phosphate preparation to the cardiac events brought on by hypoxia from over-sedation, to the sepsis that may follow perforation and the blood loss that can occur with hemorrhage. Prevention and correct management of these complications will minimize mortality.

SUMMARY

Colonoscopy is a complex process that offers several opportunities for misadventures and complications. The continuing increase in demand for colonoscopy as a way of screening for colorectal cancer, diagnosing colorectal disease, and treating colorectal mucosal lesions means that complications are certain to occur with increasing frequency. An awareness of common complications, a routine to minimize or prevent them, and a familiarity with the treatment options and how to apply them is an essential part of every colonoscopist's practice.

REFERENCES

1. Mai CM, Wen CC, Wen SH, et al. Iatrogenic colonic perforation by colonoscopy: a fatal complication for patients with a high anesthetic risk. Int J Colorectal Dis 2010;25:449–54.
2. Geenen JE, Schmitt MG, Wu WC, et al. Major complications of colonoscopy: bleeding and perforation. Dig Dis 1975;20:231–52.
3. Fruhmorgan P, Demling L. Complications of diagnostic and therapeutic colonoscopy in the Federal Republic of Germany; results of an inquiry. Endoscopy 1979;2:146–50.
4. Wexner SD, Garbus JE, Singh JJ, SAGES Colonoscopy Study Outcomes Group. A prospective analysis of 13,580 colonoscopies. Reevaluation of credentialing guidelines. Surg Endosc 2001;15:251–61.
5. Griffin JM, Hulbert EM, Vernon SW, et al. Improving endoscopy completion: effectiveness of an interactive voice response system. Am J Manag Care 2011;17(3):199–208.
6. Lee CS, McCormick PA. Telephone reminders to reduce non-attendance rate for endoscopy. J R Soc Med 2003;96(11):547–8.
7. Abuksis G, Mor M, Segal N, et al. A patient education program is cost-effective for preventing failure of endoscopic procedures in a gastroenterology department. Am J Gastroenterol 2001;96(6):1786–90.
8. Markowitz GS, Nasr SH, Klein P, et al. Renal failure due to acute nephrocalcinosis following oral sodium phosphate bowel cleansing. Hum Pathol 2004;35(6):675–84.
9. Gabel A, Muller S. Aspiration: a possible severe complication in colonoscopy preparation of elderly people by orthograde intestine lavage. Digestion 1999;60:284–5.
10. Poon CM, Lee DW, Mak SK, et al. Two liters of polyethylene glycol-electrolyte lavage solution versus sodium phosphate as bowel cleansing regimen for colonoscopy: a prospective randomized controlled trial. Endoscopy 2002;34:560–3.
11. Toledo TK, DiPalma JA. Review article: colon cleansing preparation for gastrointestinal procedures. Aliment Pharmacol Ther 2001;15:605–11.
12. Hookey LC, Depew WT, Vanner S. The safety profile of oral sodium phosphate for colonic cleansing before colonoscopy in adults. Gastrointest Endosc 2002;56:895–902.
13. Cohen SM, Wexner SD, Binderow SR, et al. Prospective randomized, endoscopic blinded trial comparing precolonoscopy cleansing methods. Dis Colon Rectum 1994;37:689–96.
14. Church JM. Pre-colonoscopy bowel preparation intolerance: a sign of upper gastrointestinal pathology. Aust N Z J Surg 1991;61:796–7.
15. Hillyer GC, Basch CH, Basch CE, et al. Gastroenterologists' perceived barriers to optimal pre-colonoscopy bowel preparation: results of a national survey. J Cancer Educ 2012;27(3):526–32.
16. Wang D, Chen C, Chen J, et al. The use of propofol as a sedative agent in gastrointestinal endoscopy: a meta-analysis. PLoS One 2013;8(1):e53311. http://dx.doi.org/10.1371/journal.pone.0053311.
17. Hull T, Church JM. Colonoscopy—how difficult, how painful? Surg Endosc 1994;8(7):784–7.
18. Garrett KA, Church J. History of hysterectomy: a significant problem for colonoscopists that is not present in patients who have had sigmoid colectomy. Dis Colon Rectum 2010;53(7):1055–60.

19. Church J. The unzygosed colon as a factor predisposing to difficult colonoscopy in slim women. Gastrointest Endosc 2002;55(7):965–6.
20. Church JM. Warm water irrigation for dealing with spasm during colonoscopy: simple, inexpensive, and effective. Gastrointest Endosc 2002;56(5):672–4.
21. Cohen LB, Ladas SD, Vargo JJ, et al. Sedation in digestive endoscopy: the Athens international position statements. Aliment Pharmacol Ther 2010;32(3):425–42.
22. Byrne MF, Chiba N, Singh H, et al, Clinical Affairs Committee of the Canadian Association of Gastroenterology. Propofol use for sedation during endoscopy in adults: a Canadian Association of Gastroenterology position statement. Can J Gastroenterol 2008;22(5):457–9.
23. Lohsiriwat V. Colonoscopic perforation: incidence, risk factors, management and outcome. World J Gastroenterol 2010;16(4):425–30.
24. Lüning TH, Keemers-Gels ME, Barendregt WB, et al. Colonoscopic perforations: a review of 30,366 patients. Surg Endosc 2007;21(6):994–7.
25. Luchette FA, Doerr RJ, Kelly K, et al. Colonoscopic impaction in left colon strictures resulting in right colon pneumatic perforation. Surg Endosc 1992;6:273–6.
26. Foliente RL, Chang AC, Youssef AI, et al. Endoscopic cecal perforation: mechanisms of injury. Am J Gastroenterol 1996;91:705–8.
27. Church J. Endoscopy of the colon and rectum. New York: Igaku Shoin/Williams and Wilkins Publishers; 1995.
28. Sumanac K, Zealley I, Fox BM, et al. Minimizing postcolonoscopy abdominal pain by using CO(2) insufflation: a prospective, randomized, double blind, controlled trial evaluating a new commercially available CO_2 delivery system. Gastrointest Endosc 2002;56:190–4.
29. Kjaergard H, Nordkild P, Geerdsen J, et al. Anaesthesia for colonoscopy. An examination of the anesthesia as an element of risk at colonoscopy. Acta Anaesthesiol Scand 1986;30:60–3.
30. Cappell MS, Ghandi D, Huh C. A study of the safety and clinical efficacy of flexible sigmoidoscopy and colonoscopy after recent colonic surgery in 52 patients. Am J Gastroenterol 1995;90:1130–4.
31. Huang C, Huang RX, Xiang P, et al. Current research status of endoscopic submucosal dissection for colorectal neoplasms. Clin Invest Med 2012;35(4):E158–64.
32. Yoshida N, Yagi N, Naito Y, et al. Safe procedure in endoscopic submucosal dissection for colorectal tumors focused on preventing complications. World J Gastroenterol 2010;16(14):1688–95.
33. Orsoni P, Berdah S, Verrier C, et al. Colonic perforation due to colonoscopy: a retrospective study of 48 cases. Endoscopy 1997;29(3):160–4.
34. Swan MP, Bourke MJ, Moss A, et al. The target sign: an endoscopic marker for the resection of the muscularis propria and potential perforation during colonic endoscopic mucosal resection. Gastrointest Endosc 2011;73(1):79–85.
35. Magdeburg R, Collet P, Post S, et al. Endoclipping of iatrogentic colonic perforation to avoid surgery. Surg Endosc 2008;22:1500–4.
36. Bleier JI, Moon V, Feingold D, et al. Initial repair of iatrogenic colon perforation using laparoscopic methods. Surg Endosc 2008;22:646–9.
37. Rumstadt B, Schilling D, Sturm J. The role of laparoscopy in the treatment of complications after colonoscopy. Surg Laparosc Endosc Percutan Tech 2008;18:561–4.
38. Schwab GC, Wetcher P, Waldenburg E, et al. Retropneumoperitoneum: an unusual case after colonoscopy. Endoscopy 1993;25:256–7.

39. McCollister DL, Hammerman HJ. Air, air, everywhere: pneumatosis cystoides coli after colonoscopy. Gastrointest Endosc 1990;36:75–6.

40. Webb T. Pneumothorax and pneumomediatinum during colonoscopy. Anaesth Intensive Care 1998;26:302–4.

41. Waye JD, Lewis BS, Yessayan S. Colonoscopy: a prospective report of complications. J Clin Gastroenterol 1992;15:347–51.

42. Waye JD, Kahn O, Auerbach ME. Complications of colonoscopy and flexible sigmoidoscopy. Gastrointest Endosc Clin N Am 1996;6:343–77.

43. Kavic SM, Basson MD. Complications of endoscopy. Am J Surg 2001;181: 319–32.

44. Rosen L, Bub DS, Reed JF 3rd, et al. Hemorrhage following colonoscopic polypectomy. Dis Colon Rectum 1993;36:1126–31.

45. Dominitz JA, Eisen GM, Baron TH, et al. Complications of colonoscopy. Gastrointest Endosc 2003;57:441–5.

46. Sorbi D, Norton I, Conio M, et al. Postpolypectomy lower GI bleeding: descriptive analysis. Gastrointest Endosc 2000;51:690–6.

47. Rabeneck L, Paszat LF, Hilsden RJ, et al. Bleeding and perforation after outpatient colonoscopy and their risk factors in usual clinical practice. Gastroenterology 2008;135:1899–906.

48. Watabe H, Yamaji Y, Okamoto M, et al. Risk assessment for delayed hemorrhagic complication of colonic polypectomy: polyp-related factors and patient-related factors. Gastrointest Endosc 2006;64:73–8.

49. Hui AJ, Wong RM, Ching JY, et al. Risk of colonoscopic polypectomy bleeding with anticoagulants and antiplatelet agents: analysis of 1657 cases. Gastrointest Endosc 2004;59:44–8.

50. Macrae FA, Tan KG, Williams CB. Towards safer colonoscopy: a report on the complications of 5000 diagnostic or therapeutic colonoscopies. Gut 1983; 24(5):376–83.

51. Kapetanos D, Beltsis A, Chatzimavroudis G, et al. Postpolypectomy bleeding: incidence, risk factors, prevention, and management. Surg Laparosc Endosc Percutan Tech 2012;22:102–7.

52. Barnert J, Messmann H. Diagnosis and management of lower gastrointestinal bleeding. Nat Rev Gastroenterol Hepatol 2009;6:637–46.

53. Buddingh KT, Herngreen T, Haringsma J, et al. Location in the right hemi-colon is an independent risk factor for delayed post-polypectomy hemorrhage: a multi-center case-control study. Am J Gastroenterol 2011;106(6):1119–24.

54. Sawhney MS, Salfiti N, Nelson DB, et al. Risk factors for severe delayed postpolypectomy bleeding. Endoscopy 2008;40(2):115–9.

55. Zuckerman MJ, Hirota WK, Adler DG, et al. ASGE guideline: the management of low-molecular-weight heparin and nonaspirin antiplatelet agents for endoscopic procedures. Gastrointest Endosc 2005;61:189–94.

56. Anderson MA, Ben-Menachem T, Gan SI, et al. Management of antithrombotic agents for endoscopic procedures. Gastrointest Endosc 2009;70:1060–70.

57. Weston AP, Campbell DR. Diminutive colon polyps: histopathology, spatial distribution, concomitant significant lesions, and treatment complications. Am J Gastroenterol 1995;90:24–8.

58. Kouklakis G, Mpoumponaris A, Gatopoulou A, et al. Endoscopic resection of large pedunculated colonic polyps and risk of postpolypectomy bleeding with adrenaline injection versus endoloop and hemoclip: a prospective, randomized study. Surg Endosc 2009;23(12):2732–7.

59. Dobrowolski S, Dobosz M, Babicki A, et al. Prophylactic submucosal saline-adrenaline injection in colonoscopic polypectomy: prospective randomized study. Surg Endosc 2004;18(6):990–3.
60. Lee SH, Chung IK, Kim SJ, et al. Comparison of postpolypectomy bleeding between epinephrine and saline submucosal injection for large colon polyps by conventional polypectomy: a prospective randomized, multicenter study. World J Gastroenterol 2007;13(21):2973–7.
61. Hong SP. How do I manage post-polypectomy bleeding? Clin Endosc 2012; 45(3):282–4.
62. Rossetti A, Buchs NC, Breguet R, et al. Transarterial embolization in acute colonic bleeding: review of 11 years of experience and long-term results. Int J Colorectal Dis 2012;28:777–82.
63. Singla S, Keller D, Thirunavukarasu P, et al. Splenic injury during colonoscopy— a complication that warrants urgent attention. J Gastrointest Surg 2012;16(6): 1225–34.
64. Ahmed A, Eller PM, Schiffman FJ. Splenic rupture: an unusual complication of colonoscopy. Am J Gastroenterol 1997;92:2101–4.
65. Michetti CP, Smeltzer E, Fakhry SM. Splenic injury due to colonoscopy: analysis of the world literature, a new case report, and recommendations for management. Am Surg 2010;76(11):1198–204.
66. Stein DF, Myaing M, Guillaume C. Splenic rupture after colonoscopy treated by splenic artery embolization. Gastrointest Endosc 2002;55:946–89.
67. Bilotta JJ, Goldenberg A, Waye JD. Colonoscopic priapism. Gastrointest Endosc 1989;35:475–6.
68. Wallner M, Allinger S, Wiesinger H, et al. Small-bowel ileus after diagnostic colonoscopy. Endoscopy 1994;26(3):329.
69. Malki SA, Bassett ML, Pavli P. Small bowel obstruction caused by colonoscopy. Gastrointest Endosc 2001;53:120–1.
70. McGovern RP, Franco RA. Acute mesenteric ischemia after colonoscopy. Am J Gastroenterol 1995;90(1):170.
71. Anderson JR, Spence RA, Wilson BG, et al. Gangrenous caecal volvulus after colonoscopy. Br Med J (Clin Res Ed) 1983;286(6363):439–40.
72. Amidon PB, Story RK Jr. Cecal volvulus after colonoscopy. Gastrointest Endosc 1993;39(1):105.
73. Thomas AW, Mitre RJ. Acute pancreatitis as a complication of colonoscopy. J Clin Gastroenterol 1994;19(2):177–8.
74. Vender R, Larson J, Garcia J, et al. Appendicitis as a complication of colonoscopy. Gastrointest Endosc 1995;41:514–6.
75. Houghton A, Aston N. Appendicitis complicating colonoscopy. Gastrointest Endosc 1988;34:489.
76. Milman PJ, Goldenberg SP. Colonoscopy cholecystitis. Am J Gastroenterol 2001;96:1666.
77. Nemeh HW, Ranzinger MR, Dutro JA. Mid-ileal perforation secondary to colonoscopy. Am Surg 1999;35:228–9.
78. Herman LL, Kurtz RC, McKee KJ, et al. Risk factors associated with vasovagal reactions during colonoscopy. Gastrointest Endosc 1993;39(3): 388–91.
79. Shore PS, Salt WB 2nd, Guthrie R. Vasodepressor reaction in an unsedated patient undergoing colonoscopy and observing the video display. Gastrointest Endosc 1993;39(2):218–9.

80. Gupta SC, Gopalswamy N, Sarkar A, et al. Cardiac arrhythmias and electrocardiographic changes during upper and lower gastrointestinal endoscopy. Mil Med 1990;155(1):9–11.

81. Alam M, Schuman BM, Duvernoy WF, et al. Continuous electrocardiographic monitoring during colonoscopy. Gastrointest Endosc 1976;22:203.

82. Davison ET, Levine M, Meyerowitz R. Ventricular fibrillation during colonoscopy: case report and review of the literature. Am J Gastroenterol 1985;80:690–3.

83. Eckardt VF, Kanzler G, Schmitt T, et al. Complications and adverse effects of colonoscopy with selective sedation. Gastrointest Endosc 1999;49:560–5.

84. Ristikankare M, Julkunen R, Mattila M, et al. Conscious sedation and cardiorespiratory safety during colonoscopy. Gastrointest Endosc 2000;52:48–54.

85. Yano H, Iishi H, Tatsuta M, et al. Oxygen desaturation during sedation for colonoscopy in elderly patients. Hepatogastroenterology 1998;45:2138–41.

86. Holm C, Christensen M, Schulze S, et al. Effect of oxygen on tachycardia and arterial oxygen saturation during colonoscopy. Eur J Surg 1999;165:755–8.

87. Cappell MS. Safety and clinical efficacy of flexible sigmoidoscopy and colonoscopy for gastrointestinal bleeding after myocardial infarction. A six-year study of 18 consecutive lower endoscopies at two university teaching hospitals. Dig Dis Sci 1994;39(3):473–80.

88. Low DE, Shoenut JP, Kennedy JK, et al. Prospective assessment of risk of bacteremia with colonoscopy and polypectomy. Dig Dis Sci 1987;32(11): 1239–43.

89. Shrake PD, Troiano F, Rex DK. Peritonitis following colonoscopy in a cirrhotic with ascites. Am J Gastroenterol 1989;84:453–4.

90. Ray SM, Piraino B, Holley J. Peritonitis following colonoscopy in a peritoneal dialysis patient. Perit Dial Int 1990;10:97–8.

91. Llach J, Elizalde JI, Bordas JM, et al. Prospective assessment of the risk of bacteremia in cirrhotic patients undergoing lower intestinal endoscopy. Gastrointest Endosc 1999;49:214–7.

92. Schembre DB. Infectious complications associated with gastrointestinal endoscopy. Gastrointest Endosc Clin N Am 2000;10:215–32.

93. Wilson W, Taubert KA, Gewitz M, et al. Prevention of infective endocarditis. Guidelines from the American Heart Association. A guideline from the American Heart Association Rheumatic Fever, Endocarditis, and Kawasaki Disease Committee, Council on Cardiovascular Disease in the Young, and the Council on Clinical Cardiology, Council on Cardiovascular Surgery and Anesthesia, and the Quality of Care and Outcomes Research Interdisciplinary Working Group. Circulation 2007;116:1736–54.

94. Dwyer DM, Klein EG, Istre GR, et al. *Salmonella newport* infections transmitted by fiberoptic colonoscopy. Gastrointest Endosc 1987;33:84–7.

95. Nelson DB, Barkun AN, Block KP, et al. Technology status evaluation report. Transmission of infection by gastrointestinal endoscopy. Gastrointest Endosc 2001;54(6):824–8.

96. ASGE Quality Assurance In Endoscopy Committee, Petersen BT, Chennat J, et al, Society for Healthcare Epidemiology of America. Multisociety guideline on reprocessing flexible gastrointestinal endoscopes: 2011. Gastrointest Endosc 2011;73(6):1075–84.

97. ASGE Standards Of Practice Committee, Banerjee S, Shen B, et al. Infection control during GI endoscopy. Gastrointest Endosc 2008;67(6):781–90.

98. ASGE Standards of Practice Committee, Banerjee S, Shen B, et al. Antibiotic prophylaxis for GI endoscopy. Gastrointest Endosc 2008;67(6):791–8.

99. Koltun WA, Coller JA. Incarceration of colonoscope in an inguinal hernia. "Pulley" technique of removal. Dis Colon Rectum 1991;3:191–3.

100. Leisser A, Delpre G, Kadish U. Colonoscope incarceration: an avoidable event. Gastrointest Endosc 1990;36(6):637–8.

101. deRoux SJ, Sgarlato A. Upper and lower gastrointestinal endoscopy mortality: the medical examiner's perspective. Forensic Sci Med Pathol 2012;8:4–12.

Training and Teaching Innovations in Colonoscopy

Victoria Gómez, MD, Michael B. Wallace, MD, MPH*

KEYWORDS

- Colonoscopy competency • Endoscopic training • Simulation-based training
- Magnetic endoscopic imaging • Retraining • Adenoma detection rate

KEY POINTS

- Competency in colonoscopy may not truly be achieved until more than 250 colonoscopies are performed by trainees.
- Because of observed disparities in quality and competence in colonoscopy across different specialties, more uniform training programs and training standards are needed.
- Computer-based simulators and magnetic endoscopic imaging tools accelerate the early phase of training and may be most useful in the early stages training.
- Improving the adenoma detection rate of trained endoscopists and maintaining this improved quality metric may be best achieved with dedicated educational interventions and training programs.

INTRODUCTION

Colonoscopy continues to be the dominant method used for colorectal cancer prevention, and optimizing training and teaching methods is critical to ensure consistent high-quality procedures in practice. Gastroenterologic and surgical societies now acknowledge the need for all trainees to master a series of motor and cognitive skills before graduating from their respective programs. High-quality supervision is important for high-quality training[1]; however, there is now evidence that the use of technology in the form of simulators and position sensors, and retraining experienced endoscopists, could further improve competency and quality in colonoscopy, a practice once seen as requiring apprenticeship-directed training. This article reviews the key studies and themes in training and teaching innovations in colonoscopy.

Disclosures/Conflicts of Interest/Funding: Dr Gómez has nothing to disclose; Dr Wallace receives research funding from Olympus Corp.
Department of Gastroenterology, Mayo Clinic, 4500 San Pablo Road South, Jacksonville, FL 32224, USA
* Corresponding author.
E-mail address: wallace.michael@mayo.edu

LEARNING CURVE OF COLONOSCOPY

The American Society for Gastrointestinal Endoscopy Training Committee most recently published a position statement on the colonoscopy core curriculum, identifying key features in motor and cognitive skills to enable endoscopists to perform colonoscopies safely and competently.[2] The core technical and cognitive skills are shown in **Box 1**.[2] These core skills can be classified within the competency outline described by the Accreditation Council for Graduate Medical Education (ACGME).

Although there is no reliable number of colonoscopies needed to complete before ensuring competency, recent studies have shown that there is a learning curve for

---

Box 1
List of the core motor and cognitive skills required to be competent in colonoscopy

Motor skills[2]

Correctly holding the colonoscope

Use of the colonoscope controls

Colonoscope insertion

Colonoscope advancement

    Tip control

    Torque

Lumen identification

Withdrawal and mucosal inspection

Loop reduction

Angulated turns

Terminal ileum intubation

Biopsy

Snare polypectomy

Cognitive skills

Anatomy

Patient selection

Preparation

Colonoscope selection

Informed consent

Sedation management

Assessment of indication and risks

Pathology identification

Therapeutic device settings

Integration of findings into management plans

Report generation and communication

Complication management

Quality improvement

Professionalism

this procedure. One of the most heavily reviewed studies is by Sedlack,[3] in which 41 gastroenterology fellows at a single center performed 6635 colonoscopies from July 2007 through June 2010. The fellows' core cognitive and motor colonoscopy skills were assessed using the Mayo Colonoscopy Skills Assessment Tool, a validation tool created to provide a valid means to objectively assess individual cognitive and motor skills throughout colonoscopy training.[4] The study concluded that a Mayo Colonoscopy Skills Assessment Tool score of 3.5, cecal intubation rates of 85%, and intubation times of less than 16 minutes were recommended as minimal competency criteria. On average, 275 procedures were needed to achieve even this conservatively defined competence in colonoscopy (**Fig. 1**). This critical number differs from the current recommendation that fellows perform a minimum of 140 colonoscopies before assessing competency. This difference is even greater when considering the threshold of 50 procedures recommended by the family practice and general surgery residency guidelines.[5,6] With such a wide range of learning curves, programs must ensure that adequate volumes of procedures be available to trainees in the outpatient and inpatient setting, and that ongoing competency assessment be performed throughout the stages of training.

IMPACT OF TYPE OF TRAINING ON QUALITY IN COLONOSCOPY

Assessment of training and competency in performing colonoscopy in general surgery has also received scrutiny. Surgical societies, the ACGME, and the Residency Review Committee require surgical residents to perform 50 colonoscopies before assessment of proficiency.[7] In a study by Spier and colleagues,[8] 21 surgical residents performed a mean of 80 ± 35 total colonoscopies during the 2-month outpatient endoscopy rotation. Average cecal intubation rate was 47%, and resident comfort level for independently performing a total colonoscopy was scored a mean 3.6 on a scale of 1 to 5 (5 = most comfortable). Thus, although surgical residents can fulfill the prescribed number of colonoscopy procedures (N = 50) during an allotted time, achieving technical competence in colonoscopy as defined by a 90% cecal intubation rate was not successful. Similarly, Selvasekar and colleagues[9] demonstrated that colorectal surgery fellows were found to achieve screening colonoscopy competency, defined by a significant reduction in total procedure and 80% cecal intubation rate within 35 minutes, after completing 94 to 114 procedures.

There is also evidence that having separate endoscopy training programs among gastroenterologists and surgeons leads to variable quality of colonoscopy performance. In a retrospective review by Leyden and colleagues,[10] all colonoscopy procedures performed in a single endoscopy unit by both gastroenterology trainees and surgical trainees with more than 2 years of endoscopy experience were audited. Among 3079 single-endoscopist colonoscopies, there was an observed disparity in endoscopic performance between surgical and gastroenterology trainees, with higher completion rates, polyp detection rates, adenoma detection rates (ADR), and greater withdrawal time correlating closely with polyp detection rate for gastroenterology trainees compared with surgery trainees.

One possible option to reduce such differences in colonoscopy competency could be to no longer mandate that all surgical trainees be trained in colonoscopy if their subspecialty interest does not involve application of endoscopy. Thus, only those whose career track requires routine use of endoscopy may need to take part in a more intense colonoscopy training program, which could be integrated into the gastroenterology trainee curriculum.

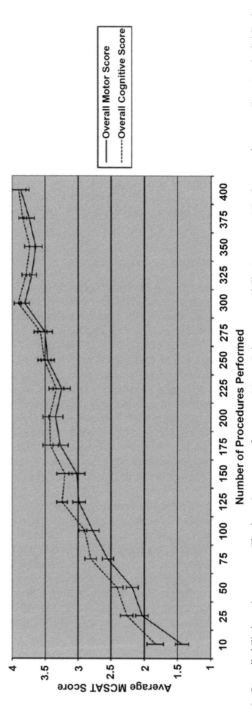

Fig. 1. Overall skills learning curves. The learning curve of average Mayo Colonoscopy Skills Assessment Tool scores for overall motor (*solid line*) and overall cognitive (*dashed line*) skills are shown. Average scores are labeled with error bars showing the 95% confidence interval. By 250 procedures, cognitive skills have achieved the 3.5 minimal competency criteria goals, with motor scores reaching this by 275 procedures. By 300 procedures, all scores and the 95% confidence interval are above this threshold. (*Adapted from* Sedlack RE. Training to competency in colonoscopy: assessing and defining competency standards. Gastrointest Endosc 2011;74(2):360; with permission.)

COLONOSCOPY SIMULATORS

Traditionally, colonoscopy is learned by hands-on training under the supervision of an experienced endoscopist. However, with increasing demands to perform more colonoscopies in a streamlined fashion with minimal interruptions and delays, significant cost considerations have been demonstrated from lost productivity at institutions where novices are being trained to perform colonoscopy.[11] In a study analyzing data from the Clinical Outcomes Research Initiative Project, involvement of fellows prolonged the procedure time by 10% to 37%, with an estimated loss of reimbursement to the academic institution of $500,000 to $1,000,000 per year.[12] Simulators have therefore been developed to potentially close the gap between increased procedure duration and financial burden.

COMPUTER SIMULATORS

Computer simulators, first developed in the 1980s, enhanced traditional endoscopy teaching. They have been the subject of much attention for possibly better preparing trainees to perform colonoscopies on real patients after completing a finite number of simulations.[13,14] Medical training has many similarities to aviation training, which catalyzed computer-based training simulators.[15] Simulators are safe, and ethical concerns are minimized when training with a mannequin. Second, simulators are multipurpose, allowing training in different environments and clinical scenarios. Third, simulators are cost-effective, providing a great deal of training for the monetary investment initially placed on the equipment.[15]

The typical electronic simulator contains a functioning colonoscope, real dials, and buttons that allow for steering and torquing of the instrument, with the exception that the hydraulic and pneumatic functions do not actually cause the scope to eject water or air. A mannequin with an anus is provided, in addition to a screen for visualization. Currently, the two commercially available simulators include the Simbionix GI Mentor (Simbionix USA Corporation, Cleveland, OH) and the CAE Healthcare AccuTouch Endoscopy Simulator (CAE Healthcare [formerly Immersion Medical], Gaithersburg, MD) (**Fig. 2**). The endoscope has a closed tip that contains forced feedback sensors, thus allowing the trainee to experience the "haptic" resistance as the endoscope is advanced through the mannequin.[16] Each case creates a different scenario with different indications for colonoscopy, vital signs, patient history, and evaluations pertaining to the chief complaint. During each simulation session, the software tracks a broad range of metrics and presents the user with a report at the end of each colonoscopy. Some of these metrics include information about looping, overinsufflation, and loss of mucosal visualization.[11] Data are collected automatically, and at the completion of the module, trainees can review their overall performance, and instructors can follow their progress longitudinally.

Several clinical trials have shown benefit with using a computer simulator early on in the fellowship training.[16–19] Sedlack and Kolars[20] developed a computer-based colonoscopy simulator course for first-year gastroenterology fellows using the Immersion Medical simulator (as of 2010, Immersion Medical is CAE Healthcare). The study demonstrated that the most benefit for trainees was during the early stages of training. One of the largest trials conducted by Cohen and colleagues,[16] a multicenter trial, randomized 45 first-year gastroenterology fellows from 16 hospitals over 2 years to 10 hours of simulation training during the first 8 weeks of fellowship. Following this, the first 200 colonoscopies performed by each fellow were graded by proctors to measure technical and cognitive success, and patient comfort level during the procedure. Results showed that the simulator-trained group demonstrated higher overall

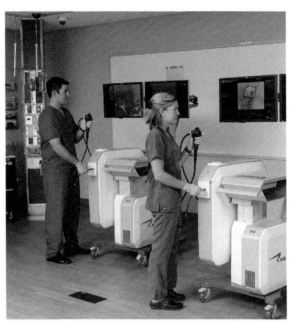

Fig. 2. CAE Healthcare (formerly Immersion Medical) Accu Touch endoscopy simulator. (*Courtesy of* CAE Healthcare. © 2012 CAE Healthcare; with permission.)

competency during the first 80 clinical cases; however, the median number of cases required to reach 90% objective competency was identical in the simulator and no-simulator groups (mean, 160). Most recently, in a multinational, randomized, blinded, controlled trial by Haycock and colleagues,[19] 36 novice colonoscopists were randomized to either 16 hours of simulator training or patient-based training and then completed three simulator cases before and after training; three live cases were assessed after training by masked experts. Results demonstrated that novices trained on the computer simulator demonstrated superior technical skills on simulated cases but no difference was observed between the groups in the live patient cases.

Several validation studies have also shown that computer colonoscopy simulators could distinguish between expert and novice endoscopists, but with varying types of measurable parameters. In the studies by Kim and colleagues[21] and Sedlack and Kolars,[22] computer-based simulators were able to discriminate levels of expertise only for parameters related to procedure time and not for actual endoscopic skills. McConnell and colleagues[23] demonstrated that the only significant differences between novice and expert endoscopists were seen in performance metrics related to procedural time, air insufflation, sedation management, endoscope force, and patient comfort. In contrast, the studies by Grantcharov and colleagues,[24] Mahmood and Darzi,[25] and Eversbusch and Grantcharov[26] demonstrated that significant differences in performance existed among endoscopists of varying levels of experience for procedure-related times and endoscopic skills. Furthermore, one validation study demonstrated that trainees failed to improve without feedback from a mentor.[27]

Although current simulators have demonstrated a benefit in skill acquisition for the first 20 to 80 cases performed by novices with an acceleration of the learning curve, no reduction in the median number of cases required to achieve technical and cognitive competency has been observed. It is in the expert opinion of the Preservation and

Incorporation of Valuable Endoscopic Innovations committee that to justify the expense and effort involved in purchasing simulators and incorporating them into the training program, a reduction in training times or procedure numbers of at least 25% is required.[28] Most recently, new ACGME training guidelines implemented in July 2012 require all gastroenterology fellows to participate in some type of simulation-based training during their fellowship.[29]

Computer-based simulators can accelerate the learning curve for trainees in colonoscopy and provide trainees with low-risk, low-stress hands-on time with endoscopic equipment before performing on real patients; however, the duration of these benefits has been shown to be limited to the very early stages of novice training.[30]

MAGNETIC ENDOSCOPIC IMAGING

Among the many challenges endoscopists face in colonoscopy, differences in the colonic anatomy can make these procedures technically challenging. Trainees and staff alike may find it difficult to learn and teach a maneuver, such as reducing. Because loop reduction is often recognized by "feel" instead of visual inspection, the trainer frequently must take over the procedure to effect progress. This can often lead to large periods of time during the procedure in which the trainee is "hands-off" and merely observing. Magnetic endoscopic imaging (MEI) is a novel technique, first developed in 1992, that avoids the use of radiation and instead provides endoscopists with positioning guidance, thus helping to overcome these issues in teaching colonoscopy.

With MEI, electromagnetic fields are detected by small coils within the colonoscope and larger ones alongside the patient. This produces a moving image of the colonoscopy configuration on a display monitor.[31] A commercially available magnetic endoscopic imager is available, the ScopeGuide (Olympus Corporation, Tokyo, Japan) (**Fig. 3**). The device consists of a unit with a receiver dish that is positioned alongside the patient and is connected to an MEI scope with built-in transmitter coils. A software program computes three-dimensional positioning and orientation of each receiver coil, and the data are displayed in real-time as a computer-delivered

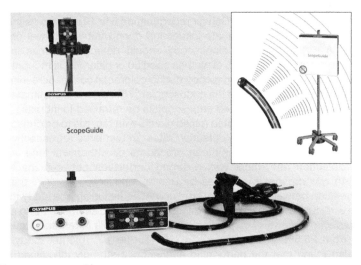

Fig. 3. Olympus scope guide.

three-dimensional image of the colonoscopy shaft configuration.[32,33] With this technology, information on looping, application of abdominal pressure, localization of the tip of the colonoscope, and instructional teaching in colonoscopy are feasible.[34]

Several studies have generated mixed results on the impact of MEI on colonoscopy performance. However, there is evidence that training with MEI has the greatest potential for benefit for trainees and inexperienced colonoscopists.[34–36] In a randomized controlled trial by Shah and colleagues,[34] a trainee endoscopist (200 previous cases) and two experienced endoscopists (>5000 previous cases) performed colonoscopies. With use of MEI, loops were straightened or controlled effectively, resulting in quick intubation times and high completion rates. The effect was greater in the trainee group when compared with the experienced group. In another pilot trial by Shah and colleagues,[35] a single novice colonoscopist, having only performed 15 prior colonoscopies, performed procedures under supervision on patients that were randomly assigned to have their procedures with or without MEI. Loop management was improved with use of MEI. After 50 cases, however, a plateau was reached, when 90% completion rates were achieved. After this number, no difference was seen comparing cases performed with and without MEI. Furthermore, in a single-center, randomized, controlled trial by Holme and colleagues,[36] inexperienced endoscopists had significantly higher cecal intubation rates using MEI compared with the standard group (no MEI use) and less need for assistance from a senior colleague. Therefore, it has been proposed that MEI may be the most beneficial in centers of endoscopy training.

MEI is a supplementary tool that can be used during colonoscopy to aid with loop reduction, application of abdominal pressure, tip localization, and localization of colonic lesions. The overall benefit of using MEI is most applicable to endoscopic trainees. Further studies are needed to address whether MEI can be reliably used in assessing competence in colonoscopy in novice and experienced endoscopists.[37]

RETRAINING EXPERIENCED ENDOSCOPISTS

The ultimate goal of a screening colonoscopy is to detect as many premalignant lesions in the safest and most efficient method possible. Quality in the field of colonoscopy has received much attention, and particularly the concept of ADR has provoked many studies evaluating the optimal method to increase ADR. Currently, the US Multi-Society Task Force on Colorectal Cancer recommends 6 to 10 minutes as the minimal amount of time needed for adequate inspection during the withdrawal phase, and furthermore, a well-performed colonoscopy should detect adenomas in at least 25% of average-risk men and 15% of women aged 50 or older.[38] It is thought that variation in clinical outcomes for colonoscopy during colorectal cancer screening is most directly related to the technique of the endoscopist.[39] Therefore, the ultimate question to be answered is: can experienced endoscopists be retrained to increase ADR?

Several studies have demonstrated mixed results with regards to colonoscopy withdrawal time and increased polyp detection rates. In two large retrospective studies that matched each endoscopist's mean procedure or withdrawal time with his or her polyp detection rate, there was a strong correlation between the two measures.[40,41] In two prospective studies by Barclay and colleagues[42,43] there was a strong correlation between withdrawal time and ADR, including one study that implemented an 8-minute withdrawal time (2 minutes per colonic segment) using an audible timer, paired with reviews of inspection techniques. In this latter study, overall ADR increased from 23.5% at baseline to 34.7% (P<.0001).[43] Another study by Chen and Rex also found that the performing endoscopist strongly influenced adenoma detection, independent of patient age or gender.[44] However, in a study by Sawhney and colleagues,[45] 42 experienced endoscopists at a single institution were asked to remain compliant with a 7-minute withdrawal time. Baseline compliance with the 7-minute withdrawal time was 65% and increased to almost 100% during the study. However, polyp detection rate did not increase for all polyps, diminutive, medium-sized, or large polyps. In another study by Lin and colleagues,[46] periodic monitoring and written, confidential feedback for experienced gastroenterologists were associated with increases in mean withdrawal times and polyp detection rates (from 33.1% to 38.1%; $P = .04$), but not patient satisfaction scores. More importantly, ADR showed a statistically nonsignificant trend toward an increase (from 19.6% to 22.7%; $P = .17$). Additional studies, outlined in a systematic review by Corley and colleagues,[47] revealed that although withdrawal times could be increased, ADR did not necessarily improve.

In two studies by Imperiali and colleagues[48] and Shaukat and colleagues,[49] multiple interventions were implemented to determine the impact on ADR. In the former study, performance data were discussed with eight gastroenterologists with varying endoscopic experience and multiple interventions were implemented, including routine sedation administered; less experienced physicians performed more examinations; less skilled physicians were periodically supervised by experienced examiners; if cecal intubation was not successful, attempts made by a second endoscopist were performed; and physicians with low polyp detection rates had personal interviews with the chief of the endoscopy unit to review polyp detection measures. Although colonoscopy completion rates increased from 84.6% at baseline to 93.1% in the final year, annual mean polyp detection rates remained unchanged.[48] In the latter study, 43 gastroenterologists with significant experience in colonoscopy were followed over time and periodic meetings reviewing individual ADR and quality measures including polyp detection and withdrawal time were held over a 3-year period. Those endoscopists that did not achieve a greater than or equal to 6-minute withdrawal time for more than 95% of examinations were fined a 1% financial penalty. Despite introduction of a financial consequence, no statistically significant changes in ADR were observed.[49] With such heterogeneity of results and studies, are there more effective methods to increase ADR besides using withdrawal time and periodic reviews of individual outcomes?

Most recently, Coe and colleagues[50] conducted a prospective educational intervention with the aim to increase ADR by implementing an endoscopist training program. Our endoscopic quality improvement program training was conducted during two training sessions in the form of teaching sets made up of videos, still images, and reference material from current literature. The first training session reviewed measures of high-quality colonoscopy, whereas the second training session reviewed measures used to identify neoplastic lesions. Overall, ADR at baseline was 36% for both groups of endoscopists. Subsequently, in the posttraining phase, the group of endoscopists randomized to endoscopic quality improvement program training had an increase in ADR to 47%, whereas the ADR for the group of endoscopists who were not trained remained unchanged at 35%. The effect of training on the endoscopist-specific ADRs was estimated with an odds ratio of 1.73 (confidence interval, 1.24–2.41; $P = .0013$). Preliminary studies suggest that the improvement in ADR is maintained beyond the initial retraining.[51] It remains to be determined if retraining can be broadly and reproducibly applied across endoscopic centers.

Endoscopist behaviors during colonoscopy vary as do personalities. Although there are little data in this regard, it is tempting to speculate that specific personality types may be more amenable to high-quality colonoscopy, and more receptive to feedback on their performance and outcomes in colonoscopy.

SUMMARY

The art of colonoscopy, once seen as a purely apprenticeship model, is now viewed as a skill that can be enhanced with the use of computer simulators and magnetic position sensors, with maximum benefits seen in the early phases of training. Although there is no set finite number of procedures needed to become certified, achieving competency in colonoscopy may not be reached until more than 250 procedures are performed, contrary to what was previously perceived as adequate training by multiple societies of different medical specialties. With the shifting paradigm of quality assurance in colonoscopy, the concept of retraining experienced gastroenterologists to improve ADR has received much attention, and will be the subject of much scrutiny and study in the years to come.

REFERENCES

1. Medical Specialist Training Streering Committee. Expanding settings for medical specialist training, a report for the Australian Health Ministers' Advisory Council (online). 2006. Cited Feb 2008. Available at: http://www.coag.gov.au/meetings/140706/index.htm. Accessed October 1, 2012.
2. Training Committee 2010-2011, Sedlack RE, Shami VM, et al. Colonoscopy core curriculum. Gastrointest Endosc 2012;76(3):482–90.
3. Sedlack RE. Training to competency in colonoscopy: assessing and defining competency standards. Gastrointest Endosc 2011;74:355–66.
4. Sedlack RE. The Mayo Colonoscopy Skills Assessment Tool: validation of a unique instrument to assess colonoscopy skills in trainees. Gastrointest Endosc 2010;72:1125–33.
5. American Academy of Family Practitioners Wed site. AAFP colonoscopy position paper. Available at: http://www.aafp.org/online/en/home/policy/policies/c/colonoscopypositionpaper.html. Accessed October 1, 2012.
6. ASGE Standards of Training Committees. Principles of training in gastrointestinal endoscopy. From the ASGE. American Society for Gastrointestinal Endoscopy. Gastrointest Endosc 1999;49:845–50.
7. ACGME Web Site. Surgery Policy Information. Available at: http://www.acgme.org/acWebsite/RRC_440/440_policyArchive.asp. Accessed October 1, 2012.
8. Spier BJ, Durkin ET, Walker AJ, et al. Surgical resident's training in colonoscopy: numbers, competency, and perceptions. Surg Endosc 2010;24:2556–61.
9. Selvasekar CR, Holubar SD, Pendlimari R, et al. Assessment of screening colonoscopy competency in colon and rectal surgery fellows: a single institution experience. J Surg Res 2012;174(1):e17–23.
10. Leyden JE, Doherty GA, Hanley A, et al. Quality of colonoscopy performance among gastroenterology and surgical trainees: a need for common training standards for all trainees? Endoscopy 2011;43(11):935–40.
11. Cohen J. Computers for colonoscopy training: where do they fit in? Gastrointest Endosc 2010;71(2):308–11.
12. McCashland T, Brand R, Lyden E, et al. The time and financial impact of training fellows in endoscopy. CORI Research Project. Clinical Outcomes Research Initiative. Am J Gastroenterol 2000;95:3129–32.
13. Williams MD, Baillie J, Gillies DF, et al. Teaching gastrointestinal endoscopy by computer simulation: a prototype for colonoscopy and ERCP. Gastrointest Endosc 1990;36:49–54.
14. Noar MD. Robotics interactive endoscopy simulation of ERCP/sphincterotomy and EGD. Endoscopy 1992;24(Suppl 2):539–41.

15. Balcombe J. Medical training using simulation: toward fewer animals and safer patients. Altern Lab Anim 2004;32(1):553–60.
16. Cohen J, Cohen SA, Vora KC, et al. Multicenter, randomized, controlled trial of virtual-reality simulator training in acquisition of competency in colonoscopy. Gastrointest Endosc 2006;64(3):361–8.
17. Clark JA, Volchok JA, Hazey JW, et al. Initial experience using an endoscopy simulator to train surgical residents in flexible endoscopy in a community medical center residency program. Curr Surg 2005;62:59–63.
18. Sedlack RE, Kolars JC, Alexander JA. Computer simulation training enhances patient comfort during endoscopy. Clin Gastroenterol Hepatol 2004; 2:348–52.
19. Haycock A, Koch A, Familiari P, et al. Training and transfer of colonoscopy skills: a multinational, randomized, blinded, controlled trial of simulator versus bedside training. Gastrointest Endosc 2010;71:298–307.
20. Sedlack RE, Kolars JC. Colonoscopy curriculum development and performance-based assessment criteria on a computer-based endoscopy simulator. Acad Med 2002;77:750–1.
21. Kim S, Spencer G, Makar G, et al. Lack of a discriminatory function for endoscopy skills on a computer-based simulator. Surg Endosc 2010;24:3008–15.
22. Sedlack RE, Kolars JC. Validation of a computer-based colonoscopy simulator. Gastrointest Endosc 2003;57(2):214–8.
23. McConnell RA, Kim S, Ahmad NA, et al. Poor discriminatory function for endoscopic skills on a computer-based simulator. Gastrointest Endosc 2012;76(5): 993–1002.
24. Grantcharov TP, Carstensen L, Schulze S. Objective assessment of gastrointestinal endoscopy skills using a virtual reality simulator. JSLS 2005;9(2):130–3.
25. Mahmood T, Darzi A. A study to validate the colonoscopy simulator. Surg Endosc 2003;17(10):1583–9.
26. Eversbusch A, Grantcharov TP. Learning curves and impact of psychomotor training on performance in simulated colonoscopy: a randomized trial using a virtual reality endoscopy training. Surg Endosc 2004;18(10):1514–8.
27. Mahmood T, Darzi A. The learning curve for a colonoscopy simulator in the absence of any feedback: no feedback, no learning. Surg Endosc 2004;18: 1224–30.
28. Cohen J, Bosworth BP, Chak A, et al. Preservation and incorporation of valuable endoscopic innovations (PIVI) on the use of endoscopy simulators for training and assessing skill. Gastrointest Endosc 2012;76(3):471–5.
29. ACGME Program Requirements for Graduate Medical Education in Gastroenterology (Section IV.A.6.b). Effective July 1, 2012. Available at: http://www.acgme.org/acgmeweb/Portals/0/PFAssets/ProgramRequirements/144_gastroenterology_int_med_07012012.pdf. Accessed October 1, 2012.
30. Sedlack RE. Incorporating simulation into the GI curriculum: the time is now. Gastrointest Endosc 2012;76(3):622–4.
31. Bladen JS, Anderson AP, Bell GD, et al. A non-radiological technique for the real-time imaging of endoscopes in 3 dimensions. Conference record of the 1993 IEEE Nuclear Science Symposium and Medical Imaging Conference. San Francisco, October 30-November 6, 1993. p. 1891.
32. Bladen JS, Anderson AP, Bell GD, et al. Non-radiological technique for three-dimensional imaging of endoscopes. Lancet 1993;341:719–22.
33. Williams CB, Guy C, Gilles D, et al. Electronic three-dimensional imaging of intestinal endoscopy. Lancet 1993;341:724–5.

34. Shah SG, Brooker JC, Williams CB, et al. Effect of magnetic endoscope imaging on colonoscopy performance: a randomized controlled trial. Lancet 2000;356: 1718–22.

35. Shah SG, Lockett M, Thomas-Gibson S, et al. Effect of magnetic endoscope imaging (MEI) on acquisition of colonoscopy skills. Gut 2002;50(Suppl 2):A41.

36. Holme Ö, Höie O, Matre J, et al. Magnetic endoscopic imaging versus standard colonoscopy in a routine colonoscopy setting: a randomized, controlled trial. Gastrointest Endosc 2011;73:1215.

37. Shah SG, Thomas-Gibson S, Brooker JC, et al. Use of video and magnetic endoscope imaging for rating competence at colonoscopy: validation of a measurement tool. Gastrointest Endosc 2002;56:568–73.

38. Rex DK, Bond JH, Winawer S, et al. Quality in the technical performance of colonoscopy and the continuous quality improvement process for colonoscopy: recommendations for the U.S. Multi-Society Take Force on Colorectal Cancer. Am J Gastroenterol 2002;97:1296–308.

39. Allen JI. Quality assurance for gastrointestinal endoscopy. Curr Opin Gastroenterol 2012;28(5):442–50.

40. Sanchez W, Harewood GC, Petersen BT. Evaluation of polyp detection in relation to procedure time of screening or surveillance colonoscopy. Am J Gastroenterol 2004;99:1941–5.

41. Simmons DT, Harewood GC, Baron TH, et al. Impact of endoscopist withdrawal speed on polyp yield: implications for optimal colonoscopy withdrawal time. Aliment Pharmacol Ther 2006;24:965–71.

42. Barclay RL, Vicari JJ, Doughty AS, et al. Colonoscopic withdrawal times and adenoma detection during screening colonoscopy. N Engl J Med 2006;355: 2533–41.

43. Barclay RL, Vicari JJ, Greenlaw RL. Effect of a time-dependent colonoscopic withdrawal protocol on adenoma detection during screening colonoscopy. Clin Gastroenterol Hepatol 2008;6:1091–8.

44. Chen SC, Rex DK. Endoscopist can be more powerful than age and male gender in predicting adenoma detection at colonoscopy. Am J Gastroenterol 2007;102:1–6.

45. Sawhney MS, Curry MS, Neeman N, et al. Effect of institution-wide policy of colonoscopy withdrawal time > or = 7 minutes on polyp detection. Gastroenterology 2008;135(6):1892–8.

46. Lin OS, Kozarek RA, Arai A, et al. The effect of periodic monitoring and feedback on screening colonoscopy withdrawal times, polyp detection rates, and patient satisfaction scores. Gastrointest Endosc 2010;71(7):1253–9.

47. Corley DA, Jensen CD, Marks AR. Can we improve adenoma detection rates? A systematic review of intervention studies. Gastrointest Endosc 2011;74(3):656–65.

48. Imperiali G, Minoli G, Meucci GM, et al. Effectiveness of a continuous quality improvement program on colonoscopy practice. Endoscopy 2007;39:314–8.

49. Shaukat A, Oancea C, Bond JH, et al. Variation in detection of adenomas and polyps by colonoscopy and change over time with a performance improvement program. Clin Gastroenterol Hepatol 2009;7:1335–40.

50. Coe SG, Crook JE, Diehl NN, et al. An endoscopic quality improvement program (EQUIP) improves detection of colorectal adenomas. Am J Gastroenterol 2013; 108(2):219–26.

51. Ussui V, Coe SG, Ngamruengphong S, et al. Long term increases in adenoma detection at colonoscopy. Follow up of a randomized controlled clinical trial. Gastrointest Endosc 2012;75(4):AB300.

New Platforms and Devices in Colonoscopy

Payal Saxena, BMBS (Hons), FRACP, Mouen A. Khashab, MD*

KEYWORDS

- Gastrointestinal endoscopy • Colonoscopy • Robotics
- Computer-assisted colonoscopy

KEY POINTS

- The Endotics System, Aer-O-Scope and Colon Capsule Endoscopy are potential alternative platforms for screening colonoscopy but lack therapeutic capabilities.
- The Invendoscope has therapeutic capabilities but further improvements are needed for reliable performance.
- Neoguide has potential for accurately identifying scope position which can assist identifying location of lesions.
- Responsive insertion technology is promising new endoscope technology which can be advantageous in patients with failed colonoscopy as a result of sharp angulations (post pelvic surgery) or a narrowed lumen.
- Colon capsule endoscopy (CCE) offers a minimally invasive and painless method of imaging the colon without the need for sedation, however optimal bowel preparation is essential. CCE is a feasible and safe tool for visualization of colonic mucosa in patients with incomplete colonoscopy attributable to difficult anatomy, however it remains a diagnostic tool without therapeutic capabilities.
- Advanced polypectomy may be facilitated by new injection solutions.
- Improved through-the-scope clips and over-the-scope clips are available to manage post polypectomy bleeding and perforations.

Gastrointestinal endoscopy is a rapidly evolving field. Techniques in endoscopy continue to become more sophisticated, as do the devices and platforms, particularly in colonoscopy and endoscopic resection. This article reviews new platforms for endoscopic imaging of the colon, and discusses new endoscopic accessories and developments in endoscopic resection.

Conflicts of Interest: M.A. Khashab is a consultant for Boston Scientific. P. Saxena has no relevant conflicts of interest to disclose.
Division of Gastroenterology and Hepatology, Department of Medicine, The Johns Hopkins Hospital Institutions, 1800 Orleans Street, Baltimore, MD 21287, USA
* Corresponding author.
E-mail address: mkhasha1@jhmi.edu

NEW PLATFORMS FOR ENDOSCOPIC IMAGING OF THE COLON

Colonoscopy is the preferred screening modality for colorectal cancer,[1] and cecal intubation rates of greater than 95% are expected.[2] However, colonoscopy can be technically difficult, owing to redundant colon or because of angulated or fixed sigmoid colon related to pelvic surgery or diverticular disease.[3] An inability to examine the entire colon undermines the benefits of screening, especially in the proximal colon.

Based on the need for better performance of screening methods and better acceptance by patients, the following devices and technology have been developed to assist navigation through the colon, some of which are equipped with therapeutic capabilities (**Box 1**).

DIAGNOSTIC PLATFORMS

Navigation through a tortuous and angulated colon can be challenging for the endoscopist. Several platforms have been devised to assist navigation by minimizing looping or by taking advantage of peristalsis to propel the device.

Endotics System

The Endotics System (ES) (Era Endoscopy, Pisa, Italy) is a disposable robotic probe with a head, steerable tip, flexible body (17 mm diameter), and tail (7.5 mm diameter, 180 cm length), connected to a control box with an electropneumatic connector. A camera, light-emitting diode light source, and channels for air and water are incorporated into the head of the device and can be steered 180° in all directions. Two vacuum anchors located in the proximal and distal ends of the device move sequentially to provide an "inchworm-like" movement of the apparatus, thereby negotiating complex contours of the colon as the probe advances through the lumen (**Fig. 1**).[4,5]

Tumino and colleagues[6] performed both standard colonoscopy and ES colonoscopy in 71 patients. Cecal intubation rate was lower in the ES group (81.6% vs 94.3%, $P = .03$). Similarly, mean procedural time was longer in the ES group (45.1 vs 23.7 minutes, $P<.0001$); however, polyp detection rates were higher when compared with standard colonoscopy (sensitivity 93.3%, specificity 100%, positive predictive value 100%, negative predictive value 97.7%). None of patients in the ES group required sedation, an advantage attributable to the inchworm-like motion of the endoscope, exerting minimal forces on the colonic wall and thereby preventing pain caused by stretching of the mesocolon.

Therefore, ES may allow performance of diagnostic colonoscopy without the need for sedation while providing a high diagnostic yield. However, it is limited by lower cecal intubation rate, lengthier procedural times, and lack of a therapeutic channel. Further improvement of the device, in addition to larger studies, are needed before incorporation into clinical practice can be considered.

Box 1	
Diagnostic and therapeutic platforms for endoscopic imaging of the colon	
Diagnostic Platforms	**Therapeutic Platforms**
Endotics System	Invendoscope
Aer-O-Scope	NeoGuide
Colon Capsule Endoscope	

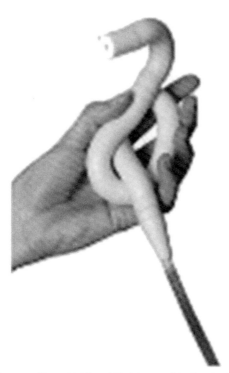

Fig. 1. The Endotics System. (*From* Valdastri P. Advanced technologies for gastrointestinal endoscopy. Annu Rev Biomed Eng 2012;14:397; with permission.)

Aer-O-Scope

The Aer-O-Scope (GI View, Ramat Gan, Israel) is a self-propelling and self-navigating diagnostic robotic colonoscope, comprising a workstation and disposable unit (**Fig. 2**). The disposable unit consists of a rectal introducer, supply cable, and endoscope embedded within a mobile balloon. The rectal introducer is a hollow tube with a balloon attached to its outer surface, which is inflated and fixed in the rectum. The endoscope is passed through the introducer. The rectal balloon provides a seal, preventing gas leakage. Carbon dioxide is insufflated between both balloons, allowing forward propulsion of the mobile balloon (which is attached to the endoscope).

The user interface is provided by a personal computer–based workstation operated by a control box, which is brought to the bedside. The workstation is connected to the scope by the disposable supply cable, and controls the gas pressure behind and within the mobile balloon. The pressures in front of, inside of, and behind the balloon are measured by sensors and automatically adjusted by a computerized algorithm. The operator can choose the operation mode (forward, backward, pause, and stop). Data from the digital camera are displayed on a screen and recorded on a compact disc. The operator can withdraw the instrument by gently pulling on the supply cable. Once the procedure is completed, the colon is deflated, the rectal seal is released, and the device is removed.

Initial proof-of-concept studies were performed in animal models[7,8] followed by clinical experiments. Vucelic and colleagues[9] studied the Aer-O-Scope in 12 healthy volunteers (age 20–43 years). The cecum was reached in 10 subjects. The instrument could not be passed beyond the hepatic flexure in the remaining 2 cases. Mean cecal

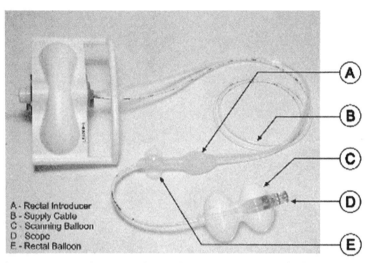

A - Rectal Introducer
B - Supply Cable
C - Scanning Balloon
D - Scope
E - Rectal Balloon

Fig. 2. The Aer-O-Scope. (*From* Vucelic B. The Aer-O-Scope: proof of concept of a pneumatic, skill-independent, self-propelling, self-navigating colonoscope. Gastroenterology 2006;130:672; with permission.)

intubation time was 14 minutes. Mild sweating and bloating was experienced by 40% of subjects. Subsequently, all subjects underwent follow-up colonoscopy, and 40% were found to have mild submucosal petechial lesions, likely a result of friction between the device and colonic mucosa.

The major limitation of this device is the lack of therapeutic capabilities. However, the device is easy to use, requires minimal training, and may have utility in helping to meet the increasing demand for screening colonoscopy.

Colon Capsule Endoscopy

Small-bowel endoscopy was revolutionized with the advent of wireless capsule endoscopy, first reported more than a decade ago.[10] Applications of the device have broadened as newer generations of the capsule continue to improve. The first generation of colon capsule endoscopy (CCE) was developed in 2006.[11] CCE offers a minimally invasive and painless method of imaging the colon without the need for sedation or gas insufflation.

Adequate colon preparation is essential for successful CCE, for several reasons. Bowel cleansing improves mucosal visualization, facilitates propulsion of the capsule through the small bowel to reach the colon, and results in filling the colonic lumen with clear liquids, which improves mucosal visualization and diminishes air bubbles.[12] The recommended bowel preparation regimen was recently modified to optimize colonic examination.[13] Patients commence a clear liquid diet the day before the procedure. Standard bowel preparation regimens should be administered, preferably in a split-dosage fashion. Booster preparations are necessary to help propel the capsule and to complete visualization of the colonic mucosa. The progression of the capsule is monitored with a real-time viewing system performed with Rapid Access Real Time Tablet DC (Given Imaging, Yoqneum, Israel). A prokinetic is recommended if the capsule is retained in the stomach for longer than 1 hour.[13] Contraindications to small bowel capsule endoscopy apply to CCE (**Box 2**).[13]

The first-generation colon capsule PillCam (Given Imaging) measured 31 × 11 mm and was equipped with dual cameras and implemented optics, with a total operating

Box 2
Contraindications to colon capsule endoscopy
Dysphagia or swallowing disorder
Prior major abdominal surgery of the gastrointestinal tract
Known or suspected bowel obstruction
Presence of cardiac pacemaker
Other implanted electromedical device
Pregnancy

time of approximately 10 hours. The angle of view from each imager was 156°. The capsule entered a "sleep" mode for the first 1 hour 45 minutes, conserving battery power for colonic examination as the capsule traversed the small bowel. Subsequently, the capsule automatically reactivated and started transmission of distal ileal images before exploring the colon.[14] The second-generation PillCam colon capsule (PCC-2; Given Imaging) is slightly larger, measuring 31.5 × 11.6 mm. The angle of view from both imagers is widened to 172°, allowing for almost 360° coverage of the colon. In addition, the capsule is equipped with an adaptable image acquisition rate, which adjusts to the speed of capsule propulsion through the intestine, helping to conserve battery energy and optimize video length. It first begins capturing at a low rate of 14 images per minute until small-bowel images are detected. The capsule also has the ability to "adapt" its frame rate. When stationary, PCC-2 captures 4 frames per second, and increases to 35 frames per second while moving. The data recorder (DR3) directs the medical staff and the patient through the procedure with vibration and noise alerts on its liquid-crystal diode screen to alert the patient to continue the preparation according to the protocol. The software (RAPID) contains additional diagnostic features for video processing and viewing.

Two meta-analyses of patients undergoing CCE have been published to date,[15,16] including 9 studies[11,17–24] examining the first-generation colon capsule. The average sensitivity and specificity for detection of significant findings (polyps ≥6 mm size or ≥3 polyps irrespective of size) was 68% to 69% and 82% to 86%, respectively.

Two studies[25,26] evaluated the second-generation capsule, with improved sensitivity for significant findings (84%–89%). The specificity varied from 64% for polyps 6 mm or larger in size to 95% for polyps 10 mm or larger. The low specificity resulted from polyps detected on capsule endoscopy but not seen at colonoscopy.

CCE was associated with no major complications in more than 1500 procedures. In addition, CCE has a very low rate of technical failures. Capsule excretion rate of about 90% is likely underestimated, as this was measured 8 hours after ingestion in most studies.[27]

Sung and colleagues[28] recently performed a multicenter prospective cohort study to investigate the accuracy of CCE for assessing the activity of colonic inflammation, using optical colonoscopy as the gold standard in 100 patients. Patients at higher risk for capsule retention (eg, Crohn disease, small-bowel tumors, radiation enteropathy, and previous intestinal surgery) were excluded. Most capsules were excreted naturally, with few (n = 9) being retrieved at colonoscopy. This study demonstrated high sensitivity for detecting mucosal inflammation (89%) but low specificity and negative predictive values of 75% and 65%, respectively. In other words, CCE failed to detect active disease in 25% of cases. The most common causes of failure to detect mucosal abnormalities were suboptimal bowel preparation, luminal bubbles, and quick colonic transit.

Recently, chromoendoscopy was incorporated into the capsule endoscopy system. Fujinon intelligent color enhancement (FICE) takes an ordinary endoscopic image and arithmetically processes the reflected photons to reconstitute virtual images for selected wavelengths. In a feasibility study by Pohl and colleagues,[29] 10 patients underwent small-bowel capsule endoscopy for evaluation of obscure gastrointestinal bleeding. Higher-quality images of polyps and angiodysplasias were obtained (**Fig. 3**). If this technology were incorporated into the CCE, perhaps further improvement in diagnostic yield would be possible.

CCE is not yet endorsed as a screening method for colon cancer. The first-generation CCE was associated with low sensitivity for polyps, but this has improved considerably with the second-generation capsule. This advance is partly due to improvements in the technology and alterations in the bowel preparation regimen. Some patients may prefer CCE over conventional colonoscopy given the lack of sedation, its noninvasive nature, and oral (rather than rectal) route of insertion. CCE is also a feasible and safe tool for visualization of the colonic mucosa in patients with incomplete colonoscopy attributable to difficult anatomy.[13] However, CCE remains a

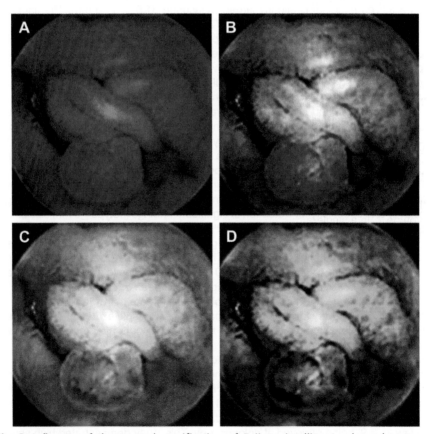

Fig. 3. Influence of the spectral specification of Fujinon intelligent color enhancement (FICE) on the vascular and mucosal contrast of a small-bowel adenoma. (*A*) Conventional imaging. (*B*) FICE set 1. (*C*) FICE set 2. (*D*) FICE set 3. (*From* Pohl J. Computed image modification for enhancement of small-bowel surface structures at video capsule endoscopy. Endoscopy 2010;42:490; with permission.)

diagnostic tool without therapeutic capabilities, and its performance depends on an optimal bowel preparation.

THERAPEUTIC PLATFORMS

Therapeutic interventions are required in up to 30% of screening colonoscopies,[30] ranging from minor polypectomy to advanced mucosal resections. Therapeutic platforms must provide an adequate working channel compatible with accessories that facilitate endoscopic resection. The following platforms provide an alternative to current standard colonoscopy, and have therapeutic capabilities.

Invendoscope

The Invendo SC20 (Invendo Medical, Kissing, Germany) uses principles of colonoscopy attached to a motor-driven device (**Figs. 4** and **5**). The design of this disposable device is similar to that of conventional endoscopes, allowing for insufflation, rinsing, and suction with a 3.1-mm working channel. Insertion and withdrawal of a colonoscope is replaced by an "inverted-sleeve" mechanism while a hand-held control unit activates all the endoscopic and software functions. The wheels grip onto the inner side of the inverted sleeve, causing the sleeve and inner sheath to drive either forward or backward. If the "forward" or "backward" key is not pressed by the operator, the wheels in the endoscope driving unit automatically stop. The endoscope tip can be flexed electrohydraulically 180° in any direction by moving a joystick on the hand-held device. The latest version of the Invendo SC20 is CE marked (Conformité Européenne).[31]

Two studies examined the use of the Invendoscope.[31,32] A pilot feasibility study of 39 healthy volunteers aimed to achieve cecal intubation without the need for sedation.[32] During the study, 2 prototypes of the instrument were used. The first was 170 cm in length and the second was 180 to 200 cm in length, with slight improvements in stiffness of the device tip. There were 5 cases of technical failures related to the instrument, 4 of which occurred while using the initial prototype. Of the remaining 34 patients, complete sedationless colonoscopy was achieved in 82% of patients, with a mean cecal intubation time of 26 minutes for prototype 1 and 20 minutes for prototype 2. In a single-arm prospective study[31] of screening colonoscopy in 61 patients older than 50 years, cecal intubation was achieved in 98.4% of patients with

A   **B**

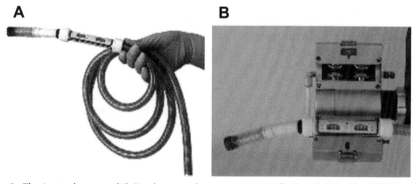

Fig. 4. The Invendoscope. (*A*) Single-use colonoscope controlled with hand-held device. (*B*) Instrument tip in the driving unit. (*From* Rosch T. A motor-driven single-use colonoscope controlled with a hand-held device: a feasibility study in volunteers. Gastrointest Endosc 2008;67:1139–46; with permission.)

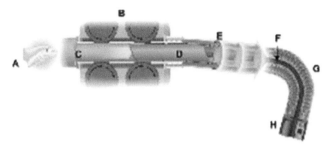

Fig. 5. Schematic of the Invendoscope and the propulsion mechanism. (*A*) The hand-held device that performs all the endoscopic and software functions. (*B*) The driving unit with 8 wheels that moves the endoscope in and out of the colon. (*C*) The inverted sleeve that causes the endoscope to grow or shrink only at the tip. (*D*) The inner endoscope sheath. (*E*) The inner layer of the inverted sleeve, when driven forward, unfolds here and becomes part of the outer layer, which then stays in position. There is therefore no relative movement, and only minimal forces are exerted on the wall of the colon. (*F*) The working channel for biopsies and treatment. (*G*) Electrohydraulic deflection of the endoscope tip, which can move 180° in any direction. (*H*) The single-use high-resolution camera with 3 light-emitting diodes. (*From* Rosch T. A motor-driven single-use colonoscope controlled with a hand-held device: a feasibility study in volunteers. Gastrointest Endosc 2008;67:1139–46; with permission.)

the Invendoscope prototype 2. Colonoscopy was commenced without sedation or analgesia, but participants were allowed to elect to receive sedation at any point during the examination. Only 4.9% of patients received intravenous sedation, and the average cecal intubation time was 15 minutes. In addition, the adenoma-detection rate was 18%. Abdominal pressure and patient repositioning were used in two-thirds of patients to assist in advancing the colonoscope. Endoscope malfunction occurred in 7% of cases owing to problems with tip deflection and clogging of the accessory channel.

The instrument has both diagnostic and therapeutic capabilities, with the major advantage being its ability to perform unsedated colonoscopy by minimizing the forces exerted by the instrument on the colonic wall. It is a single-use device that can eliminate the cost of labor and equipment associated with endoscope reprocessing, and achieves cecal intubation in a reasonable time. The optics of the current device use a complementary metal-oxide semiconductor chip. Although the image resolution has allowed an adenoma detection rate in line with expectations, the performance of the device compared with high-definition colonoscopes is yet to be evaluated. The incidence of equipment malfunction was notably reduced (from 13% to 7%) with modifications in the second prototype, but further improvements are needed for reliable equipment performance.

NeoGuide

The NeoGuide Endoscopy System (Intuitive Surgical, Sunnyvale, CA) is a computer-assisted colonoscope that was designed to limit patient discomfort during colonoscopy by avoiding loop formation. The insertion tube is computer controlled. The position and angle of the tip of the instrument are encoded into an algorithm, such that a 3-dimensional map of the position and shape of the insertion tube can be displayed on a video monitor with a simultaneous view of the colonic lumen. The colonoscope is 173 cm long and comprises 16 independent vertebrae, each of which is 8 cm in length. It tapers from a diameter of 20 mm at the base to 14 mm at the tip. The device has therapeutic capabilities, with a 3.2-mm working channel (**Figs. 6**

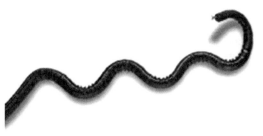

Fig. 6. NeoGuide. The insertion tube of the NeoGuide system has multiple segments that are controlled by the system, allowing the endoscope to follow the shape of the colon. (*From* Eickhoff A. Computer-assisted colonoscopy (the NeoGuide Endoscopy System): results of the first human clinical trial ("PACE study"). Am J Gastroenterol 2007;102:261–6; with permission.)

and **7**).[5,33] As the operator advances the endoscope, each 8-cm segment assumes a circular shape in the required direction, as instructed by computer control. Each segment bends where the prior segment turned and, thus, the shaft follows the trajectory of the tip in a "follow-the-leader" manner while, theoretically, preventing loop formation.

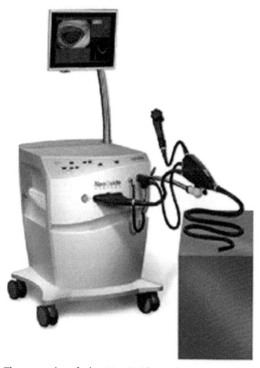

Fig. 7. NeoGuide. The console of the NeoGuide endoscopy system contains the video control, light and insufflation functionality in addition to motors that control the segments in the insertion tube. (*From* Eickhoff A. Computer-assisted colonoscopy (the NeoGuide Endoscopy System): results of the first human clinical trial ("PACE study"). Am J Gastroenterol 2007;102:261–6; with permission.)

The first clinical study included 10 patients (median age 43 years).[34] The cecum was successfully reached in all cases with a median insertion time of 20.5 minutes. Although the instrument can be operated by 1 person, colonoscopy was performed as a 2-person procedure. Sigmoid loops occurred in 40% of patients, but sedation requirements were not reported.

The advantages of the NeoGuide appear to be 2-fold: prevention of loop formation and accurate identification of scope position. However, loop formation was only prevented in 60% of cases in the only published clinical study.[34] Nonetheless, the instrument has great promise for accurately identifying scope position, which is clinically useful in accurate reporting of lesion location. In addition, real-time imaging has great potential for teaching colonoscopy to trainees. Large-scale clinical trials are needed to assess these potential indications for the device.

RESPONSIVE INSERTION TECHNOLOGY

Responsive insertion technology (RIT) was recently introduced by Olympus (Tokyo, Japan) and was incorporated into their EVIS EXERA III 190 series colonovideoscopes. RIT consists of "passive bending" and use of a "high force transmission insertion tube." The passive-bending colonoscope increases ease of insertion through flexures or hairpin bends in the colon, by way of its flexible tip with a narrow turning radius. The colonoscope insertion tube has a 3-layered structure consisting of a metal flex tube (the innermost layer), a mesh tube, and a polymer resin (the outermost layer). By altering the composition, the response of the tube can be changed. The new high force transmission insertion tube enables fine manipulation and torque applied by the endoscopist to be precisely transmitted through the insertion section to the distal end of the colonoscope, even when the endoscope is in a looped conformation (**Fig. 8**).[35]

Mizukami and colleagues[36] presented a case series of 11 patients who underwent initial colonoscopy with a conventional colonoscope and then a second colonoscopy using colonoscopes equipped with RIT 1 week later. There was a significant reduction in cecal intubation time (10.1 ± 3.2 min vs 5.1 ± 2.8 min, $P<.05$) and self-reported pain scores (3.7 ± 0.6 vs 2.3 ± 0.9, $P<.01$).

Sato and colleagues[37] compared performance efficiency of a small-caliber colonoscope equipped with RIT (PCF PQ260L; Olympus) with a standard colonoscope (CF-Q260AI; Olympus). A total of 330 patients were randomized to either the small-caliber colonoscope (outer diameter 9.2 mm) or standard colonoscope (outer diameter 12 mm). There was no significant difference in cecal intubation times or rates. However, women reported significantly lower pain scores. Level of sedation administration was similar between both groups. The smaller-caliber instrument did allow successful intubation in 4 patients with severe angulations caused by diverticulosis or adhesions, and in 3 of 4 patients with stenosis caused by an obstructing tumor. In this study, it is plausible that the decreased pain in the small-caliber group was due to the smaller size of the instrument rather than the RIT.

Further studies comparing colonoscopes of identical diameter, and with and without RIT, are needed to assess the benefits of this promising new technology, including its effect on postprocedural pain, and cecal intubation rates and times. The narrow-caliber instrument will most likely be advantageous in patients with failed colonoscopy as a result of sharp angulations (post pelvic surgery) or a narrowed lumen.

ACCESSORIES

Aside from skillful complete navigation, endoscopists have risen to every challenge thrown by the colon, which has been made possible by the array of tools provided

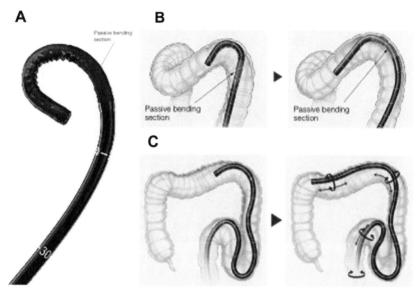

Fig. 8. (*A*) The passive-bending section is located proximal to the tip of the colonoscope. (*B*) The passive-bending section helps the endoscope move through acute bends in the colon. When the endoscope meets with resistance, the pressure is redistributed so that the insertion tube automatically bends to adjust to the contours of the colon. (*C*) High force transmission: When the endoscope is pushed forward or rotated, the pushing force or rotational torque is transmitted down the length of the insertion tube even when the endoscope is in a looped conformation.

by medical technology. This section describes the latest resection and closure devices.

Novel Lifting Gel

Conventional saline-assisted colonic endoscopic mucosal resection (EMR) allows en bloc resection of small (<20 mm) lesions.[38] Endoscopic submucosal dissection (ESD) is a technique that allows en bloc resection of large lesions in the hands of highly skilled endoscopists. The benefits of en bloc resection include negligible risk of neoplasia recurrence, more accurate histologic assessment, and potential cure of low-risk submucosal disease.[39] A major limitation is the lengthy time required to perform submucosal dissection.

The authors recently described their experience with a new endoscopic lifting gel (Cook Medical, Winston-Salem, NC).[40] The gel is a novel injectate for submucosal lift of polyps or other gastrointestinal lesions before excision. It is composed of a proprietary material, which is hydrated and prefilled in a 10-mL syringe provided with the device. The gel is an effective lifting solution that facilitates tissue resection by maintaining a long-lasting submucosal cushion. The syringe containing the gel is connected to a 19-gauge needle, which is attached to a gauge for monitoring pressure and is delivered to the tissue by a rotatable handle. The nominal working pressure generated from injecting the gel is approximately 1000 psi. The material has been validated to be able to withstand up to 1500 psi. The gel has received regulatory clearance in the United States and is registered in Europe (**Figs. 9 and 10**).

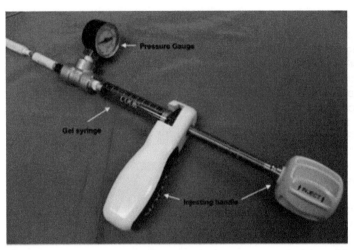

Fig. 9. Gel syringe attached to delivery device with pressure gauge and rotatable handle.

In addition to providing a submucosal cushion, the gel has tissue-dissecting properties and, thus, has the potential to simplify and increase efficiency of resection of wide-field colonic lesions. The gel has been used to perform ESD in simulated lesion within the gastrointestinal tract. Unpublished data have shown that the gel allowed en bloc resections of lesions 3 to 5 cm in size. Autodissection of submucosal fibers was a key feature, reducing procedural times by 50% when compared with conventional ESD of similar-sized lesions. In addition, bleeding was negligible and endoscopic hemostatic methods were rarely required. Human studies are needed to validate the clinical utility of the gel.

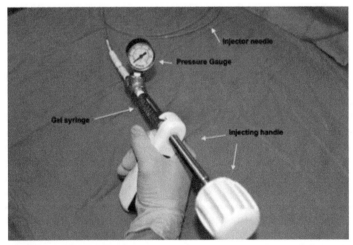

Fig. 10. Gel-injection apparatus. The gel syringe is attached to a delivery device with pressure-gauge monitor and rotatable handle, which is used to inject the gel through a 19-gauge needle.

Endoscopic Clips

Endoscopic clips have been shown to be effective for the control of acute gastrointestinal hemorrhage. Various models are available, which offer simplicity of use with relatively few complications. Recently endoscopic clips have been used for a variety of nonhemorrhagic conditions, including closure of polypectomy sites for prevention of postpolypectomy bleeding, and closure of perforations and fistulas.[41]

Endoscopic clips can be divided into 2 categories: through-the-scope clips (TTSC) and over-the-scope clips (OTSC). Three commonly used TTSC are the Resolution clip (Boston Scientific, Natick, MA), Quickclip2 and Quickclip2 Long (Olympus), and Instinct clip (Cook Medical) (**Table 1**).

Resection of large polyps leaves behind a large mucosal defect. The mucosal ulcer that forms after polyp resection can take several weeks to heal. Bleeding complications are frequent,[42] typically occur within 7 to 10 days, and often require hospital admission, repeat colonoscopy and, possibly, blood transfusions. There are no randomized trials that have examined whether clip application would affect complications after resection of large polyps. A small retrospective study on mucosal resection of large polyps in the duodenum showed that closing the resection defect with clips reduced the risk of bleeding from 75% (no-clip group) to 28% (clip group).[43] A study of colon polyps did not find a similar benefit.[44] However, this study was limited by inclusion of patients with smaller polyps (mean size 8 mm) with a low expected absolute risk of bleeding. A recent study presented as an abstract at a national meeting assessed the effects of clip closure of large colonic polypectomy sites.[43] Clip closure was associated with a significantly reduced risk of delayed bleeding (3% vs 9%) when compared with historical controls.[45] A randomized study is needed to examine the cost-effectiveness of prophylactic clip closure after large polypectomies.

The incidence of colonic perforations during diagnostic and therapeutic colonoscopy ranges from 0.07% to 0.1%.[46] The risk increases to 0.2% after EMR and is as high as 5% after ESD. If a perforation is immediately recognized and endoscopic closure can be achieved, surgery can be avoided, provided there is absence of generalized peritonitis and sepsis.[46]

Both TTSC and OTSC clips produce results comparable with those of hand-sewn colostomy closure in terminal animal studies.[47,48] TTSC are useful in the closure of small (1 cm) nongaping perforations.[46,49] These clips can be deployed anywhere in the colon and are ideal for immediate closure of postpolypectomy perforation, without leaving the site of perforation.[46] However, their relatively small open jaw span limits the size of mucosal defect that can be closed, and multiple clips are often required. TTSC are reported to be unsuccessful in the closure of large, gaping perforations with everted edges and defects after full-thickness resection.[50]

Table 1
Characteristics of TTSC

Clip	Jaw Span (mm)	Opening Angle (°)	Rotatable	Reopening Capability	MR Imaging Compatible
Resolution Boston Scientific	11	72	Partial	Yes	Yes
Instinct Cook Medical	16	125	Yes	Yes	Yes
QuickClip2 QuickClip2 Long Olympus	9 11	85 85	Yes	No	No

The OTSC (Ovesco Endoscope AG, Tubingen, Germany) is different in design from TTSC. The clip is preloaded on a cap, which is loaded onto the tip of the endoscope, in a fashion similar to band-ligation devices. The clip is available in 3 styles of teeth with 3 different sizes (8.5–11 mm, 10.5–12 mm, 11.5–14 mm) to fit most commercially available endoscopes. It comes in 2 different cap lengths (3 mm and 6 mm), the larger cap allowing more tissue to be grasped and approximated for closure. The Twin Grasper and Anchor (Ovesco Endoscope AG) are accessories that pass through the working channel, and can assist tissue approximation and withdrawal into the cap if required, especially in the case of larger defects. The OTSC is capable of grasping larger amounts of tissue than the TTSC, and provides more durable closure because of greater compressive forces.[51,52] Few studies have examined the use of OTSC for the closure of colonic perforations.[52,53] The OTSC does have some limitations. First, the endoscope must be removed from the patient to load the clip. Once the endoscope is reinserted, visibility is somewhat limited owing to the narrower field of view with the clip and cap positioned at the tip of the endoscope. Second, the OTSC is relatively bulky and stiffens the tip of the endoscope, thereby making access to proximal colon difficult and potentially risky, especially if acute angulations are encountered. Lastly, if the clip is misdeployed, removal can be difficult. Nonetheless, a recent technique for OTSC removal was described whereby a guide wire was passed through the oval hole of the OTSC at the 6 o'clock position and the clip prized off at the hinges, in an atraumatic fashion.[54] Argon plasma coagulation at high power has also been used to section the clip.[53]

There are at least 28 cases of iatrogenic colonic perforations, up to 30 mm in size, which have been treated with OTSC.[52,53,55–57] All described defects were located in the left colon. Although closure was successful in most cases, 5 patients required subsequent surgery.[52,55,57] Therefore, closure of left-sided colonic defects can be successfully achieved using the OTSC in most patients. OTSC may provide more durable closure than TTSC, especially in cases of large defects; however, comparative data are lacking.

ROBOTICS

The use of robotics in surgery has increased over the last decade, and has evolved from devices capable of performing tasks by mechanical manipulation to interfaces between the patient and provider. The evolution has been characterized by a variety of self-navigating endoscopes such as those already described.

The major current limitation of robotic tools is their inflexibility, making movement in and out of small openings difficult. To eliminate this obstacle, "programmable matter"[58] has been conceptualized and is under development. Any material that can change its physical attributes by stimulus from its surroundings or user input is defined as programmable matter. Claytronics has been the most extensively described medium with potential endoscopic applications, and is currently being investigated by Carnegie Mellon University and Intel Research. The aim of the project is to create a programmable material composed of millions of cooperating submillimeter particles (catoms) that can sense the surrounding environment, including adjacent catoms. This material would perform programmed computations within itself to form new shapes capable of executing diagnostic or therapeutic interventions. In this manner, Claytronics material could be injected distant from a desired target site, operated via remote control to facilitate delivery to the desired site, and instructed to form a desired shape to perform the task at hand. The participants in the Claytronics project have proposed colonoscopic examination as a reasonable first step in realizing this goal.[58] A wireless suppository with the capability to traverse the entire colon, gather images, and conform its shape and characteristics based on identified lesions has been envisaged. Such a suppository would be compiled from millions of cooperating catoms. By communicating with each other, these will transform shapes and obtain 360° images. If a polyp is identified, the device will transform to encapsulate the lesion and remove it through heat ablation.[58] In addition, the device would be able to change its shape in order to pass through narrowed lumen or navigate around fecal matter.

The concept is extraordinary, though still in its early stages of development. Significant advances in software and hardware are required before realization of the technology.

SUMMARY

This article reviews the latest developments in endoscopic technology that facilitates navigation through the colon, accessories to perform mucosal and submucosal resection, and various closure devices. Colonoscopy is a field in dynamic evolution that is not limited by a set of unchanging tools. New options, including very imaginative ones, continue to push the boundaries and advance the field, ultimately for the greater benefit of patients.

REFERENCES

1. Levin B, Lieberman DA, McFarland B, et al. Screening and surveillance for the early detection of colorectal cancer and adenomatous polyps, 2008: a joint guideline from the American Cancer Society, the US Multi-Society Task Force on Colorectal Cancer, and the American College of Radiology. Gastroenterology 2008;134:1570–95.
2. Rex DK, Petrini JL, Baron TH, et al. Quality indicators for colonoscopy. Gastrointest Endosc 2006;63:S16–28.
3. Vemulapalli KC, Rex DK. Water immersion simplifies cecal intubation in patients with redundant colons and previous incomplete colonoscopies. Gastrointest Endosc 2012;76:812–7.
4. Cosentino F, Tumino E, Passoni GR, et al. Functional evaluation of the Endotics System, a new disposable self-propelled robotic colonoscope: in vitro tests and clinical trial. Int J Artif Organs 2009;32:517–27.
5. Valdastri P, Simi M, Webster RJ 3rd. Advanced technologies for gastrointestinal endoscopy. Annu Rev Biomed Eng 2012;14:397–429.
6. Tumino E, Sacco R, Bertini M, et al. Endotics system vs colonoscopy for the detection of polyps. World J Gastroenterol 2010;16:5452–6.
7. Pfeffer J, Grinshpon R, Rex D, et al. The Aer-O-Scope: proof of the concept of a pneumatic, skill-independent, self-propelling, self-navigating colonoscope in a pig model. Endoscopy 2006;38:144–8.
8. Arber N, Grinshpon R, Pfeffer J, et al. Proof-of-concept study of the Aer-O-Scope omnidirectional colonoscopic viewing system in ex vivo and in vivo porcine models. Endoscopy 2007;39:412–7.
9. Vucelic B, Rex D, Pulanic R, et al. The Aer-O-Scope: proof of concept of a pneumatic, skill-independent, self-propelling, self-navigating colonoscope. Gastroenterology 2006;130:672–7.
10. Iddan G, Meron G, Glukhovsky A, et al. Wireless capsule endoscopy. Nature 2000;405:417.
11. Eliakim R, Fireman Z, Gralnek IM, et al. Evaluation of the PillCam Colon capsule in the detection of colonic pathology: results of the first multicenter, prospective, comparative study. Endoscopy 2006;38:963–70.

12. Spada C, Hassan C, Sturniolo GC, et al. Literature review and recommendations for clinical application of colon capsule endoscopy. Dig Liver Dis 2011;43: 251–8.

13. Spada C, Hassan C, Galmiche JP, et al. Colon capsule endoscopy: European Society of Gastrointestinal Endoscopy (ESGE) guideline. Endoscopy 2012;44: 527–36.

14. Riccioni ME, Urgesi R, Cianci R, et al. Colon capsule endoscopy: advantages, limitations and expectations. Which novelties? World J Gastrointest Endosc 2012;4:99–107.

15. Rokkas T, Papaxoinis K, Triantafyllou K, et al. A meta-analysis evaluating the accuracy of colon capsule endoscopy in detecting colon polyps. Gastrointest Endosc 2010;71:792–8.

16. Spada C, Hassan C, Marmo R, et al. Meta-analysis shows colon capsule endoscopy is effective in detecting colorectal polyps. Clin Gastroenterol Hepatol 2010;8:516–22.

17. Van Gossum A, Munoz-Navas M, Fernandez-Urien I, et al. Capsule endoscopy versus colonoscopy for the detection of polyps and cancer. N Engl J Med 2009; 361:264–70.

18. Schoofs N, Deviere J, Van Gossum A. PillCam colon capsule endoscopy compared with colonoscopy for colorectal tumor diagnosis: a prospective pilot study. Endoscopy 2006;38:971–7.

19. Sieg A, Friedrich K, Sieg U. Is PillCam COLON capsule endoscopy ready for colorectal cancer screening? A prospective feasibility study in a community gastroenterology practice. Am J Gastroenterol 2009;104:848–54.

20. Lewis B, Rex D, Leiberman D. Capsule colonoscopy: an interim report of a pilot 3 arm, blinded trial of capsule colonoscopy versus virtual colonoscopy and colonoscopy [abstract]. Am J Gastroenterol 2006;101:A1470.

21. Sacher-Huvelin S, Le Roun M, Sebile V. Wireless capsule endoscopy compared to conventional colonoscopy in patients at moderate or increased risk for colorectal cancer: interim analysis of a prospective multicenter study [abstract]. Gastroenterology 2009;136:A276.

22. Costamagna G, Spada C, Riccioni ME. Evaluation of bowel preparation and procedure for PillCam Colon capsule: an interim analysis [abstract]. Gastroenterology 2009;136:A276.

23. Spada C, Riccioni M, Petruzziello L. Evaluation of bowel preparation and procedure for Pillcam colon capsile. An interim analysis. Endoscopy 2009; 41:A40.

24. Pliz JB, Portmann S, Peter S. A new method for colorectal cancer screening: capsule endoscopy compared to conventional colonoscopy. Gut 2008;57:A357.

25. Eliakim R, Yassin K, Niv Y, et al. Prospective multicenter performance evaluation of the second-generation colon capsule compared with colonoscopy. Endoscopy 2009;41:1026–31.

26. Spada C, Hassan C, Munoz-Navas M, et al. Second-generation colon capsule endoscopy compared with colonoscopy. Gastrointest Endosc 2011;74: 581–589.e1.

27. Spada C, De Vincentis F, Cesaro P, et al. Accuracy and safety of second-generation PillCam COLON capsule for colorectal polyp detection. Therap Adv Gastroenterol 2012;5:173–8.

28. Sung J, Ho KY, Chiu HM, et al. The use of Pillcam Colon in assessing mucosal inflammation in ulcerative colitis: a multicenter study. Endoscopy 2012;44: 754–8.

29. Pohl J, Aschmoneit I, Schuhmann S, et al. Computed image modification for enhancement of small-bowel surface structures at video capsule endoscopy. Endoscopy 2010;42:490–2.
30. Gurudu SR, Ramirez FC, Harrison ME, et al. Increased adenoma detection rate with system-wide implementation of a split-dose preparation for colonoscopy. Gastrointest Endosc 2012;76:603–8.e1.
31. Groth S, Rex DK, Rosch T, et al. High cecal intubation rates with a new computer-assisted colonoscope: a feasibility study. Am J Gastroenterol 2011; 106:1075–80.
32. Rosch T, Adler A, Pohl H, et al. A motor-driven single-use colonoscope controlled with a hand-held device: a feasibility study in volunteers. Gastrointest Endosc 2008;67:1139–46.
33. Striegel J, Jakobs R, Van Dam J, et al. Determining scope position during colonoscopy without use of ionizing radiation or magnetic imaging: the enhanced mapping ability of the NeoGuide Endoscopy System. Surg Endosc 2011;25: 636–40.
34. Eickhoff A, van Dam J, Jakobs R, et al. Computer-assisted colonoscopy (the NeoGuide Endoscopy System): results of the first human clinical trial ("PACE study"). Am J Gastroenterol 2007;102:261–6.
35. Saito Y, Kimura H. Responsive insertion technology. Dig Endosc 2011;23(Suppl 1): 164–7.
36. Mizukami T, Ogata H, Hibi T. "Passive-bending colonoscope" significantly improves cecal intubation in difficult cases. World J Gastroenterol 2012;18: 4454–6.
37. Sato K, Ito S, Shigiyama F, et al. A prospective randomized study on the benefits of a new small-caliber colonoscope. Endoscopy 2012;44:746–53.
38. Sakamoto T, Matsuda T, Nakajima T, et al. Efficacy of endoscopic mucosal resection with circumferential incision for patients with large colorectal tumors. Clin Gastroenterol Hepatol 2012;10:22–6.
39. Moss A, Bourke MJ, Metz AJ, et al. Beyond the snare: technically accessible large en bloc colonic resection in the West: an animal study. Dig Endosc 2012;24:21–9.
40. Khashab M, Sharaiha RZ, Saxena P. Novel technique of auto-tunneling during peroral endoscopic myotomy (POEM) (with video). Gastrointest Endosc 2013; 77(1):119–22.
41. Raju GS, Kaltenbach T, Soetikno R. Endoscopic mechanical hemostasis of GI arterial bleeding (with videos). Gastrointest Endosc 2007;66:774–85.
42. Khashab M, Eid E, Rusche M, et al. Incidence and predictors of "late" recurrences after endoscopic piecemeal resection of large sessile adenomas. Gastrointest Endosc 2009;70:344–9.
43. Lepilliez V, Chemaly M, Ponchon T, et al. Endoscopic resection of sporadic duodenal adenomas: an efficient technique with a substantial risk of delayed bleeding. Endoscopy 2008;40:806–10.
44. Shioji K, Suzuki Y, Kobayashi M, et al. Prophylactic clip application does not decrease delayed bleeding after colonoscopic polypectomy. Gastrointest Endosc 2003;57:691–4.
45. Liaquat H, Rohn E, Rex DK. Large sessile colorectal polyps: reduction in delayed bleeding with prophylactic clipping. Gastrointest Endosc 2012;75: AB348.
46. Raju GS, Saito Y, Matsuda T, et al. Endoscopic management of colonoscopic perforations (with videos). Gastrointest Endosc 2011;74:1380–8.

47. Agrawal D, Chak A, Champagne BJ, et al. Endoscopic mucosal resection with full-thickness closure for difficult polyps: a prospective clinical trial. Gastrointest Endosc 2010;71:1082–8.

48. Voermans RP, Vergouwe F, Breedveld P, et al. Comparison of endoscopic closure modalities for standardized colonic perforations in a porcine colon model. Endoscopy 2011;43:217–22.

49. Saito Y, Uraoka T, Yamaguchi Y, et al. A prospective, multicenter study of 1111 colorectal endoscopic submucosal dissections (with video). Gastrointest Endosc 2010;72:1217–25.

50. von Renteln D, Schmidt A, Vassiliou MC, et al. Endoscopic full-thickness resection and defect closure in the colon. Gastrointest Endosc 2010;71:1267–73.

51. Parodi A, Repici A, Pedroni A, et al. Endoscopic management of GI perforations with a new over-the-scope clip device (with videos). Gastrointest Endosc 2010; 72:881–6.

52. Seebach L, Bauerfeind P, Gubler C. "Sparing the surgeon": clinical experience with over-the-scope clips for gastrointestinal perforation. Endoscopy 2010;42: 1108–11.

53. Baron TH, Song LM, Ross A, et al. Use of an over-the-scope clipping device: multicenter retrospective results of the first U.S. experience (with videos). Gastrointest Endosc 2012;76:202–8.

54. Neumann H, Diebel H, Monkemuller K, et al. Description of a new, endoscopic technique to remove the over-the-scope-clip in an ex vivo porcine model (with video). Gastrointest Endosc 2012;76:1009–13.

55. Voermans RP, Le Moine O, von Renteln D, et al. Efficacy of endoscopic closure of acute perforations of the gastrointestinal tract. Clin Gastroenterol Hepatol 2012;10:603–8.

56. Kirschniak A, Subotova N, Zieker D, et al. The Over-The-Scope Clip (OTSC) for the treatment of gastrointestinal bleeding, perforations, and fistulas. Surg Endosc 2011;25:2901–5.

57. Gubler C, Bauerfeind P. Endoscopic closure of iatrogenic gastrointestinal tract perforations with the over-the-scope clip. Digestion 2012;85:302–7.

58. Smith K, Goldstein SC. Programmable matter: applications for gastrointestinal endoscopy and surgery. Gastroenterology 2011;140:1884–6.

Index

Note: Page numbers of article titles are in **boldface** type.

Gastroenterol Clin N Am 42 (2013) 689–699
http://dx.doi.org/10.1016/S0889-8553(13)00072-1
0889-8553/13/$ – see front matter © 2013 Elsevier Inc. All rights reserved.

gastro.theclinics.com

Printed and bound by CPI Group (UK) Ltd, Croydon, CR0 4YY

03/10/2024

01040409-0007